SCHOOL VIOLENCE

■

Assessment,
Management,
Prevention

SCHOOL VIOLENCE

■

Assessment, Management, Prevention

EDITED BY

Mohammad Shafii, M.D.
Sharon Lee Shafii, R.N., B.S.N.

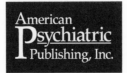

American **P**sychiatric Publishing, Inc.

Washington, DC
London, England

MT

Copyright © 2001 American Psychiatric Publishing, Inc.
ALL RIGHTS RESERVED
Manufactured in the United States of America on acid-free paper

04 03 02 01   4 3 2 1
First Edition

American Psychiatric Publishing, Inc.
1400 K Street, N.W.
Washington, DC 20005
www.appi.org

Library of Congress Cataloging-in-Publication Data
School violence : assessment, management, prevention / edited by Mohammad
    Shafii, Sharon Lee Shafii
            p. cm.
    Includes bibliographical references and index.
    ISBN 1-58562-009-2 (alk. paper)
        1. School violence. 2. Violence in adolescence. 3. Violence in children. I. Shafii,
    Mohammad. II. Shafii, Sharon Lee.

    LB3013.3 .S3765 2001
    371.7'82—dc21

                                                                                    00-042163

British Library Cataloguing in Publication Data
A CIP record is available from the British Library.

Cover photo: Digital Imagery© Copyright 2000, PhotoDisc, Inc.

7/15/03

To our grandchildren,
Liam Arie Kreiss
and
Mitra Alyce Shafii

We hope that they
and all children
will grow up
in a tolerant, peaceful, and inspiring
school and society.

Contents

Contributors XI

Preface XV

I
CONTRIBUTING FACTORS

1 Making Sense of School Violence: Why Do Kids Kill? 3
   JAMES GARBARINO, PH.D.

2 School Violence and the School Environment 25
   LOIS T. FLAHERTY, M.D.

3 Biological and Social Causes of School Violence 53
   PAUL KETTL, M.D.

4 Trends in School Violence: Are Our Schools Safe? 73
   KATHLEEN M. FISHER, PH.D., C.R.N.P.
   PAUL KETTL, M.D.

II
ASSESSMENT AND MANAGEMENT

5 Diagnostic Assessment, Management, and Treatment of
   Children and Adolescents With Potential for School Violence . . . 87
   MOHAMMAD SHAFII, M.D.
   SHARON LEE SHAFII, R.N., B.S.N.

6   Coping With School Violence: An Eyewitness Account 117
BECKY ROWAN, M.ED.

7   Columbine High School Shootings: Community Response. 129
PHILIPPE WEINTRAUB, M.D.
HARRIET L. HALL, PH.D.
ROBERT S. PYNOOS, M.D., M.P.H.

8   Wounded Adolescence: School-Based Group Psychotherapy for
Adolescents Who Sustained or Witnessed Violent Injury 163
CHRISTOPHER M. LAYNE, PH.D.
ROBERT S. PYNOOS, M.D., M.P.H.
JOSE CARDENAS, PSY.D.

III
LEGAL ASPECTS

9   Duty to Foresee, Forewarn, and Protect Against
Violent Behavior: A Plaintiff Attorney's Perspective. 189
MICHAEL BREEN, J.D.

10   Duty to Foresee, Forewarn, and Protect Against
Violent Behavior: A Psychiatric Perspective 201
ROBERT I. SIMON, M.D., P.A.

IV
PREVENTION

11   Prevention of Firearm Fatalities and Injuries:
Public Health Approach 219
GEORGE J. COHEN, M.D.

12   Problems With and Solutions for School Violence:
The Philadelphia Experience. 231
PAUL J. FINK, M.D.

13   Strategies for the Prevention of Youth
Violence in Chicago Public Schools 251
CARL C. BELL, M.D., F.A.C.PSYCH.
SUE GAMM, J.D.
PAUL VALLAS, M.A.
PHILLIP JACKSON, B.A.

14 A Social Systems–Power Dynamics
Approach to Preventing School Violence 273
STUART W. TWEMLOW, M.D.
PETER FONAGY, PH.D., F.B.A.
FRANK C. SACCO, PH.D.

15 The School in a Multicultural Society:
Teaching Tolerance and Conflict Resolution 291
JAN ARNOW, B.F.A.

Index 303

Contributors

Jan Arnow, B.F.A.
Institute for Intercultural Understanding, Louisville, Kentucky

Carl C. Bell, M.D., F.A.C.Psych.
Professor, Psychiatry and Public Health, University of Illinois in Chicago;
Chief Executive Officer, Community Mental Health Council, Chicago,
Illinois

Michael Breen, J.D.
Attorney-at-Law, Certified Trial Specialist, Bowling Green, Kentucky

Jose Cardenas, Psy.D.
Private Practice, San Fernando, California

George J. Cohen, M.D.
Clinical Professor of Pediatrics, George Washington University,
Washington, D.C.; Attending Pediatrician, Children's National Medical
Center, Washington, D.C.

Paul J. Fink, M.D.
Professor of Psychiatry, Temple University, Philadelphia, Pennsylvania

Kathleen M. Fisher, Ph.D., C.R.N.P.
Assistant Professor, School of Nursing, The Pennsylvania State University,
Hershey, Pennsylvania

Lois T. Flaherty, M.D.
Adjunct Associate Professor, Department of Psychiatry, University of Maryland School of Medicine; Consultant, Center for School Mental Health Assistance, University of Maryland, Baltimore, Maryland

Peter Fonagy, Ph.D., F.B.A.
Director, Child and Family Center and Clinical Protocols and Outcomes Center, The Menninger Clinic, Topeka, Kansas; Freud Memorial Professor of Psychoanalysis, University College, London, England; Director of Research, The Anna Freud Centre, London, England

Sue Gamm, J.D.
Chief Specialized Services Officer, Chicago Public Schools, Chicago, Illinois

James Garbarino, Ph.D.
Co-Director, Family Life Development Center; and Elizabeth Lee Vincent Professor of Human Development, Cornell University, Ithaca, New York

Harriet L. Hall, Ph.D.
President and Chief Executive Officer, Jefferson Center for Mental Health, Arvada, Colorado

Phillip Jackson, B.A.
Chief for Education, Office of the Mayor, Chicago, Illinois

Paul Kettl, M.D.
Chair and Joyce D. Kales Professor of Community Psychiatry, Penn State University College of Medicine, Hershey, Pennsylvania

Christopher M. Layne, Ph.D.
Assistant Professor of Psychology, Department of Psychology, Brigham Young University, Provo, Utah; Trauma Psychiatry Program, Department of Psychiatry and Biobehavioral Sciences, University of California School of Medicine, Los Angeles

Robert S. Pynoos, M.D., M.P.H.
Professor of Psychiatry and Director, Trauma Psychiatry Program, Department of Psychiatry and Biobehavioral Sciences, University of California School of Medicine, Los Angeles

Becky Rowan, M.Ed.
Counselor, Pearl High School, Pearl, Mississippi

Frank C. Sacco, Ph.D.
President, Community Services Institute, Springfield, Massachusetts

Mohammad Shafii, M.D.
Professor of Psychiatry and Director, Child and Adolescent Psychiatry
Residency Training Program, Department of Psychiatry and Behavioral
Sciences, University of Louisville School of Medicine, Louisville, Kentucky

Sharon Lee Shafii, R.N., B.S.N.
Editor-in-Residence, Louisville, Kentucky; formerly Assistant Head Nurse,
Adolescent Service, Neuropsychiatric Institute, University of Michigan
Medical Center, Ann Arbor, Michigan

Robert I. Simon, M.D., P.A.
Clinical Professor of Psychiatry and Director, Program in Psychiatry and
Law, Georgetown University School of Medicine, Washington, D.C.

Stuart W. Twemlow, M.D.
Clinical Professor of Psychiatry, University of Kansas School of Medicine,
Wichita, Kansas; Teaching Faculty, Topeka Institute for Psychoanalysis;
Co-Director Peaceful Schools Project Research Investigator, Childhood
Family Center, The Menninger Clinic, Topeka, Kansas

Paul Vallas, M.A.
Chief Executive Officer, Chicago Public Schools, Chicago, Illinois

Philippe Weintraub, M.D.
Associate Professor of Psychiatry, Division of Child Psychiatry, Department
of Psychiatry, University of Colorado Health Sciences Center, Denver,
Colorado

Preface

In the United States, acts of violence have been decreasing among adults but increasing among children and adolescents, particularly in schools. Acts of violence include vandalism, physical and sexual assault, rape, bodily injury, and homicide. Between 8% and 10% of U.S. high school students carry guns to school every day. In a typical middle-sized city, 30–50 cases of school violence are reported daily, and in half of these cases guns are involved.

Each year in the United States, more than 30,000 people die from gunshot wounds. Between 4,500 and 5,000 of these deaths occur in children and adolescents age 19 years and younger. Two-thirds of these deaths are homicides and one-third are suicides. The chance of a student dying a violent death in an American high school is five times higher than in other developed, industrialized countries. In Japan, for instance, with half the population of the United States, the annual death rate by guns for all ages is 170 persons or fewer per year.

Every day in the United States, 12–13 children and adolescents die a violent death either from homicide or from suicide. In addition, thousands of physical injuries occur from gunshot wounds. The spread of endemic school violence from urban centers to suburban and smaller communities has brought this major public health problem to national attention.

The incidence of school shootings across the country—in Pearl, Mississippi; Paducah, Kentucky; Springfield, Oregon; Jonesboro, Arkansas; Littleton, Colorado; Conyers, Georgia; and Fort Gibson, Oklahoma—has awakened the nation to the endemic nature of violence in our society, our communities, our schools, and our homes. Educators and health and mental health professionals need to take a more proactive role in understanding, dealing with, and preventing school violence. Not only have many youths, teachers, and parents been killed or maimed, but thousands are suffering and will continue to suffer for years to come from the physical and psychological traumas of school violence.

School Violence: Assessment, Management, Prevention is an examination by leading clinicians, researchers, school counselors, and legal authorities with special interest or experience in the area of youth violence, particularly violence in a school setting. This book comprises four parts.

PART I: CONTRIBUTING FACTORS

James Garbarino, Ph.D., internationally known expert on human development, child abuse, and family violence, shares some of his sociological and developmental data-based observations on making sense of school violence and the psychology and ecology of children who kill. He discusses the multiple factors involved in creating a violent child and a school setting prone to violence. Lois T. Flaherty, M.D., an experienced and nationally known child and adolescent psychiatrist and academician, lucidly and comprehensively discusses the nature and context of school violence and the school environment. Paul Kettl, M.D., interested for many years in the area of electronic media and television violence and their effect on children and youth, reviews the biological and cultural causes of violence. Kathleen M. Fisher, Ph.D., in her review of national data on school and youth violence, reports that although the number of actual deaths by shooting in schools was stable during the 1990s, the number of violent acts, especially those against female students, increased significantly. Fisher also reports a significant increase in gangs in schools and in the availability of guns.

PART II: ASSESSMENT AND MANAGEMENT

The editors, who have extensive clinical experience with and have done extensive research and scholarly work in child and adolescent depression and suicide, discuss diagnostic assessment, management, and treatment of children and adolescents who have the potential for or have threatened school violence. Similarities between violent youths and suicidal youths are a point of focus. Becky Rowan, M.Ed., a counselor at Pearl High School in Pearl, Mississippi, relates her harrowing and deeply touching eyewitness account of the school shooting there, bringing to life this tragic event. Philippe Weintraub, M.D., Harriet L. Hall, Ph.D., and Robert S. Pynoos,

M.D., M.P.H., describe the aftermath of school violence as experienced in the school shootings in Littleton, Colorado. They discuss the in-depth measures taken to decrease the traumatic effect of these violent acts on children and adolescents and their families, their educators, and the community at large.

Dr. Pynoos, an internationally known trauma expert on violence in war and in the community, with his colleagues Christopher M. Layne, Ph.D., and Jose Cardenas, Psy.D., describes an effective school-based group psychotherapy program for adolescents who sustained or witnessed violent injuries. This time-limited, cognitive-behavioral group therapy could be adopted as a model in other settings.

A question arises about the relation between personality disorders and violent behavior in youths. Because of ongoing developmental changes in children and adolescents, clinicians and researchers are often reluctant to make the diagnosis of personality disorder. Consequently, there are limited data-based studies currently available in this area.

PART III: LEGAL ASPECTS

Clinicians, educators, peers, and others who become aware of the possibility of an act of violence by a youth need to know that they have a legal responsibility to warn the potential victim(s) or to alert others who can warn or protect the potential victim(s).

Michael Breen, J.D., a practicing lawyer in Bowling Green, Kentucky, who is the plaintiff lawyer for the victims of school violence in Paducah, Kentucky, discusses the Tarasoff case and its ramifications for the duty to warn and to protect as it applies to having knowledge of a possible act of violence. Robert I. Simon, M.D., P.A., a nationally known forensic psychiatrist, discusses the Tarasoff case and the duty to warn and to protect from a clinical and psychiatric perspective. The delicate issue of deciding whether to warn a potential victim, while weighing the risks versus the benefits of such a decision, is examined.

PART IV: PREVENTION

At the present time, our knowledge of the prediction and the prevention of violence by an individual in a community, particularly in a school setting, is limited. George J. Cohen, M.D., an experienced pediatrician and academician, looks from a public health perspective at the epidemic of firearm injuries and the resulting physical, psychological, and economic costs. He proposes effective public health methods to decrease and prevent such injuries.

Two nationally known psychiatrists, Paul J. Fink, M.D., in Philadelphia, and Carl C. Bell, M.D., in Chicago, cogently discuss their extensive experience in the effective prevention of youth violence in the school and the community. Hopefully, various aspects of their experiences can be applied by school authorities and mental health professionals in other communities for the prevention of violence.

Stuart W. Twemlow, M.D., a practicing psychiatrist and training psychoanalyst at the Menninger Foundation, Topeka, Kansas, and his colleagues Peter Fonagy, Ph.D., F.B.A., and Frank C. Sacco, Ph.D., discuss an innovative and effective violence prevention program from a social system and power dynamic perspective—one that focuses on the school as a whole rather than on individuals.

Jan Arnow, the former manager of Multicultural Education for the Kentucky Department of Education and the founder of the Institute for Intercultural Understanding, makes an effective argument for incorporating teaching tolerance and conflict resolution in the curriculum of our multicultural school environment.

Resources and effort should be devoted to all aspects of school violence, a multifaceted public health problem, in order to decrease or, it is hoped, prevent this national tragedy. The involvement of health and mental health professionals in the school setting is essential to assess and to help our troubled youths and their families. Teaching tolerance, avoiding scapegoating and bullying, limiting the availability of guns, and providing close parental supervision of children's and adolescents' behavior, peer relationships, and use of electronic media may help to curtail this major national epidemic.

From the inception to the conclusion, *School Violence: Assessment, Management, Prevention* has been a joint effort, with many hours of discussion, planning, writing, rewriting, and editing. We hope that this book will become a vehicle for increasing understanding, improving management and treatment, and implementing effective prevention programs for the endemic public health problem of youth violence and particularly school violence.

Heartfelt thanks to Bryan Warren, M.D., of St. Mary's, Georgia, a good friend and colleague, whose inquiries and concerns about school violence ultimately led us to plan, organize, and edit this book. We also are appreciative for the support and encouragement of Rodrigo Munoz, M.D., then President of the American Psychiatric Association, and Pedro Ruiz, M.D., then Chair of the Scientific Program Committee of the American Psychiatric Association. The enthusiastic reception and constructive suggestions of Carol Nadelson, M.D., Editor-in-Chief of American Psychiatric Publishing, Inc., and Claire Reinburg, Editorial Director, made the idea for this book a reality. We are deeply grateful for their efforts. We appreciate the work of Amy Willard, B.A., Program Assistant, for her computer skills, cross-referencing, and helpful suggestions.

Mohammad Shafii, M.D.
Sharon Lee Shafii, R.N., B.S.N.

I

CONTRIBUTING FACTORS

Making Sense of School Violence

Why Do Kids Kill?

JAMES GARBARINO, PH.D.

PROLOGUE: CHICAGO, JANUARY 1994

I lived and worked in Chicago for almost 10 years, from the mid-1980s until the mid-1990s. My two children grew up there. Throughout 1993, the *Chicago Tribune* published a long series of stories that consisted of in-depth profiles of every kid who was killed in Chicago that year. As an expert on violence and trauma, I spent a lot of time talking with reporters, trying to help them make sense of what they had found during their investigation of each individual story. Having worked on the project all through 1993, they published, at the beginning of 1994, the photo and name of every single child and teenager who had been murdered during the previous 12 months. It was a chilling and haunting sight to see the rows and rows of names and faces—61 in all.

This chapter is from Chapter 1, "The Epidemic of Youth Violence," from *Lost Boys: Why Our Sons Turn Violent and How We Can Save Them*, by James Garbarino, Ph.D. Copyright © 1999 by James Garbarino. Reprinted with permission of The Free Press, a division of Simon & Schuster, Inc.

The same night the *Tribune* published the death toll from 1993, my 17-year-old son, Josh, was heading out for an evening on the town with his friends. "Be careful," I said, "it's dangerous out there and I worry about you." He turned to me, with the *Tribune* in hand, and said, "Don't worry, dad. Just how many white faces and names like mine do you see in the newspaper?" The reality was that in 1994 he could reassure me by this simple reference to the facts of the matter: you had to look long and hard to find a white teenage face with a non-Hispanic surname. Even though we lived in the city, within walking distance of some of the most violent streets in America, *he* felt safe.

When his observation forced me to confront this fact, I recalled a meeting I had attended just weeks before. I was the lone white person on a panel of African American and Hispanic professionals addressing a community forum on violence. During the coffee break, we panel members began chatting among ourselves, and it turned out that all of us had teenage sons. As we talked about being parents of teenagers in the city, it became clear to me that while I *worried* when my son went out at night, my African American and Hispanic colleagues felt *dread*, because they thought of their boys as part of an endangered species, even though the actual number of children killed that year was fewer than 100 in a city of 3 million. But that number is a compelling feature of the violence problem—the fact that even a relatively small number of deaths can stimulate a profound sense of threat and insecurity. Homicide *is* the leading cause of death for minority male youth. Each new death creates tremendous psychological reverberations, so that this feeling of tremendous apprehension my colleagues experienced was neither paranoid nor far-fetched. That was 1994. Fast forward to 1998.

By May 1998, I was living and working in Ithaca, a small university town located in the rolling hills of central New York State. Ithaca is a lovely place, mostly known for being the home of Cornell University. For many years and for most of Ithaca's citizens, it has been a kind of idyllic paradise where the big local news is likely to be a faculty member receiving a prize or the local school board meeting. Among vegetarians, it is famous as the home of the Moosewood Restaurant and the cookbooks it inspired.

On May 22, 1998, my 15-year-old daughter Joanna and my 14-year-old stepson Eric sat at the kitchen table reading the newspaper, which that morning was filled with accounts of the shooting of 24 students in Springfield, Oregon, by 15-year-old Kip Kinkel. Looking up from the front-page story, Joanna, shaking her head, said, "I wonder who it's going to be at our school."

No One Is Immune

The 1997–1998 school year will go down in American history as the turning point in our country's experience and understanding of lethal youth violence. *October 1, 1997, Pearl, Mississippi:* After killing his mother, 16-year-old Luke Woodham opens fire at his high school, killing three and wounding seven (see Chapter 6, this volume). *December 1, 1997, West Paducah, Kentucky:* 14-year-old Michael Carneal kills three students at a high school prayer meeting (see Chapter 9, this volume). *March 24, 1998, Jonesboro, Arkansas:* 13-year-old Mitchell Johnson and 11-year-old Andrew Golden open fire on their schoolmates, killing four of them and a teacher. *April 24, 1998, Edinboro, Pennsylvania:* 14-year-old Andrew Wurst kills a teacher at a school dance. *May 21, 1998, Springfield, Oregon:* After killing his parents, 15-year-old Kip Kinkel walks into the school cafeteria and shoots 24 classmates—two fatally. American consciousness was shaken by these events. But the 1998–1999 school year was the coup de grace: *April 20, 1999, Littleton, Colorado:* Eric Harris and Dylan Klebold assault their school, killing 13 before they take their own lives (see Chapter 7, this volume).

These cases made the national and international news, and each produced assailants identifiable by the fact that all were middle-class, white teenagers from small towns and suburbs. But these headline-grabbing shooting sprees reminded some other families and victims of youth violence of similar crimes, which did not seem to merit the attention of the national and international media. Standing just off screen, beyond our gaze, were hundreds of other kids, the same age as the assailants in the well-publicized cases, who committed acts of lethal violence. Most of us never heard about the adolescents who shot and killed other kids in the inner-city neighborhoods of Houston, Chicago, New York, Los Angeles, or Detroit during that same 1997–1998 school year. They remained mostly anonymous. The acute, one-day massacres eclipse in the public consciousness the long, slow massacre that occurs day in and day out in incidents across the country.

What about the 14-year-old African American kid who shot an 18-year-old convenience store clerk? The 15-year-old Hispanic kid who opened fire with an assault rifle on a street full of kids? The 16-year-old African American who gunned down three teens outside his apartment building? The 15-year-old Asian boy who executed a 16-year-old with a single shot to the head? Rarely do cases like these make the national news, and when they do, it is usually as dehumanized images—"cold blooded," "remorseless," "vicious"—that lead observers to speculate on whether these kids are even human. Rarely do we hear or see inquiries into their inner emotional lives and efforts to make sense of their acts. Why is that?

Is it because the high-visibility cases all involved white kids from small towns and suburbs in the American heartland, while the anonymous killings involved poor, predominantly African American and Hispanic kids living in inner-city neighborhoods? Is it easier for the media and the general public to forget or demonize these kids who kill? Some informed observers of the role of race and class in our society have said publicly that they think the answer to both of these questions is "yes." Given our society's history of institutional and interpersonal racism, it would be naive to think that poor minority kids automatically get the same attention and concern as white and middle-class kids do.

But the lack of interest among mainstream white America has its origins in more than racism and class bias. Until recently, most American parents *could* count on the fact that acts of random youth violence were not "our" problem, it was "their" problem. After all, in 1995, 84% of the counties in the entire country recorded no youth homicides at all (Office of Juvenile Justice and Delinquency Prevention 1997). Parents and children in most places must have felt a kind of immunity—if they thought about it at all—because, like my son in 1994, they didn't see themselves in the pictures of the killers and the killed. But that was before Jonesboro and Paducah and Springfield, and especially before Littleton, before the cast of characters expanded and my daughter saw that this could happen to her and her schoolmates.

Now, new voices of concern are heard, new faces appear in the newspaper, and new people show up for my lectures and workshops on violence, trauma, and kids who kill. The killings in small towns and suburbs during the 1997–1998 and 1998–1999 school years served as a kind of wake-up call for America. But it is also an opportunity for America to wake up to the fact that the terrible phenomenon of youth violence has been commonplace for the past 20 years. And it is an opportunity to learn from the experiences of those who have lived with this problem for the last two decades.

WHAT CAN WE LEARN FROM THE PAST?

What do the large number of anonymous killings and kids have to do with the highly publicized killings and the kids in Jonesboro and Paducah and

Springfield? What do they have in common? Answers come by moving beyond the surface differences between these two groups of violent boys—principally poverty and race—to see the profound and tangible emotional and psychological similarities that link them together. By getting to know the people and places where the epidemic of youth violence first took hold—among minority youth from low-income families in inner-city areas—we can begin to gain some insight into the lives of the boys in places like Jonesboro, Paducah, Springfield, and Littleton.

Certainly there are individuals and cases that defy explanation; some youth violence is the result of kids who have totally lost touch with reality. But these instances truly are the exceptions. I believe we can make some sense of youth violence "from the inside out" by looking deeply into the lives of kids who kill, listening closely to their own stories, and seeing the accumulating problems and the sequence of events in the life of a child that lead from childhood play to lethal violence, whether it be in urban war zones or in the cities, small towns, and suburbs of the heartland.

How Much Killing Is There?

The Federal Bureau of Investigation (FBI) reports that there are about 23,000 homicides each year in the United States. In about 10% of these cases, the perpetrator is under 18 years of age (U.S. Federal Bureau of Investigation 1995). If we extend the age cut-off to include youths up to the age of 21, the figure is about 25%. But even the reliable homicide statistics that are used widely for comparative purposes are not transparent and their meanings are not unambiguous. There are many complexities and subtleties to be considered in making sense of the numbers. For one thing, improved medical trauma technology has meant that an injury that would have been fatal just 20 years ago is today much less likely to result in death. The same injuries, such as being shot or stabbed in the stomach, that once were usually fatal are now often survivable, just as some diagnoses of childhood cancer that 40 years ago promised a nearly certain early death are now curable in 90% of cases.

An example of this change with respect to homicide is seen in Chicago, where from the mid-1970s to the mid-1990s, the number of serious assaults—attacks that could lead to death of the victim—increased 400%, while the homicide rate remained about the same (Garbarino et al. 1992). This factor is particularly important when we try to look at long-term historical trends and compare rates of violence, such as by comparing the homicide rate in the nineteenth century with that in the twentieth century, or the rate in the first half of this century with that in the last 10–20 years. Further, any consideration of the overall homicide rate should be tempered by an appreciation for the role of age and sex in these numbers. For instance, it is well known that young men are about 10 times more likely than young women to commit murder (see Chapter 2, this volume). Thus, historical comparisons may be skewed by changes in the population's age and sex profile. For example, if a society with an average age of 15 has the same total homicide rate as a society with an average age of 30, it probably means that the first society has much less lethal *youth* violence than the second one.

This kind of distortion is evident in the American homicide data, as reflected in two facts. First, the average age of perpetrators of homicide in the United States decreased from 33 years in 1965 to 27 years in 1993 (Bronfenbrenner et al. 1996). Second, whereas the overall homicide rate has been relatively constant over the last 30 years, the youth homicide rate has more than doubled (Bronfenbrenner et al. 1996). The period of greatest growth was from the mid-1980s to the mid-1990s, when the youth homicide rate increased by 168% (Bronfenbrenner et al. 1996). So changes in the youth homicide rate may be obscured when the total national picture is considered because more and more of the population is older. These increased numbers of older Americans dilute the effect of rising youth homicide rates on the overall rate for the country as a whole.

Nonetheless, we can see some distinct patterns in the growth of severe youth violence in the United States. Much has been made in the press and in city halls around the country of the welcome news that the total national homicide rate took a dip from 1991 to 1997 (Heide 1998). Similarly, after more than a decade of steady increase, homicides by juveniles dropped 17% between 1994 and 1995 (which still leaves the number more than 50% higher than it was in 1980) (Heide 1998). Does this mean the problem is under control? Not necessarily, according to criminologist James Fox of Northeastern University's College of Criminal Justice. For one thing, homicide rates in general, and juvenile homicide rates in particular, remain much higher in the United States than they are in other industrialized societies, such as the countries of Europe (Fox 1996). Closer to home, Canada reports a youth homicide rate about one-tenth as high as that in the United States.

Moreover, criminologists expect fluctuations because of the many influences on how many murders occur each year. For example, higher rates of incarceration for lesser offenses take some likely killers out of circulation for a period of years. The lethal violence associated with highly competitive illegal drug dealing has been associated with the extraordinary levels of youth homicide reported for some inner-city neighborhoods. But since the mid-1990s, in some cities the drug business has settled down, becoming better organized, resulting in a decrease in the youth homicide rate. And several communities have been undertaking a major campaign to curtail violence in their inner-city areas. In the mid-1990s, Boston was able to cut its youth homicide rate to zero for a period of 2 years (Metaksa 1997; see also Chapter 13, this volume).

So to reach a true, deep understanding of why children kill, we need to look beyond short-term trends. Certainly, the long-term trends are very disturbing. According to the FBI, juvenile arrests for possession of weapons, aggravated assault, robbery, and murder rose more than 50% from 1987 to 1996 (U.S. Federal Bureau of Investigation 1997). Looking back still further, we can see a sevenfold increase in serious assaults by juveniles in the United States since World War II. But perhaps the most disturbing trend is that whereas the overall youth homicide rate dropped in 1997, the rate among small-town and rural youth increased by 38% (Fields and Overberg 1998). That change highlights my conviction that no longer can any of us outside inner-city areas believe that we and our children are immune to lethal youth violence, because almost every teenager in America goes to school with a kid who is troubled enough to become the next killer, and chances are that kid has access to the weapons necessary to do so.

KIDS WHO KILL . . . THEMSELVES

While thinking about kids who kill others, we shouldn't lose sight of the young people who turn their violence inward, the kids who kill themselves. Suicide among juveniles is a serious problem (see Chapter 5, this volume). According to statistics from the early 1990s, each murder committed by an adolescent is matched by a suicide—about 2,300 each year. And just as youth homicide rates have risen dramatically in recent decades, youth suicide rates have skyrocketed 400% since 1950 (Norton 1994).

According to a Centers for Disease Control and Prevention (CDC) survey of youth, in 1997 15% of high school boys seriously considered suicide. About 12% of boys made a suicide plan, and 5% of boys actually attempted suicide (Centers for Disease Control and Prevention 1998). Two percent of the boys attempted suicide in ways that required medical attention. The CDC study shows that whereas girls are more likely to contemplate, plan, and attempt suicide, boys are more likely than girls to complete the act. This difference reflects the more lethal methods chosen by boys: boys use guns, whereas girls tend to use pills.

Harvard University psychiatrist James Gilligan points out in his in-depth look at the world of incarcerated violent men that acts of self-destruction and the destruction of others often have similar roots in the psychology of men involved in lethal violence—namely, the sense that life is intolerable (Gilligan 1996). Thus, the links between suicide and homicide for boys are an important part of the problem we are facing. Sometimes only at the last minute does a boy choose between killing himself and killing others; sometimes he does both (see Chapter 5, this volume).

In some cases, the act of killing others is itself intended as a suicide attempt. When an individual arranges a confrontation with the intent of causing himself to be killed by the police—for example, by taking hostages or pointing a loaded gun at a police officer—it is called "suicide by cop." The first words spoken by 15-year-old Kip Kinkel when he was wrestled to the ground by fellow students after his shooting spree in Springfield, Oregon, were reportedly, "Kill me! Kill me!" Understanding the frequent self-destructive impulses in kids who kill is a necessary element of the overall task before us. Eric Harris and Dylan Klebold killed themselves to complete the massacre at Columbine High School (see Chapter 7, this volume).

Where Did The Epidemic of Youth Violence Start?

In 1995, as noted earlier, 84% of all counties in the United States had no juvenile homicides and 10% reported only one (Office of Juvenile Justice and Delinquency Prevention 1997). Twenty-five percent of all known juvenile homicides were committed in five cities: Chicago, New York, Los Angeles, Detroit, and Houston (Office of Juvenile Justice and Delinquency Prevention 1997). Together these cities contain about 10% of the nation's population. Why was there such a geographic concentration of youth violence in these places?

Think about the characteristics that increase a teenager's risk of joining the ranks of the boys who kill. Chicago-based psychologists Robert Zagar and Jack Arbit and colleagues offer the following picture of this risk, based on their research (Zagar et al. 1991). They find that a boy's chances of committing murder are *twice* as high if he experiences these risk factors:

- Comes from a family with a history of criminal violence
- Has a history of being abused
- Belongs to a gang
- Abuses alcohol or drugs

The odds *triple* when

- he uses a weapon.
- he has been arrested.
- he has a neurological problem that impairs thinking and feeling.
- he has difficulties at school and has poor attendance.

The odds increase when the number of risk factors increases. This is a general principle in understanding human development: Rarely, if ever, does one single risk factor tell the story or determine the future. Rather, it is the buildup of negative influences and experiences that accounts for differences in how youth turn out. And it is one of the most important things we must remember in understanding boys who kill. If we try to find *the* cause of youth violence, we will be frustrated and confused. We may even decide the violence is completely unpredictable and incomprehensible. But our view changes if we recognize the central importance of risk accumulation. Understanding comes from seeing the whole picture of a boy's life, whether the individual is a troubled middle-class boy in a town like Springfield, Oregon, or a troubled poor child in inner-city Los Angeles.

Chicago, New York, Los Angeles, Detroit, and Houston have in common large and numerous inner-city "war zone" neighborhoods where many children experience a buildup of the risks identified by Zagar et al. (1991). These areas have been known as the places with the highest rates of adult criminality, child maltreatment, gang activity, illicit drug sales, illegal handguns in the possession of kids, health problems that affect newborns, and school failure. In addition, most of these children have experienced the ravages of racism. Sociologists have long recognized that the experience of racial discrimination provokes feelings of rage and shame that play a potent role part in stimulating violence. Interestingly, the populations most affected by the epidemic of youth violence are the ones that have been disproportionately influenced by the particular historical and cultural patterns found in the southern region of the United States.

Social analyst and journalist Fox Butterfield, who explored this southern effect, reported that the highest homicide rates in the United States are found among those who have roots in the Old South. For example, in 1996, all of the states that constituted the Confederacy during the Civil War were on the list of the 20 states with the highest homicide rates (Butterfield 1995). The 10 states with the lowest rates were located in New England and the northern Midwest. Thus, for example, in 1996 Louisiana had a rate of murders 12 times that of South Dakota. This pattern was as much in existence in the 19th century as it is today.

In his book *The History of Murder*, historian Roger Lane of Haverford College points out that until the 1960s, America's big cities had murder rates lower than the national average because southern states had the highest rates and were predominantly rural (Lane 1997). What is the reason for this connection between southern culture and violence? Historian Samuel Hyde at Southeastern Louisiana University, who has explored this phenomenon, concluded that it reflects the special cultural and political history of the southern region, notably the system of slavery and the violence associated with the prosecution and aftermath of the Civil War (Butterfield 1998).

Institutionalized violence plays a role in perpetuating a cycle of violence across the generations. But religious tradition is important as well. Sociologist Christopher Ellison at Duke University finds that the public religious culture of the South plays an important role in legitimizing violence by making revenge a moral requirement (Butterfield 1998). Those who transgress against one's honor or kin and dependents must be punished. Psychologist Richard Nisbett at the University of Michigan has also studied this phenomenon. He confirms that it is the code of honor that is passed on from generation to generation through childrearing that accounts for this cultural susceptibility to homicide. In his research, he found that when a young man from the South encounters an insult (someone bumping into him in a hallway and then calling him "a jerk"), he shows a different pattern of response than do young men from the Northeast (Nisbett and Cohen 1996). The southern young men tend to react with anger and show an increase in stress-related hormones in their bodies. The northeastern young men are more likely to respond with laughter, without any detectable rise in hormones. Fox Butterfield has detailed these issues in his work, and it is beyond the scope of this chapter to explore any further the cultural and social forces in southern history except to say that they do play a role in lethal youth violence. How?

One place to look for answers is the fact that the African American populations that constitute the bulk of the population in inner-city neighborhoods have their origins in the Old South. This is not simply a matter of long-ago generations making the trip from the South to the cities of New York, Chicago, Los Angeles, and Detroit. It is common for children to spend time in their family's ancestral homes in the Old South. I hear it often when I interview boys in prison, as they speak about taking summer trips to Alabama or Mississippi or being sent back to Louisiana or South Carolina when they get in trouble "up North."

It is not *race* per se, but rather the *role of race* in the situation created by all the other influences that makes the difference in homicide rates. In 1994, the homicide rate among African American youths was eight times the rate among white youths (Fox 1996). Butterfield's (1998) analysis is important to us because he makes clear that this disparity has much more to do with the southern origins of black youth than their African heritage. Speaking to this point, psychiatrist James Gilligan reports that the homicide rates among blacks living in Africa are generally no higher than the rates in other countries (Gilligan 1996). In the United States, the homicide rate for African Americans outside inner-city neighborhoods is no higher than the rate for the rest of the population. The combination of racism and cultural values that promote violence as a response to dishonor exerts a devastating impact on children wherever it is geographically concentrated and coupled with economic deprivation—as is the case with blacks in South Africa, who have been shaped by apartheid, and the aboriginal peoples of Australia, who suffered through generations of cultural genocide. These two groups have some of the highest homicide rates in the world.

What I have attempted to show is that the origins of lethal youth violence lie in a complex set of influences. Southern culture as a single influence does not explain everything, of course. Honor by itself, no matter its origins, does not explain everything. Neither racism nor economic deprivation nor child abuse alone can provide the answer to the question of why kids kill. No one factor explains everything. But this does not mean we are powerless to make sense of what is happening. Quite to the contrary, we have at our disposal ideas and concepts that can take us far in our efforts to understand why our sons turn violent and how we can save them. Most importantly, these ideas shed light on the influences at work that are spreading the epidemic of youth violence.

By all measures, the risks that Zagar et al. (1991) identified continue to increase.

- *Child abuse.* According to the best study we have on the rate of child maltreatment (Sedlak and Broadhurst 1996), from 1986 to 1993 child abuse and neglect rose from 14 per 100,000 to 23 per 100,000, if the standard used is actual experience of harm. If the standard used in defining maltreatment is risk of imminent harm—what the study calls "endangerment"—the increase is even larger, with the rate nearly doubling, from 22 per 100,000 in 1986 to 42 per 100,000 in 1993.

- *Gangs.* According to research compiled by the federal government, more and more communities are facing the problem of youth gangs. Nationwide, surveys find that more children and youths report there are gangs active in their schools and community—up 50% from 1989 to 1995 ("Gangs," *Minneapolis Star Tribune* 1998).
- *Substance abuse.* Hard drugs have spread throughout the United States; virtually every community in the country has a drug subculture. The CDC, in its annual report on youth risk behavior surveillance for 1997, reported that 9% of all high school age males reported having used cocaine (Centers for Disease Control and Prevention 1998). Fifty percent of these adolescent boys had used marijuana, and 30% had used it in the last month. After a decline in overall drug use among teenagers that started in 1976 (when 45% admitted to some drug use) to 1994, the reported overall rate is increasing again and now stands at 36%. Moreover, heavy alcohol use among teenage boys is common. Thirty-seven percent of the boys reported they had drunk five or more drinks on one occasion at least once in the previous month.
- *Weapons.* Surveys attest to an extraordinary increase in the likelihood that kids will carry weapons, primarily because they feel threatened and feel they cannot count on adults to protect them. The most recent data from the same CDC survey reveal that 28% of the adolescent boys had carried a weapon—a gun, a knife, or a club—in the previous month. Nearly 13% had carried a weapon to school in the previous month. Fascination with guns often begins at a very young age. Eleven-year-old Andrew Golden, of Jonesboro, Arkansas, and 15-year-old Kip Kinkel of Springfield, Oregon, spent much of their lives immersed in the gun culture.
- *Arrests.* Arrests of youths under 18 have increased dramatically since 1980—up 50% from 1980 to 1994 for serious offenses (Fox 1996). In addition, law enforcement agencies in many communities have taken a much more active approach to arresting juveniles in response to community pressures, political directives, and court rulings that limit their discretion and their authority to use informal means of redirecting delinquent juveniles (e.g., taking kids home and confronting parents, or ordering kids to make restitution without arrests that lead to court sanctions).
- *Neurological problems.* Surveys point to a significant increase in conditions in childhood such as attention-deficit disorder (ADD) that may reflect neurological problems and certainly result in behavioral difficulties (see Chapters 2, 3, and 5, this volume). Because of improvements in medical care for highly vulnerable babies, more premature infants who might have died in previous decades are surviving today. For example,

in 1960, only 10% of babies born weighing less than 2 pounds survived. By the early 1990s, that figure had risen to 50%. Ironically, this appears to mean that more kids are, as a result of their prematurity, living with neurological difficulties that can impair the processes of thinking and feeling. Studies show that the rate of learning difficulties in premature infants is about 25% higher than the rate in infants not born prematurely. Use of drugs and alcohol by pregnant women compounds this problem.

• *Difficulties at school.* Data show that about one in three high school students report having skipped school at least 1 day in any 30-day period (Bronfenbrenner et al. 1996). The likelihood of skipping is greatest among youth who live in family forms other than two-parent households (30% for two-parent households, 24% for mother-only households, and 37% for all others). The declining proportion of children and youth living in two-parent households signals an increase in skipping school. Moreover, research documents increasing rates of behavioral, emotional, and intellectual problems that affect children's and youths' ability to succeed in school. Since 1969, the percentage of high school students who have cheated on a test increased from 34% to 68% (Bronfenbrenner et al. 1996). According to the CDC, 20% of all high school boys reported that they had been in a physical fight on school property in the past year, and 26% of the boys said their property had been stolen or deliberately damaged on school property in the past year (Centers for Disease Control and Prevention 1998). Four percent of high school boys reported that on at least one day in the past month they had felt too unsafe to go to school.

More children and youth across the country experience the specific negative influences that increase the risk of youth violence. Where and when these negative influences show themselves in actual acts of aggression may differ from group to group. For example, the youth who committed the infamous school shootings in 1997–1998 and 1998–1999 killed and injured multiple victims in a single incident and did not have some secondary criminal motive such as robbery or drug dealing. This scenario is different from most of the lethal violence committed by inner-city youth. But the net result is the same for parents, friends, teachers, and civic leaders who must cope with the aftermath of the shooting.

Epidemics tend to start among the most vulnerable segments of the population and then, like ripples in a pond, work their way outward. These vulnerable populations do not cause the epidemic. Rather, *their disadvantaged position makes them a good host for the infection.* That the exact nature of the problem may change a bit as it spreads is not surprising. It is not uncommon for infections to mutate as they spread, with one strain being particularly successful in invading a particular host.

The Black Plague of the Middle Ages started in the poorest and most deprived homes and neighborhoods, where sanitation conditions and nutrition were most primitive, but eventually reached into the palaces of the nobility. Unmarried teenage pregnancy over the past 30 years has shown the same pattern. The high rates observed among minority girls from low-income families in the inner city in the 1960s are to be found throughout America today, among small-town, suburban, and rural girls. The same is true of the phenomenon of "latchkey children." Finding young children at home without adult supervision was once common among low-income families but almost unknown among middle-class families. Now it is common everywhere.

The same epidemic model describes what is happening with boys who kill. The first wave of lethal youth violence in schools peaked in 1992–1993, when 50 people died, mostly in urban schools, and involved minority youth from low-income families (Fox 1996). In response to what we now call stage 1 of the epidemic, inner-city high schools scrambled to devise and implement measures to teach teenagers nonviolent conflict resolution techniques, to disarm students before they could enter school, and to remove them if they did enter the school with weapons. American high schools became the major market for worldwide sales of metal detectors. We are now in stage 2, the spread of youth violence throughout American society. How did we get there?

How Do Epidemics of Violence Spread?

My use of the word *epidemic* to describe what's been happening with youth violence is deliberate. Epidemiology provides some useful tools for analyzing and understanding the situation of violent boys. For one thing, it helps explain how conditions can change so dramatically and quickly. One of these tools is the concept of *tipping point,* the moment in the development of an epidemic at which only a small change in the presence of the germ produces a big change in the rate of infection. Characteristic of physical illness epidemics, it is true of social epidemics as well.

Jonathan Crane, a geographer in Illinois, identified the tipping point in the social decline of neighborhoods (Crane 1991). He reported that when the proportion of "affluent leadership class" families in a neighborhood drops below 6%, there is a rapid increase among teens of social pathologies such as delinquency, out-of-wedlock pregnancy, and dropping out of high school. Once this tipping point is reached, the neighborhood is ripe for becoming an "inner-city war zone." This is clearly what happened in many of the neighborhoods in cities like Chicago in the 1950s and 1960s, setting the stage for the dramatic upsurge of youth violence that occurred during the 1980s.

Harvard University sociologist William Julius Wilson documented this phenomenon in Chicago and other cities as an end to strict racial segregation allowed affluent and middle-class African American families to leave the ghettos to which they had been confined by segregationist laws and policies. They were able to find a home in middle-class and integrated communities, leaving behind an ever poorer and more isolated population to deal with the decline of the industrial-sector jobs that had sustained them in earlier times (Wilson 1993). Neighborhoods that were once complete and resilient communities became homogeneously poor and socially troubled environments, the perfect "host" for an epidemic of violence.

Public policies have played a direct part in this process, for example, by clustering public housing in large projects, rather than dispersing it as scattered-site housing, and then forcing middle-class families out of public housing by setting income limits. I know this from firsthand experience. When I was 3 years old, I lived in a large public housing project in New York City, a racially integrated project that included families of many varieties. Five years later, my family was forced to move out because my father's income exceeded the ceiling set by short-sighted policy-makers and administrators. As a result of such policies, what had been a very livable community in the 1950s joined the ranks of the urban war zones by the 1960s. Unfortunately, that story has been repeated over and over again, in city after city around our country.

War-zone neighborhoods are places where almost every 14-year-old has been to the funeral of a playmate who was killed, where two-thirds of the children and youth have witnessed a shooting, and where young children play a game they call "funeral" with the toy blocks in their preschool classroom. Since the 1960s, such war zones in the most troubled cities have been the primary sites for kids who kill, but in the last two decades additional cities have spawned war-zone–like neighborhoods (Garbarino et al. 1992).

The change came first with the addition of a second tier of large- to medium-sized cities like Denver and Minneapolis–St. Paul, which have long been held up as models of civic virtue and social well-being. These cities have increasingly sported microenvironments exhibiting the plague of gunfire in a climate of fear and pervasive insecurity that has come to symbolize inner-city life. In some cities these areas may be only a few square blocks, but they are there nonetheless. Even Salt Lake City, Utah, the home of the Mormon Church, is not immune, as I learned when I was invited there to address a gang violence task force in 1994. Over time, smaller cities have joined the ranks. Now, even places like Battle Creek, Michigan, the home of Kellogg Cornflakes, have had drive-by shootings. And in my own small town of Ithaca, New York, there is a small section of town characterized by regular reports of shootings, stabbings, gangs, drug dealing, and the other accoutrements of the urban war zone. My own home, the idyllic college town, had a drive-by shooting in August 1999.

This development has a special significance for little cities, small towns, and rural areas. In big cities, the large population base has allowed for multiple large public high schools and for the maintenance of private high schools by affluent families and by others who wished to escape from the threat of inner-city youth violence. This has meant that "trouble spots" could largely be avoided by most affluent families. But outside the largest cities, this is not possible. Every teenager in Ithaca goes to one public high school. This brings the problems of the micro war-zone home to my daughter going to high school in Ithaca in a way that was not experienced by my son going to high school in Chicago. Ironically, she feels more threatened going to school in small-town Ithaca than he did going to school in big bad Chicago.

But this account of the rise of micro war-zones in small cities and towns is not the whole story. Another implication of the tipping point is that conditions in families and neighborhoods throughout a society may deteriorate for years before suddenly achieving a critical mass for lethal youth violence. I have witnessed this in my professional lifetime. In 1970, as a young graduate student, I accompanied my mentor, psychologist Urie Bronfenbrenner, on a trip to the American heartland. We attended a community meeting in Racine, Wisconsin, a small city nestled in the Midwest. Dr. Bronfenbrenner was there to talk to a group of civic leaders and parents about the trends he was detecting in American society that he thought boded ill for coming generations of children and youth, trends he had described in his book *Two Worlds of Childhood* (Bronfenbrenner 1970). The assembled group listened politely to what Urie had to say, but when he had finished, their questions and comments revealed that their overall reaction to his analysis had been, "This is all very interesting, but what does it have to do with us here in Racine?"

A quarter of a century later, I was invited to speak to a similar group of community leaders and parents in Racine. The meeting was held in the same room where Urie had spoken 25 years earlier. I was there to talk about my 1995 book *Raising Children in a Socially Toxic Environment* (Garbarino 1995), in which I had taken Urie's analysis into the 1990s. The audience listened avidly as I described the unfortunate changes that were occurring in American life, changes that I said were "poisoning" more and more kids. At the end of my speech outlining the problem and what it would take to turn things around, there was sustained, loud applause. I then asked the group, "How many of you think what I have said today is relevant for the situation you face in Racine?" Every hand went up. One man spoke up, "Yes. This is exactly what we are dealing with here. We have to act now!"

When I reported back to Urie, now retired but still active, his response was not a smug "I told you so," but rather one of sadness as he said, "Twenty-five years ago when this was just starting, how much easier it would have been to turn things around. Now . . ." He sighed. Now we have come to the tipping point and gone beyond it in many places in our country: in almost every community in America growing numbers of children and youths live in a socially toxic environment.

Though they may weight the odds in one direction or the other, social conditions alone do not cause boys to kill. Those conditions must be incorporated into the way kids think and feel about the world, about their world, and about themselves. Ultimately, it is on the inner lives of boys that the environmental influences take their toll and set in motion the chain of events that results in the horror of Jonesboro, Springfield, and Paducah.

The surface conditions that we find associated with the inner damage to kids in Washington, D.C., and Detroit may not be entirely the same as the conditions that play a critical role when the epidemic comes to the suburbs and small towns. For this reason, it is crucial to explore the links between the social conditions outside and the psychological conditions inside boys, such as the role played by depression, shame, rage, alienation, and bloated self-centeredness in the origins of youth violence (see Chapters 2, 3, and 5, this volume). I am concerned first and foremost with understanding why kids kill. I know that many individuals are desperate for answers, but do we *as a society* really want to know?

WHO CARES ABOUT THE CHILD INSIDE THE KILLER?

In 1995, I was called to testify as an expert witness in the trial of a Denver teenager charged with murder. The defense wanted my testimony to explain how this boy's history of abuse and exposure to violence in the community was relevant to understanding his motives and actions. By then I had become accustomed to hearing about the violent acts boys commit, so I was prepared to deal with the details of this boy's crime. What surprised me most about my experience in the courtroom was the prosecutor's response to my testimony.

He had access to the same records I did and had heard the boy's account of life in his family and on the street. Nonetheless, the prosecutor denied the relevance of the boy's childhood experience, saying indignantly, "Who cares what happened to him when he was a child?" As the prosecutor saw it, the only thing that mattered now was the crime the boy had committed, nothing more. The only relevant question for him was, "Did he do the crime?" It's not enough.

Each of the violent teenage boys I meet moves and intrigues me, as I come to know him as a human being rather than just as a "host" to an epidemic virus of violence. Many have committed monstrous acts. Their victims are testimony to that. And yet when I meet one of these boys, I can see beyond the facts of his crime. He is a sad woman's son, a young girl's brother, and a baby boy's cousin. While never forgetting about the victims of his violence, I always seek to see him as more than a perpetrator, as more than his crimes. He is a boy, a dangerous boy to be sure, but still a boy. Sometimes I discover that boy loves basketball or baseball as I did as a teenager. Some boys excel in a particular school subject that was particularly dear to my heart when I was in school. One boy I spoke with shares my love of mystery novels. Another shares my birthday.

Some of these boys appear so tough on the outside. But when I get a glimpse of their inner lives, I am deeply touched by their vulnerability and their pain, and I come to see their toughness as a survival strategy, something that helps them get through another day. In many ways, their cold exterior is a defense against overwhelming emotions inside. These boys puzzle me: seeming in some ways so much like my own teenage son, yet in other ways so alien. They are incarcerated as criminals, and they sometimes have long records that include multiple lethal assaults and armed robberies. Yet young or old, they often seem naive and childlike as they talk about their lives. More than one of the boys I have interviewed even sucked their thumb as they recalled the events of their life for me.

It was these experiences that led me to refer to them as "lost boys." Some boys get lost because they are systematically led into a moral wilderness by their experiences at home and on the streets, left there to fend for themselves. These are the boys on whose behalf I testify in court, trying to help judge and jury see the injustice of their experiences—how they have been robbed of their childhood by abusive and neglectful parents, by malevolent drug dealers, by the sheer viciousness of their daily experience. I argue that to simply punish them with death or decades of incarceration only compounds the injustice imposed on them by the world in which they grew up.

Other boys are better understood as having gotten lost through unfortunate accidents of human development. In their cases, no one set out to abuse or neglect them, but they ended up feeling rejected and humiliated nonetheless. Adults in their lives made ordinary efforts to teach them how to live in society, but these ordinary efforts were not enough, and they failed. Sometimes it is the absence or withdrawal of positive adults from their lives, not through some plan, but through the adults' own fumbling efforts as they dealt with their own lives through divorce and their own disappointment. It is always something outside that becomes deadly when filtered through the lens of these boys' tormented inner lives.

These boys fall victim to an unfortunate synchronicity between the demons inhabiting their own internal world and the corrupting influences of being awash in modern American culture. They lost their way in the pervasive experience of vicarious violence, crude sexuality, shallow materialism, competitiveness, and spiritual emptiness that affect us all to some degree but poison these especially vulnerable kids. The unforgiving nature of modern life puts so much pressure on kids to grow up perfectly—perfectly powerful, perfectly sexy, perfectly rich, and perfectly resistant to day-to-day pressures. It is always something. However, whether deliberately misled or just unintentionally lost, some boys find their way to lethal violence. Every boy has his limit; some reach it earlier than others. With at least one gun in nearly half the households in the country, with two-thirds of our teenagers reporting they could get a gun in an hour (Fields and Overberg 1998), with virtually every kid exposed to vivid movie and television scenarios legitimizing violence, we live in dangerous times.

PSYCHOLOGICAL AND LEGAL REALITIES

One thing I have learned from talking to violent boys is that "homicide" is just part of the violence in their lives. Legally, there is a world of difference between violent assaults that end in death and violent assaults that fail to produce a dead body. I see this in the cases of boys I know. Michael shot two police officers; one died after being hit by one bullet, and the other survived four bullets to the chest. Michael now faces the death penalty.

Larry shot a police officer seven times, and the man spent two nights in the hospital. Larry is serving two years. Conneel fired an assault rifle into a crowded playground and killed no one. He served three months on a weapons charge. Thomas fired a single "warning shot" from his .22 caliber pistol and felled a 16-year-old boy with that one small bullet. He was sentenced to 25 years in prison.

The legal system feasts on these distinctions, but I find them to be of very limited psychological significance in most cases. Thus, my concern is with potentially lethal violence as much as it is with homicide. We must look at kids who engage in assaults that *can* kill, even if they do not actually end a human life. It is very hard to predict with precision which boy will end up taking a life. Much more practical is to identify the boys who are at greatest risk for engaging in potentially lethal violence.

As I noted earlier, according to the surveys conducted by the CDC, in any 30-day period nearly 30% of our boys attending high school have carried a potentially lethal weapon around with them as they go about their business in the community, and nearly 13% of our boys have carried a weapon to school (Centers for Disease Control and Prevention 1998). Recent research suggests that less than 10% of all juvenile killers are psychotic, meaning they had symptoms of severe mental illness such as delusions and hallucinations (Cornell et al. 1989). The rest commit acts of lethal violence in roughly equal proportions in connection with conflicts, such as disputes or arguments that get out of hand or crimes such as robbery or rape.

These findings indicate there is a lot of potential for lethal violence every day in the day-to-day world of boys who attend American high schools. The elements are there, even if hidden from view, as they often are in the case of the white, middle-class school shooters whose acts have terrified schools and parents across the country. The elements are often hidden and muted when a boy is from Springfield or Littleton rather than from the inner city. But white boys from the American heartland mostly reveal many of the same patterns in their most intimate and important relationships and in their inner lives as their poor, minority, inner-city brothers. They may come from what appears on the surface to be a "good family" from the right side of the tracks rather than one that is obviously dysfunctional. They may appear to be doing well in school rather than dropping out for life on the streets. But the accumulation of risk factors is there to be found if we look carefully, deeply, and without prejudice. They are all our sons.

It is there to be found in the more subtle forms of psychological maltreatment, in alienation from positive role models, in a spiritual emptiness that spawns despair, in adolescent melodrama, in humiliation and shame, in the video culture of violent fantasy that seduces many emotionally vulnerable boys, and in the gun culture that arms our society's troubled boys. There is an epidemic of youth violence, and no community is immune. This is the starting point for efforts to prevent school violence.

REFERENCES

Bronfenbrenner U: Two Worlds of Childhood: U.S. and USSR. New York, Russell Sage Foundation, 1970

Bronfenbrenner U, McClelland P, Wethington E, et al: The State of Americans: This Generation and the Next. New York, Free Press, 1996

Butterfield F: All God's Children: The Basket Family and the American Tradition of Violence. New York, Knopf, 1995

Butterfield F: Southern curse: why America's murder rate is so high. New York Times, July 26, 1998, section 4, pp 1, 16

Centers for Disease Control and Prevention: Youth Risk Behavior Surveillance—United States, 1997. Washington, DC, U.S. Department of Health and Human Services, 1998

Cornell DG, Benedek EP, Benedek DM: A typology of juvenile homicide offenders, in Juvenile Homicide. Edited by Benedek EP, Cornell EG. Washington, DC, American Psychiatric Press, 1989, pp 59–84

Crane J: The epidemic theory of ghettos and neighborhood effects on dropping out and teenage childbearing. American Journal of Sociology 96:1226–1259, 1991

Fields G, Overberg P: Juvenile homicide arrest rate on rise in rural USA. USA Today, March 26, 1998, A11

Fox JA: Trends in Juvenile Violence. Washington, DC, U.S. Department of Justice, Bureau of Justice Statistics, 1996. Available at http://www.ojp.usdoj.gov/bjs/pub/pdf/tjvfox.pdf

Gangs: violence on the rise in U.S. schools. Minneapolis Star Tribune, April 13, 1998, A5

Garbarino J: Raising Children in a Socially Toxic Environment. San Francisco, CA, Jossey-Bass, 1995

Garbarino J, Dubrow N, Kostelny K, et al: Children in Danger: Coping With the Consequences of Community Violence. San Francisco, CA, Jossey-Bass, 1992

Gilligan J: Violence: Our Deadly Epidemic and Its Causes. New York, Putnam, 1996

Heide KM: Young Killers: The Challenge of Juvenile Homicide. Thousand Oaks, CA, Sage, 1998

Lane R: Murder in America: A History. Columbus, Ohio State University Press, 1997

Metaksa TK: Attacking gangs not civil rights. 1997. Available at http://www.nra.org/politics/1197tar.html, 1997. Accessed November 1998

Nisbett RE, Cohen D: Culture of Honor: The Psychology of Violence in the South. Boulder, CO, Westview Press, 1996

Norton RD: Adolescent suicide: risk factors and countermeasures. Journal of Health Education 25:358–361, 1994

Office of Juvenile Justice and Delinquency Prevention: Juvenile Offenders and Victims: 1997 Update on Violence (NCJ 165703). Washington, DC, U.S. Department of Justice, 1997. Available at http://www.ojjdp.ncjrs.org/pubs/juvoff/index.html

Sedlak AJ, Broadhurst DD: The Third National Incidence Study of Child Abuse and Neglect (NIS-3): Final Report. Washington, DC, U.S. Department of Health and Human Services, National Center on Child Abuse and Neglect, 1996

U.S. Federal Bureau of Investigation: 1994 Uniform Crime Report: Supplemental Homicide Reports. Washington, DC, U.S. Department of Justice, 1995

U.S. Federal Bureau of Investigation: 1996 Uniform Crime Report. Washington, DC, U.S. Department of Justice, 1997

Wilson WJ: The Ghetto Underclass: Social Science Perspectives. Newbury Park, CA, Sage, 1993

Zagar R, Arbit J, Sylvies R, et al: Homicidal adolescents: a replication. Psychol Rep 67:1235–1242, 1991

2

School Violence and the School Environment

Lois T. Flaherty, M.D.

Violence in urban school systems has been a focus of concern for at least the past two decades. The view that this problem is limited to large inner-city schools has been challenged by recent school shootings in predominantly well-to-do American suburbs. School violence has been termed "the tip of the iceberg" in American society, viewed as a symptom of a pervasive undercurrent of violence that is part of the basic American cultural identity. Youth violence has been termed a national epidemic and hence a public health problem. It has become a priority of the Departments of Education and of Justice, through the Office of Juvenile Justice and Delinquency Prevention. The U.S. Congress and state legislatures around the country have passed legislation in attempts to control youth violence, and President Clinton called a summit conference and spoke out about the need for effective interventions. (The White House Conference on School Safety, held October 15, 1998, resulted in two grant programs: The Safe Schools/Healthy Students Initiative and the School Action Grant Program.)

Center for School Mental Health Assistance supported in part by project no. MCJ24SH02-01-0 from the Office of Adolescent Health, Maternal and Child Health Bureau (Title V, Social Security Act), Health Resources and Services Administration, U.S. Department of Health and Human Services.

Students have marched to protest youth violence, parents have voiced alarm, and schools have adopted ever more stringent security measures.

School violence can be understood both as a problem of the social environment of schools and as a problem of violence-prone individuals and those youngsters likely to be victimized. In this chapter, I consider the context within which school violence occurs by focusing on characteristics of schools and of high-risk youngsters that predispose them to higher rates of violence. I discuss the implications for intervention of what we know about risk, including the social environment of the school and its contribution, and briefly summarize successful approaches to changing this milieu to reduce the likelihood of school violence.

EXTENT AND SCOPE OF THE PROBLEM

Definition of Violence

The Centers for Disease Control and Prevention (CDC) has defined violence as "the threatened or actual physical force or power initiated by an individual that results in, or has a high likelihood of resulting in[,] physical or psychological injury or death" (Youth Violence and Suicide Prevention Team 1999). Suicidal acts are included in this definition. *Severe violence* includes a range of assaultive behavior, from assault with a weapon, forcible robbery, and rape to actual homicide (Office of Juvenile Justice and Delinquency Prevention 1996). Other forms of violence are also significant in terms of their impact on victims, although they are more likely to be unreported and perhaps less a focus of public concern. These include fighting, cursing, name calling, bullying, and harassment, which are much more prevalent than the violence that captures the headlines (Furlong et al. 1994).

Data on Youth Violence

Ongoing tracking of youth violence has been done by the U.S. Office of Juvenile Justice and Delinquency Prevention since 1980. Until recently, statistics were not collected specifically on school-associated violence. One of the earliest efforts to collect data was a survey of school administrators done by the National School Boards Association (1993). The 1994 Safe and Drug-Free Schools and Communities Act included a requirement for the Departments of Education and Justice to collect data on the "frequency, seriousness, and incidence of violence in elementary and secondary schools." Two surveys were done as a result: one of students' reports of violent victimization (Chandler et al. 1998) and the other of reports by school principals/school disciplinarians (Heaviside et al. 1998). Because it defined violence-related injuries and deaths as a public health problem for adolescents, the CDC began, in 1991, to track high-risk youth behaviors, including those related to school violence, via biannual surveys of nationally representative samples of U.S. adolescents in grades 9 through 12. The CDC also undertook a special study of school-related violent deaths from 1992 through 1994, using newspaper and police reports as sources (Kachur et al. 1996). Since the 1992 school year, the National School Safety Center also has tracked, through newspaper reports, school-associated violent deaths (National School Safety Center 1999).

The principal sources of data from which the statistics are compiled are newspaper reports, public records, and surveys of school administrators, teachers, and school students. While homicides and assaults with injuries leading to hospital treatment are likely to be reflected in news and police reports, as well as in the schools' reporting systems, less physically damaging incidents may not be recorded in a way that is retrievable. It is widely believed, for example, that school administrators have tended to underreport fights between students and assaults on teachers because these incidents reflect negatively on their schools. Classification of what constitutes violent incidents varies among studies, and surveys differ in whom they query and how questions are asked. Some studies include only events inside the school building, while others also count incidents on school grounds outside the building, on the school bus, or on trips or athletic events away from the school. Nevertheless, the data are convergent in many respects.

Types of School Violence

Interpersonal disputes are by far the most frequent reason for both fatal and nonfatal violence. The most common forms of reported violence in schools involve assaults without weapons—in other words, beatings or fights (Heaviside et al. 1998; National School Boards Association 1993). In a National Center for Education Statistics survey, 190,000 physical attacks or fights without weapons were reported, compared with 214,000 incidents of theft, larceny, or vandalism and 21,000 incidents of serious violent crime (rape, robbery, or assaults with weapons) (Heaviside et al. 1998). The percentage of school principals reporting physical conflicts among students as a moderate to serious discipline problem in this survey ranged from 14% in rural schools to 25% in city schools.

School-associated violent deaths are rare (see Chapter 4, this volume). The National School Safety Center, using newspaper reports, reported a total of 253 school-associated deaths from September 21, 1992, through April 20, 1999, the date of the Littleton, Colorado, shootings (National School Safety Center 1999). Their data include killings of and by adults on school property, going to and from school, and at athletic events. The three most frequent reasons for school-associated violent deaths were interpersonal disputes (26%), gang activity (13%), and suicides (14%), with most deaths caused by shooting (77%). During the period studied, only 1% of violent deaths of juveniles took place on school grounds.

SCHOOL VIOLENCE IN PERSPECTIVE

Involvement of Youths Outside Schools

Most violence involving youths does not occur on school grounds and does not involve youth-on-youth incidents. In 1996, students ages 12 through 18 were victims of about 255,000 incidents of nonfatal serious violent crime (rape, sexual assault, and robbery and/or aggravated assault) at school and about 671,000 such incidents away from school (Kaufman et al. 1998). Fewer than 1 percent of all homicides of school-age children occur in or around school grounds or on the way to and from school (Kachur et al. 1996). For all types of communities, the vast majority of violence involving school-age youngsters occurs outside school settings and during the hours when they are not in school. Children and adolescents are much more likely to be victimized by adults, including family members, than by their peers. A Justice Policy Institute study using multiple data sources estimated that the risk of a child being killed in school was one in a million (Donohue et al. 1998).

Higher Risk of Violence at Urban Schools

Urban schools are much more prone to violence than are their suburban or rural counterparts. Although media attention focuses on school violence in suburban areas, in actuality these schools are relatively safe. Violence is much more prevalent in urban schools than in their suburban or rural counterparts. Urban, urban fringe, and rural schools reported serious crimes at schools, including murder, rape or other sexual battery, physical attack or fight with or without a weapon, robbery, theft or larceny, or vandalism, as well as suicide, at a rate of approximately 90 per 100,000 students; the rate was 28 per 100,000 for towns (Heaviside et al. 1998). Statistics from 1992–1994 indicate that the rate of school-associated violent death in urban schools is about nine times greater than the rate in rural schools and twice the rate in suburban schools (Kaufman et al. 1998).

Safety of Urban Schools Relative to Their Neighborhoods

Urban schools, even with their higher risk of violence relative to schools in other areas, are much safer than the neighborhoods in which they are located. Schools are a part of the larger neighborhood and reflect the characteristics of that community. Because adolescents who attend school spend a significant proportion of their day in school, school is a place where teens are in contact with other teens; violence related to interpersonal disputes is likely to be played out there. It has been known for some time that the exposure of children and adolescents living in inner cities to violence, either as victims or witnesses, is appallingly high, with as many as 80% witnessing or being direct victims of violence (Gladstein and Slater 1988; Shakoor and Chalmers 1991). Homicide is the leading cause of death for black males between the ages of 15 and 24 (National Vital Statistics Report 2000). Urban schools, even with their higher rates of violence, have an incidence of fewer than 1 violent incident per 1,000 students during the course of a school year. Violence in urban schools is in reality just one aspect of urban violence, and schools are the safest places for urban children to be (see Chapter 4, this volume).

Decrease in Youth Violence

Youth violent crime in general—and serious violence and weapon-carrying in schools in particular—is actually decreasing, although the rates remain high. After peaking in 1981, rates of victimization, based on self-report, have actually declined in the United States. The youth homicide rate actually fell 33% between 1993 and 1997, from 20.5 to 13.64 per 100,000 (Bureau of Justice Statistics 1999). Many large urban school districts—for example, Boston, Chicago, and Los Angeles—have experienced significant declines in youth violence both in and out of school (Bell 1999; Office of Juvenile Justice and Delinquency Prevention 1996). These declines are probably related to the early-intervention programs implemented in these areas. The CDC, in its data analysis from the four biennial surveys it conducted between 1991 and 1997, found significant linear decreases in the percentages of students who reported carrying a weapon (26.1% to 18.3%), engaging in a physical fight (16.2% to 14.8%), and being injured in a physical fight (4.4% to 3.5%) (Brener et al. 1999). There were also decreases in some violence-related behaviors on school property between 1993 and 1997. Despite these encouraging findings, the CDC concluded that the rates of youth violence remain unacceptably high. Little change occurred in the percentages of students who reported feeling too unsafe to go to school, being threatened or injured with a weapon on school property, or having property stolen or deliberately damaged at school. Youths ages 12 to 17 are three times more likely than adults to be victims of serious violent crimes (Sickmund et al. 1997).

Access to Guns and Youth Violence

Guns are a major factor in youth violence. Given the ubiquitousness of physical fights, the ready availability of weapons adds a dimension of lethality to an already volatile situation. In fact, all the increase in youth homicide during the last three decades can be traced to firearms. In each year since 1988, more than 80% of homicide victims 15 to 19 years of age were killed with a firearm (National Center for Injury Prevention and Control 1999). A very significant finding of Resnick et al. (1997) in their study of more than 12,000 adolescents from a nationally representative sample was that 24.2% of respondents reported that guns were easily accessible at home. The availability of firearms was positively correlated ($P<0.001$) with suicidality among students in grades 9 to 12 and with violence among all students.

The implementation of effective measures to restrict access of youth to guns is a sine qua non of violence prevention. Even though taking away all firearms from children and teens would not stop other forms of assault, which, though not necessarily fatal, can be severely emotionally and physically damaging, it would go a long way in preventing fatalities and disabling injuries.

Times and Places Where School-Associated Violence Is More Likely

School violence does not occur randomly during the school day. Violent episodes are most likely to occur before and after school and during transitions between classes or activities. These and any other relatively unstructured times are periods when words or perceived slurs can quickly escalate into fights or threats. Crowded places, likewise, are more likely to serve as a breeding ground for conflicts. Places where there is less supervision also are possible locales for students or teachers to be victimized; these include isolated places, such as bathrooms or near building entrances and exits, and on the grounds outside the school building (Dwyer et al. 1998; Warner et al. 1999).

Other Youth and School Problems

A high rate of violence is only one of many problems that beset troubled adolescents and poorly functioning schools. Other problems are high drop-out rates, underachievement, teen pregnancy, and substance abuse (Dryfoos 1998; Flaherty and Weist 1999). Taylor and Adelman (1999) assert that over 50% of the students in many large urban schools manifest significant learning, behavior, and emotional problems. These authors have called for integrated school and community approaches to address what they term "barriers to learning" and have criticized school reform efforts that focus only on imposing standards for academic achievement and reorganizing administrative structure. Jonathan Kozol, in his book *Savage Inequalities*, details the appalling lack of resources of urban schools attended by poor children (Kozol 1991). He points out that many of these children were doomed to failure and stresses the futility of trying to improve schools simply by testing students. Although there are some signs of hope, we are far from offering all children a chance to succeed.

CORRELATES OF SCHOOL VIOLENCE

Characteristics of Schools With Higher Rates of Violence

Several characteristics are consistently associated with higher rates of student violence. These include large school size, overcrowding of classrooms, large number of transient students, changes in leadership, and poor resources for learning (Warner et al. 1999). Students who report the presence of gangs, drugs, and guns in the school are more likely than those who do not to report having been victims of violence (Chandler et al. 1998). Public schools on the whole have higher rates of violence than private ones (Chandler et al. 1998). Having a large percentage of minority students is also a risk factor (Heaviside et al. 1998).

School and Class Size

Larger school size makes it more difficult for students to feel that they are part of their school and to have a sense that their participation makes a difference. Larger school size also makes it more difficult for school administrators to be aware of potential problems among students. Smaller schools are especially important for poor and minority students, for whom positive attitudes toward school are most strongly correlated with school size. For students from all backgrounds, negative behaviors are less prevalent in smaller schools. Additional characteristics of smaller schools are better attendance, lower dropout rates, more participation in co-curricular activities, more positive attitudes toward school, and an increased sense of belonging.

The average school size in the United States has increased greatly over the past several decades. From 1940 to 1990, there was a 70% decrease in the total number of United States public schools with kindergarten through grade 12. During the same period, the population in the United States rose 70%. The average school enrollment increased more than five times. Although an optimal number of students per school size is generally considered to be 400 to 600, 30% of U.S. schools have more than 800 students (Galletti 1998). There is a movement to reduce the effective school size by subdividing some of the larger schools into smaller components, each with its own administrative structure and defined student body, creating schools within schools. However, it is unclear that this alone would make a difference.

Large classes make it difficult for teachers to know their students and to offer any individualized attention—a situation that negatively affects the student-teacher relationship. Teachers routinely have classes of 35–40 students, even in elementary school. There is good evidence that reducing class size enhances academic achievement (Pritchard 1999). Under the Class Size Reduction Program, an initiative sponsored by President Clinton, federal funding is being made available to school districts to recruit, hire, and train new teachers, beginning with the 1999–2000 school year. This initiative is anticipated to provide $12.4 billion over 7 years to help schools hire 100,000 new teachers and reduce class size in the early grades to a nationwide average of 18.

Student-Teacher Relationships and School Social Climate

The social climate of the school, though seemingly difficult to measure, is a very important factor in the level of violent behavior in a school (see Chapter 15, this volume). In a survey conducted by Louis Harris and Associates in 1995–1996 of 2,524 public school students in grades 7 through 12, students who perceived their teachers as treating students with respect tended to report that students got along with each other and that there was less "social tension," as manifested by fewer hostile or threatening remarks between different groups of students, turf battles, and physical fights and less gang violence in their schools (Metropolitan Life Insurance Company 1996).

Furlong et al. (1994) interviewed older high school students in the Los Angeles area about their perceptions of teachers. The students, many of whom had histories of gang involvement, characterized teachers in three ways: 1) strict and distant, 2) inconsistent and afraid, and 3) tough and caring. The students felt that the teachers in the last-mentioned group genuinely cared about them and wanted them to succeed. The teenagers said that these teachers "picked on" them and kept after them but also challenged them and used appropriate, consistent, and fair discipline. Sadly, these teachers were the fewest in number in these students' experience. Much more common were teachers who were perceived as indifferent about the students and who either adhered rigidly to rules in attempting to maintain order or allowed the students to do whatever they wanted and who appeared fearful and timid. These authors made a strong plea for teacher training and education that empowers teachers to connect with students in meaningful ways and includes effective behavior management techniques.

In schools with lower rates of violence, administration and teachers work together. These schools have clear and enforced rules, and teachers are able to manage behavior in their classrooms and are engaged enthusiastically in their roles.

Clearly, the most effective means of addressing the problems discussed earlier involve structural changes within the school, the school administration, and teacher training and supervision. Obviously, strong administrative support is necessary to enable teachers to work effectively, and teachers' skills in classroom management are important. Changes in leadership at the school make it difficult for rules to be clearly and consistently articulated and enforced, so consistent leadership is important. Many teachers lack prior training in classroom behavior management, but these skills can be taught (Bell 1999).

Neighborhood Influences

The Project on Human Development in Chicago Neighborhoods, using a sophisticated data analysis, showed that the degree of social cohesion in a community, defined as the willingness of neighbors to act on behalf of the common good, had an impact on youth crime by virtue of the "informal social control" exerted by adults on adolescents (Sampson et al. 1997). Even in neighborhoods beset by poverty, where adults monitored youth activity and were willing to confront youths who were hanging out on street corners or truant from school, delinquency was reduced. These findings have implications not only for urban communities but for all communities. Affluent suburban communities, in which homes are spaced far apart to give a sense of privacy, are equally in need of the kind of "collective efficacy" cited by the urban researchers.

Characteristics of Students Prone to Violence

Violent students tend to be males from problem families (i.e., those characterized by instability, family violence, and/or mental illness) (see Chapter 1, this volume). Factors that contribute to violence among boys include involvement with gangs, substance abuse, carrying weapons, and previous arrests (Garbarino 1999). These youngsters often have histories of abuse and neglect, as well as of school failure and/or delinquent behavior (Dryfoos 1998). In terms of psychological profile, they tend to have attention problems, impulsive behavior, poor frustration tolerance, and poor self-control and tend to be sensation seeking (see Chapter 5, this volume). Clearly, this constellation of qualities suggests that many of these youngsters might meet the diagnostic criteria for attention-deficit/hyperactivity disorder and/or learning disabilities—conditions that are responsive to appropriate medical, psychosocial, and educational interventions.

Bullying and harassment, long considered an inevitable part of the school milieu, are beginning to be viewed as pathological behaviors that are indicative of psychiatric disorder and that have profound effects on those victimized (Olweus 1993). Bullying is a manifestation of aggression, and youngsters who engage in bullying others are at risk of becoming violent later on. Conversely, students who are habitually bullied or harassed because they are different from their peers may retaliate in a violent manner to get revenge (DeBernardo and McGee 1999; Dwyer et al. 1998).

Since 1993, there has been a series of much-publicized school shootings involving multiple victims. The shootings were perpetrated by white, male students who were seeking vengeance for discipline or rejection; a strong suicidal dynamic was involved in these homicides (see Chapter 5, this volume). The perpetrators have been termed "classroom avengers" by DeBernardo and McGee (1999) on the basis of their review of 14 multiple-victim school shootings between 1993 and 1999. In contrast to the typical profile of violent urban youth, these teenagers were from suburban or rural areas and grew up in middle-class or affluent communities. They were not failing in school and may even have performed well academically, although there was usually some decline prior to the incident. They lacked histories of extensive involvement in the juvenile justice system, although some received mental health services. The youngsters all have been described as isolated loners who were ostracized by other students, often having experienced harassment or bullying at school for several years. Some formed ties with other outcast students. What they do have in common with other violent youth is a lack of normal social bonding, including close ties with significant adults.

DeBernardo and McGee (1999) formulated a psychological profile of the classroom avenger as having atypical depression and mixed personality disorder with paranoid, narcissistic, and antisocial features. They describe these youngsters as chronically angry, sullen, and irritable with a long-standing interest in violence. These youths spend a long time planning the shooting. Access to guns provides them with a means to carry out their violent fantasies. And, finally, extensive media coverage of prior shootings appears to have a contagion effect, much like that seen in media coverage of suicide (see Chapter 5, this volume).

Student Victims of Violence

Males and teenagers ages 12–14 are most at risk of experiencing violent victimization at school, according to self-report data (Chandler et al. 1998). The rate of victimization declines with increasing age. A possible reason for this decline is that youthful perpetrators do not remain in school as they get older, but instead either drop out or are incarcerated or killed.

Just as there is a profile of violent students, certain characteristics seem consistent in those who are victimized. Victimized students tend to be socially isolated, unpopular, and insecure youngsters. They are often smaller and thinner than their classmates. Transient students and those who are in the racial minority, as well as those who are in transition to middle or high school, are more vulnerable (Warner et al. 1999). Levels of depression and concomitant symptoms such as dysphoric mood, low self-esteem, and excessive fears and worries about death or injury have been found to be prevalent in urban school children who have experienced violence perpetrated against either themselves or a friend or relative (L. Freedman et al. 1993).

Teacher Victims of Violence

Not only students but also teachers can be victims of violence. Between 1992 and 1996 there were, on average, 18,000 serious violent crimes (rape or sexual assault, robbery, and aggravated assault) against teachers per year. This translates to an average of 4 incidents per 1,000 teachers. However, during the 1993–1994 school year, 12% of all teachers reported that they had been threatened with injury by a student from their school, and 4% said that they had been physically attacked by a student (Heaviside et al. 1998).

The most common form of violence against teachers is simple assault. Middle school teachers are most at risk, followed by those in high schools. Male teachers are more likely than female teachers to be attacked. Just as for students, urban and public schools pose the highest risk for teachers (Heaviside et al. 1998).

Teachers who have unclear rules for classroom behavior and/or inconsistent enforcement of rules are more prone to be victimized. Punitive attitudes and differential treatment of students are also risk factors for victimization of teachers. Teachers may avoid setting limits out of fear of being attacked; such avoidance creates a climate of fear, which increases the likelihood of violence.

Normalization of Violence With Psychiatric Sequelae

Fatalism and a heightened acceptance of death are two outcomes of chronic exposure to violence. In communities where exposure to violence is common, individuals adapt by developing an expectation that violence may occur at any moment and that it is a part of day-to-day life. This adaptation does not mean that individuals are not impacted by the violence or that they develop a kind of immunity to its effects. Rather, they experience a sense of helplessness and futility about their present lives and the possibility that they could actively work to make things change. This kind of pessimism is strongly associated with depression as well.

Other effects of chronic exposure to violence are depersonalization and emotional distancing, which can be understood as psychological defenses against anxiety and other painful affects. Depersonalization is linked to dehumanization or objectification of others, making it easier to victimize them. From a psychiatric standpoint, these symptoms can be understood as part of the spectrum of posttraumatic stress disorder, additional features of which include "futurelessness," numbing, constricted affect, and dissociation (see Chapter 8, this volume).

Coping mechanisms include acting as if nothing has really happened and trying to forget or ignore the violence. These avoidant defenses, though adaptive in the immediate context, are not helpful in resolving problems or promoting change. This kind of coping occurs in children and adolescents as well as in adults and can affect both students and teachers in a school. This in turn leads to apathy and lack of active coping to prevent violence. School avoidance and dropping out are not uncommon (Weist and Warner 1997). Aggressive behavior, including violence, may also be an outcome as youngsters feel a need to protect themselves against real or perceived threats. In one study, students who reported multiple forms of violent victimization were 22 times more likely to score high on a hostility measure than those who were not victims (Furlong et al. 1995). Thus, violence begets more violence, either through apathy and lack of appropriate activity to decrease it or through efforts at retaliation and/or self-defense.

The "Conspiracy of Silence"

In several of the multiple victim shootings, other students later talked about having heard threats, which they did not take seriously, or having had some concerns about which they had not told anyone (see Chapters 5, 9, and 10, this volume). In some cases, the student perpetrator had actually shown a gun to classmates in the days prior to the shooting. A high school sophomore, interviewed about school safety at his school in the wake of the Littleton, Colorado, school shootings in April 1999, said, "You want to keep your mouth shut, or you might end up dead somewhere" ("What Can the Schools Do?" *Time* 1999). The silence surrounding threats of interpersonal violence is like the silence around suicide (see Chapter 5, this volume). The silence results in part from denial, a psychological defense against the anxiety such threats evoke, and in part from lack of trust that telling someone would not result in retaliation.

The teenage ethic not to tell on each other also plays a role. A high school essay contest, "When Not to Keep a Secret," a project sponsored by the American Psychiatric Association Alliance (formerly the APA Auxiliary), produced writings from ninth- and tenth-graders throughout the country. Many youngsters focused on the conflicts they experience over revealing information, but many also made the point that students bore some responsibility. As one student put it, "I think that all of these school shootings could have been prevented if any of these kids' friends had just told someone about what was going to happen. If kids don't step forward, I'm sure there will be even more school shootings. It's our responsibility to make sure that nobody has a gun or knife in their locker" ("Teens Share Poignant Thoughts" 1999). The conspiracy of silence also applies to witnessing of bullying or harassment. The tendency of students to remain silent must be counteracted by efforts to educate them about the importance of coming forward with information.

Barriers to Help Seeking

Numerous studies suggest that the teenagers who most need mental health services do not receive them (Dubrow et al. 1990; Offer et al. 1991). In the context of traditional service delivery systems, mental health professionals are among those least likely to be consulted when adolescents have problems. Youngsters with greater impairment are actually less likely to ask for help than those who are better functioning. Adolescents' help-seeking behavior is affected by developmental processes, cultural norms, and accessibility of services. To confide in an adult, a teenager must trust that the information shared will be acted on in a way that is helpful. Our own experience is that concerns about confidentiality are paramount. Students can be assured that, although the information must be shared with the appropriate adults, the source will be kept confidential. Assuring the availability and accessibility of appropriately trained mental health professionals will increase utilization of counseling services.

Cultural norms against emotional expression—for example, against expressing a sense of fear or vulnerability—are strong in many cultures, especially among males. These tendencies both increase the likelihood that an aggressive stance will be taken if the individual feels threatened and inhibit help-seeking behavior.

A Culture of Disrespect

Violent behavior is the ultimate act of disrespect, at the extreme end of a continuum that includes many forms of "dissing." Lack of respect for others is shown in daily incidents of pushing, shoving, hitting, and kicking, which can be seen even in preschoolers. It is also manifested in obscene language, name calling, and insulting others. The prevalence of these protean manifestations of disrespect blurs the line between violence and nonviolence and makes it easier to cross this line. The American Medical Association (Walsh et al. 1996), in its report on media violence, concluded, "We have redefined how it is that we should treat one another," noting that "a steady diet of violent entertainment aimed at children . . . has created and nourished a culture of disrespect" (p. 17). The AMA urged physicians to take an active role in assessing violence exposure in their patients and educating parents about the effects of media violence on children.

However, in addition to the media, modeling of these behaviors by adults in their homes and communities is undoubtedly a strong influence. One has only to shop in the neighborhood supermarket to hear instances of parents calling their children names, yelling, threatening, and sometimes even striking them. Many teachers, undoubtedly feeling that they have no other recourse, yell at and demean students.

Individual Risk and Protective Factors

An important contribution to our understanding of adolescent mental health comes from the growing body of knowledge on risk and protective factors. Some youngsters are quite resilient and do not get in trouble despite growing up in poverty and in communities with high levels of violence. Others from affluent communities have problems despite growing up in what outwardly appear to be good environments. It is necessary to understand both risk factors and protective factors in order to design appropriate interventions. The research in this area strongly supports the concept that problem behaviors in adolescents arise from an interaction between stress and vulnerability, as well as a relationship between risk and the level of what Garbarino (1999) has termed "toxicity" of the individual's social, genetic/biological environment.

One of the implications of this conceptualization for the design of school-based mental health programs is that different kinds of programs are appropriate for different kinds of communities and schools. For example, in schools in less "toxic" communities, a primary focus on identification, assessment, and treatment of youngsters with psychiatric disorders that place them at risk for violent behaviors is appropriate. Although this kind of intervention is needed in schools in high-risk communities as well, there should also be an emphasis on interventions that improve the functioning of these communities (see Chapter 15, this volume).

School Connectedness

An important study by Resnick et al. (1997) involved a survey of a large sample of high school students from throughout the United States. The authors looked at relations between various parameters of adolescent health and morbidity (emotional distress, suicidal thoughts and behaviors, violence, substance abuse, and sexuality), risk factors in the family and school context, and individual characteristics. Two parameters, "school connectedness" and perceived student prejudice, were found to be significant. School connectedness was associated with lower levels of emotional distress and suicidal involvement, and perceived student prejudice was associated with emotional distress.

School connectedness involves a sense that teachers care and have high expectations for student performance. Questions that pertained to a sense of connectedness were 1) Do you feel that teachers treat students fairly? 2) Are you close to people at your school? and 3) Do you feel part of your school? No other aspects of the school environment measured in this study predicted either emotional distress or suicidality. Noting that most schools spend more effort on trying to control students' behavior than on trying to improve students' sense of belonging to the school, the authors commented, "While much emphasis is placed on school policies governing adolescent behaviors, such policies appear in the present analysis to have limited associations with the student behaviors under study" (Resnick et al. 1997, p. 831). These findings are consistent with those from other studies that have supported the idea of school engagement as protective against risk.

Indicators of Psychological Resiliency

Findings of many studies of normative populations of adolescents point in the direction of self-esteem, social support, coping strategies, and participation in social activities as the major factors associated with psychological well-being and good adaptation. Conversely, involvement in negative social activities, such as stealing, bullying, or illegal substance use, is associated with depression and stress, as well as with violent behavior. These findings point to a need for programs to improve coping skills and self-esteem and to foster participation in school activities as a way of improving children's psychological functioning as one component of violence prevention efforts.

APPROACHES AND SOLUTIONS TO SCHOOL VIOLENCE

Given the level of concern over school violence, interventions are being implemented widely in schools and communities to decrease violence in schools as well as in communities. The best of these are based on what we know from empirically based studies. These interventions can be broadly grouped in two categories: those designed to improve school safety through security measures and those designed to reduce violent tendencies in students. Although many of these interventions are too recent to be fully evaluated, there is an emerging body of knowledge about what is effective. What works best are programs that involve an array of interventions that are targeted not only at students but also at teachers, parents, and communities. The focus must be on improving students' coping skills as well as school environments. Support of school administrators is crucial, as is proper training for those who deliver the interventions. Many of the risk factors for violence, such as poverty, abuse and neglect, and drug and alcohol use, are part of societal problems that can be changed only by concerted and long-term efforts to improve the quality of life in communities and to support child-rearing. The following is a brief overview of interventions that have demonstrated effectiveness.

School Security

Restricted access to the school building is the most common form of school security; 84% of schools reported this as their only security measure during the 1996–1997 school year (Heaviside et al. 1998). Metal detectors, drug sweeps, increased security personnel, and use of police officers in the school are the most frequently used security measures. It is generally believed that the use of metal detectors, either daily for everyone entering the school building or for random checks, has reduced the prevalence of weapon carrying. More recently, schools have been requiring see-through book bags and proscribing baggy clothing that can serve to conceal weapons. School uniforms and bans on gold jewelry are other approaches in use in many areas. Three percent of all public schools in the National Center for Education Statistics survey required uniforms in 1996–1997, and three-quarters of these had instituted this policy in 1994 or later (Heaviside et al. 1998). Although such measures are now widely accepted by the public and seen as necessary by students, parents, and school staffs, they alone are not enough to prevent violence.

School Safety Plans

School safety plans involve procedures for staff and students to follow in case of threatened or actual violence. A third-grader in a local suburban school told me matter of factly about having drills in which the students evacuate the school as they would if someone were to come to the school and start shooting. A sizeable industry of selling school safety plans to school systems has developed, suggesting that this is a profitable area. It is worth noting that Columbine High School, scene of the Littleton, Colorado, school shooting in 1999 that resulted in 15 deaths, had a detailed school safety plan in effect (see Chapter 7, this volume). Although such plans may help to decrease the number of casualties in the case of an actual shooting, they do not necessarily affect the emotional climate of the school in a positive manner and may, in and of themselves, do little to affect the risk factors for school violence.

The National School Boards Association recommends that all schools (1) establish reporting procedures for safety and security concerns, (2) enforce policies consistently, (3) train staff, and (4) conduct periodic emergency preparedness drills. The National School Boards Association also recommends periodic assessments by coalitions of parents, teachers, school security personnel, school administrators, and representatives of local government to evaluate how the policies are working (National School Boards Association 1999).

Identification of potentially violent students is another area of school safety plans. After a multiple-victim school shooting in Oregon, the U.S. Department of Education produced the document *Early Warning, Timely Response: A Guide to Safe Schools,* developed by a task force of experts from various fields of education and mental health, with input from parent and student representatives (Dwyer et al. 1998). This document included a list of 16 warning signs, ranging from social withdrawal, isolation, victimization, and feelings of rejection and persecution, to uncontrolled anger, history of violent behavior, intolerance and prejudice, threats, impulsivity, drug and alcohol use, gang involvement, and access to firearms. The document urged schools to obtain comprehensive evaluations for youngsters so identified and to ensure that they receive appropriate treatment, including alternative schooling when needed (see Chapter 5, this volume). The pitfall of using warning signs to label and stigmatize children instead of helping them was emphasized.

Zero-Tolerance Policies

Zero tolerance refers to predetermined consequences for various student offenses, such as violence, weapon carrying, and tobacco, alcohol, or drug use. The 1994 Safe and Gun-Free Schools Act mandated state laws requiring expulsion for at least 1 year and referral to the criminal or juvenile justice system for any student bringing a firearm to school, for states receiving federal funding under the Elementary and Secondary Education Act. Zero-tolerance policies have been widely implemented in schools throughout the country. The National Center for Education Statistics study found that 79%–94% of schools surveyed had zero-tolerance policies in place (Heaviside et al. 1998).

The state laws are required to include a provision for case-by-case exceptions, but, in practice, they have sometimes been administered in a heavy-handed manner. Although unequivocal policies regarding weapons do send an important message to students, the use of inflexible consequences can cause problems. These policies have been criticized for resulting in the "dumping" of problem students outside of the educational system and into the streets, where they potentially are exposed to influences that can increase their violent tendencies. Parents and other advocates for children with serious and persistent psychiatric disorders have been particularly concerned that youngsters in need of special education services may be denied the necessary support of the school system and their behavior criminalized. In some cases, such behaviors as bringing a nail file to school have resulted in expulsions.

The negative consequences of zero-tolerance policies illustrate the difficulties inherent in trying to solve social problems with purely legislative and punitive approaches. On the other hand, if comprehensive assessment and treatment are available, including good alternative schools for youngsters who cannot function in the regular school system, such programs, if used in conjunction with zero-tolerance policies, can form part of an effective community approach to violence prevention.

PROGRAMS FOR IMPROVING THE SCHOOL'S EMOTIONAL CLIMATE

Structured Curricula

Typically, components of curricular approaches to violence prevention involve attempting to convince youngsters that violence does not pay and giving them alternative methods of dealing with provocations. So-called anger management is widely used as part of these approaches. Conflict resolution is another approach commonly used. Negotiation of disagreements so that neither side loses or is humiliated is the goal. Promoting empathy and awareness of others' feelings is a logical strategy when violations of the basic rights of others are understood as linked to a lack of empathy. Finally, it is crucial to convey to students the importance of reporting their own concerns about violence as a measure that can save not only their own lives but the lives of others as well. Curricular approaches are often part of peer mediation programs.

An approach developed by our group involves classroom presentations by a team of two mental health professionals, with a focus on giving information about the effects of violence and how to cope with it. The team members discuss strategies for avoiding involvement in violence, such as traveling in groups, not wearing gold or expensive jewelry, and avoiding isolated places in the school. They also emphasize ways that students can get help, thereby linking information to services (Weist and Warner 1997).

Probably the best known violence prevention curriculum is the 10-session curriculum for high school students developed by Prothrow-Stith (1987), which has been widely used in the Boston city school system. This curriculum combines didactic and experiential approaches with a goal of giving teens the wherewithal to deal with violence in nonviolent ways. The initial sessions involve imparting information about violence and homicide, and the later sessions focus on practicing alternative behaviors through skits and role-playing. Students are encouraged to consider the consequences of reacting to violence with violence, to develop a kind of cost-benefit analysis, and then to enact alternative coping.

Psychotherapists will of course recognize these approaches as basic to many psychotherapeutic techniques, particularly those used in family therapy. Mental health professionals understand that maladaptive defenses may be part of personality distortions and developmental psychopathology, which are not easily modifiable and are unlikely to respond to educational techniques alone. However, it is at least conceivable that for many youngsters the learned patterns of behavior are the result of adaptations of healthy individuals to an unhealthy social environment and that, when presented with alternative views and options, these persons can choose and learn different behaviors without having to undergo intensive treatment.

Peer Mediation and Conflict Resolution

Peer mediation involves using students as negotiators to help other students resolve conflicts peacefully (see Chapter 13, this volume). Mediation may involve informal meetings or a structured process akin to a court proceeding. The goal is for both sides to use constructive ways to resolve disagreements, as opposed to the more usual strategies of verbal threats, withdrawal, telling the teacher, or repeating demands (Johnson and Johnson 1995). Rather than trying to bring about a distributive outcome, in which one side wins and the other loses, an integrative approach seeks to maximize gains on both sides, a win-win outcome (Johnson and Johnson 1995).

Peer mediation is becoming a widely used approach in schools. The usual method of implementation involves training for children, including didactic sessions and role-playing. Some programs have involved training all the students in the school, whereas others have focused on high-risk youngsters. Some programs include teachers and parents as well as children. Peer mediation programs have been implemented at all grade levels, even with young children. Outcomes beyond the intervention period or the school year in which the intervention takes place have not generally been studied. Benefit has not always been demonstrated; these programs are most successful when they are embedded in a school and community-wide effort that involves intervention at multiple levels (Bell 1999).

Mentoring

The strength of a bond with a caring adult in preventing delinquency and other high-risk behaviors in youth is one of the most robust findings in the prevention literature. For this reason, mentoring programs have received increasing attention (M. Freedman 1993). These programs involve pairing high-risk youth with adults recruited from the business community, professional organizations, and schools. Perhaps the best known is Big Brothers/Big Sisters of America, an organization in existence since 1904. Mentoring programs work by "helping shift the balance between protective and risk factors present in the young person's life" (M. Freedman 1993, p. 72). Although limited in their effectiveness without a societal infrastructure to support them, these programs can be an important part of a community-wide prevention effort.

Counseling for Victims and Witnesses

In addition to being important in reducing pain and suffering and preventing the sequelae of psychiatric morbidity, victim counseling and a variety of less intensive interventions may be thought of as part of the violence prevention spectrum, because violent trauma can engender violent behavior (see Chapter 8, this volume). Weist and Warner (1997) described a structured approach for school-based mental health teams to intervening in school settings in the aftermath of tragedies such as the violent death of a student or teacher. First the principal announces the death over the public address system and requests a moment of silence. He or she then announces classrooms where counselors will be available to talk with any students who wish to. Teams of two counselors (social workers, psychologists or school counselors) meet two to three times per week for 2–3 weeks with groups of seven or eight students. At the initial session, the counselors share public information about the death, and students are encouraged to express feelings of sadness and anger. Subsequent sessions focus on sharing stories about the deceased, developing and reinforcing coping skills, discussing survival skills, and fostering group support. Emotional expression is encouraged throughout. Although the focus is time-limited, some groups evolve into ongoing support groups.

School-Based Mental Health Services

School-based mental health services are part of a growing national movement to provide services in schools for high-risk youngsters who would
not normally avail themselves of this kind of help (Weist 1998). Locating
programs in schools can greatly decrease the stigma associated with seeking help and reduce barriers to care. The presence of a strong school counseling component is an important contributor to an atmosphere of caring
in a school and encourages connectedness and close personal contact between students and adults (Kist-Klene and Quantz 1998). Professionals
from several disciplines are trained to provide mental health services in
schools. Traditionally this role has been filled by school counselors and
school psychologists, but nurses, clinical psychologists, and psychiatrists
are also in a position to work in school settings if they have the appropriate
training and education (Flaherty et al. 1998).

Weist (1998) has referred to programs created by the placement of
mental health professionals from the mental health system who comple-
ment the services already in place as "Expanded School Mental Health"
services. Successful programs are linked to the community as well as the
school and require careful planning and joint funding and administrative
support (Flaherty and Weist 1999). One of the main contributions mental
health professionals working in school settings can make is assisting
schools in identifying youngsters for whom educational programs are unlikely to be successful and who are in need of more intensive approaches.

DeBernardo and McGee (1999) outlined a treatment approach to the
would-be "classroom avenger," or a youngster who is referred because of
threats, boasts, or warnings and who meets the psychological profile the
authors have described. DeBernardo and McGee advocate a coercive strategy to treatment that involves the family as well as the teenager. This approach makes it clear that the youngster's behavior is taken very seriously
and that threats of violence will not be tolerated. Preferred treatment mo-
dalities are cognitive-behavioral therapy and social skills training, together
with medication when indicated. Close parental monitoring and increased
limits on behavior, and, of course, prevention of access to firearms, are essential. DeBernardo and McGee advocate for referral to the criminal justice
system as a way of "sending a message" to the youth and his family, as
well as expulsion from the school setting as part of a "zero tolerance" policy,
which they feel should apply to threats in addition to actual behavior.
Their recommendations are based on extensive experience working with
the Baltimore County and Maryland State Police and are clearly based on
a model of working with violent adults with personality disorders. Al-

though such an approach may be an effective way of reducing the likelihood that a youngster identified as having violent fantasies will act them out, we do not yet have data to show that the classroom avenger can be helped to become a productive young adult through such measures.

Comer School Development Program

The essential aspect of this model, one of the first and most widely replicated, is modification of the school to create a climate supportive to learning through intensive family-school partnerships as well as improved teaching. This program, developed by child and adolescent psychiatrist James Comer in the 1960s, has demonstrated effectiveness in terms of improved academic achievement, behavior, and retention of students and teachers. The curriculum is integrated, with its major emphasis on academic subjects, social skills, and the arts and athletics (Comer 1996).

Full-Service Schools

Researcher and child advocate Joy Dryfoos noted the importance of incorporating health and social services within schools to create a "one-stop shopping" approach (Dryfoos 1994). The goal is to increase the effectiveness of services to support children's educational and social and emotional growth by integrating them and making them more accessible to parents as well as teachers. In addition to providing education that challenges and engages youngsters to learn, these schools attempt to meet the health, mental health, and social service needs of the enrolled youngsters, either through on-site services or by coordination with community agencies. These schools—really much more than schools—are open beyond the traditional 9:00 to 3:00 school day and often year-round, 7 days a week. Dryfoos estimated the cost of such an ideal school per pupil is $5,000 per year out of the education budget, plus $1,000 from additional sources, such as departments of health or mental health, community agencies, and foundations (Dryfoos 1994).

Initiatives of the Centers for Disease Control and Prevention

Because of concern about youth violence as a significant cause of mortality and morbidity, and therefore a public health problem, the National Center for Injury Prevention and Control of the CDC has funded 17 violence prevention projects in schools around the country (National Center for Injury Prevention and Control 1999). Most of the participating schools are located in low-income areas. The programs are designed with control groups and measurable outcomes so that the efficacy of interventions can be tested. Outcomes measured include fighting, weapon carrying, verbal insults and threats, disciplinary actions, injuries, and prosocial behavior. Programs in elementary schools involve cognitive-behavioral interventions, social skills training, peer mediation, conflict resolution, and modification of the school climate. Programs in high schools focus on mentoring, academic achievement, victim counseling, and job training.

Preliminary results indicate that, in order to be successful, programs must be developmentally appropriate, involve training of teachers, and provide administrative support within the school, as manifested by allocation of time and resources for the program. Programs in middle schools tend to be the least successful. The degree of effect of the program is correlated with its level of intensity (Potter 1999).

CONCLUSION

Youth violence can best be understood as a result of the impact of social and cultural forces on vulnerable children. School violence is but one aspect of youth violence, which has multiple etiologies. A comprehensive approach involving schools, families, and communities is necessary for effective prevention and intervention. Youngsters at high risk of violence, either as perpetrators or as victims, can be identified. Effective intervention can be done at all age levels and should target risk factors. Since schools are where youngsters spend so much of their day and are charged with so much of a child's cognitive, social, and emotional development, they have an opportunity to serve as safe havens where children can grow to become well-functioning adults. In well-functioning schools, teachers have adequate resources for teaching and class sizes are small to moderate; these conditions should characterize all schools. Simply having school safety policies in place is not sufficient; the most important aspect of school safety and security is consistent enforcement of rules and policies. Although school safety measures such as security personnel and metal detectors are necessary in some schools, measures to improve school safety must address the need for a social climate in which children feel valued and respected without a need to resort to violence to solve interpersonal conflicts or to maintain a sense of identity.

Psychiatrists can identify vulnerable and high-risk youth through psychiatric assessment and assist in developing treatment and intervention plans for those in need of mental health services. Mental health professionals can also provide invaluable consultation to school staffs in their efforts to make their schools a safe and healthy environment for learning. And finally, as experts on child development and psychopathology, psychiatrists and mental health professionals can advocate that schools be guaranteed the resources they need to do what our society asks them to do.

REFERENCES

Bell CC: Violence prevention in Chicago public schools. Paper presented at the 152nd annual meeting of the American Psychiatric Association, Washington, DC, May 15–20, 1999

Brener ND, Simon TR, Krug EG, et al: Recent trends in violence-related behaviors among high school students in the United States. JAMA 282:440–446, 1999

Bureau of Justice Statistics: National Crime Victimization Survey: Criminal Victimization 1997: Changes 1996–97 With Trends 1993–97. Washington, DC: U.S. Department of Justice, 1999

Chandler KA, Chapman CD, Rand MR, et al: Students' Reports of School Crime: 1989 and 1995 (NCES 98-241/NCJ-169607). Washington, DC, U.S. Departments of Education and Justice, 1998

Comer JP: Rallying the Whole Village: The Comer Process for Reforming Education. New York, Teachers College Press, 1996

DeBernardo CR, McGee JP: Preventing the classroom avenger's next attack: safeguarding against school shootings. The Forensic Examiner 8:16–18, 1999

Donohue E, Schiraldi V, Zeidenberg J: School House Hype: School Shootings and the Real Risks Kids Face in America. Washington, DC, Justice Policy Institute, 1998

Dryfoos J: Full Service Schools: A Revolution in Health and Social Services for Children, Youth, and Families. San Francisco, CA, Jossey-Bass, 1994

Dryfoos J: Safe Passage: Making It Through Adolescence in a Risky Society. New York, Oxford University Press, 1998

Dubrow EF, Lovko KR, Kausch DF: Demographic differences in adolescent health concerns and perceptions of helping agents. J Clin Child Psychiatry 19:44–54, 1990

Dwyer K, Osher D, Warger C, et al: Early Warning, Timely Response: A Guide to Safe Schools. Washington, DC, U.S. Department of Education, 1998

Flaherty LT, Weist MD: School-based mental health services: the Baltimore models. Psychology in the Schools 36:379–389, 1999

Flaherty LT, Garrison EG, Waxman R, et al: Optimizing the role of school mental health professionals. J Sch Health 68:420–424, 1998

Freedman L, Mokros H, Poznanski E: Violent events reported by normal urban school-aged children: characteristics and depression correlates. J Am Acad Child Adolesc Psychiatry 32:419–423, 1993

Freedman M: The Kindness of Strangers: Adult Mentors, Urban Youth, and the New Volunteerism. San Francisco, CA, Jossey-Bass, 1993

Furlong M, Morrison G, Dear J: Addressing school violence as part of schools' educational mission. Preventing School Failure 38:10–17, 1994

Furlong MJ, Chung A, Bates M, et al: Who are the victims of school violence? Education and Treatment of Children 18:1–17, 1995

Galletti S: School size counts. Schools in the Middle: Theory and Practice 8:25–27, 1998

Garbarino J: Lost Boys: Why Our Sons Turn Violent and How We Can Save Them. New York, Free Press, 1999

Gladstein J, Slater EJ: Inner-city teenagers' exposure to violence: a prevalence study. Md Med J 37:951–954, 1988

Heaviside S, Rowand C, Williams C, et al: Violence and Discipline Problems in U.S. Public Schools: 1996–97 (NCES 98-030). Washington, DC, U.S. Department of Education, National Center for Education Statistics, 1998

Johnson DW, Johnson R: Teaching Students to Be Peacemakers, 3rd Edition. Edina, MA, Interaction Book Company, 1995

Kachur SP, Stennies GM, Powell KE, et al: School-associated violent deaths in the United States, 1992–1994. JAMA 275:1729–1733, 1996

Kaufman P, Chen X, Choy SP, et al: Indicators of School Crime and Safety, 1998 (NCES 98-251/NCJ-172215). Washington, DC, U.S. Departments of Education and Justice, 1998

Kist-Klene GE, Quantz RA: Understanding a school-based mental health program: creating a caring environment. Journal for a Just and Caring Education 4:307–322, 1998

Kozol J: Savage Inequalities: Children in America's Schools. New York, Crown Publishers, 1991

Metropolitan Life Insurance Company: The Metropolitan Life Survey of the American Teacher 1996: Students Voice Their Opinions On: Violence, Social Tension and Equality Among Teens, Part 1. New York, Metropolitan Life Insurance Company, 1996

National Center for Injury Prevention and Control: NCIPC Cooperative Agreements on Youth Violence. Atlanta, GA, Centers for Disease Control and Prevention, 1999

National School Boards Association: Violence in the Schools. Alexandria, VA, National School Boards Association, 1993

National School Boards Association: Keeping Our Schools Safe: A Challenge to Our Communities (Web site). 1999. Available at http://www.nsba.org. Accessed September 1999

National School Safety Center: National School Safety Center's Report on School Associated Violent Deaths. Westlake, CA, National School Safety Center, 1999

National Vital Statistics Report, 48(11), July 24, 2000, pp 26–36 (tables)

Offer D, Howard KL, Schonert KA, et al: To whom do disturbed adolescents turn for help? Differences between disturbed and non-disturbed adolescents. J Am Acad Child Adolesc Psychiatry 30:623–630, 1991

Office of Juvenile Justice and Delinquency Prevention: Youth Violence: A Community-Based Response. One City's Success Story. Washington, DC, U.S. Department of Justice, September 1996

Olweus D: Bullying in Schools: What We Know and What We Can Do. Cambridge, MA, Blackwell Publishers, 1993

Potter LB: Implementing and evaluating violence prevention programs, Paper presented at the 152nd annual meeting of the American Psychiatric Association, Washington, DC, May 15–20, 1999

Pritchard I: Reducing Class Size: What Do We Know? Washington, DC, U.S. Department of Education, 1999

Prothrow-Stith D: Violence Prevention Curriculum for Adolescents. Newton, MA, Education Development Center, 1987

Resnick MA, Bearman PS, Blum RW, et al: Protecting adolescents from harm: findings from the National Longitudinal Study of Adolescent Health. JAMA 278:823–832, 1997

Sampson RJ, Raudenbush SW, Earls F: Neighborhoods and violent crime: a multilevel study of collective efficacy. Science 277:918–924, 1997

Shakoor BH, Chalmers D: Co-victimization of African-American children who witness violence: effects on cognitive, emotional and behavioral development. J Natl Med Assoc 83:233–238, 1991

Sickmund M, Snyder HN, Poe-Yamagata E: Juvenile Offenders and Victims: 1997 Update on Violence (CJ165703). Washington, DC, U.S. Department of Justice, Office of Juvenile Justice and Delinquency Prevention, 1997, p 4

Taylor L, Adelman H: School Reform Is Failing to Address Barriers to Learning. Los Angeles, CA, UCLA Center for Mental Health in Schools, 1999

Teens share poignant thoughts about tragedy of youth violence. Psychiatric News, August 6, 1999, p 6

Walsh D, Goldman LS, Brown RL: Physician Guide to Media Violence. Chicago, IL, American Medical Association, 1996

Warner BS, Weist MD, Krulak A: Risk factors for school violence. Urban Education 34:52–58, 1999

Weist MD: Mental health services in schools: expanding opportunities, in Handbook of Child and Adolescent Outpatient, Day Treatment and Community Psychiatry. Edited by Ghuman HS, Sarles RM. New York, Brunner/Mazel, 1998, pp 347–358

Weist MD, Warner BS: Intervening against violence in the schools, in Adolescent Psychiatry, Vol 21. Edited by Flaherty LT, Horowitz HA. Hillsdale, NJ, Analytic Press, 1997, pp 349–360

What can the schools do? Time, April 26, 1999, pp 38–39

Youth Violence and Suicide Prevention Team: Preventing Violence and Suicide (Web site). Atlanta, GA, Centers for Disease Control and Prevention, National Center for Injury Prevention and Control, 1999. Available at http://www.cdc.gov/ncipc/dvp/yvpt/yvpt.htm. Accessed September 1999

3

Biological and Social Causes of School Violence

PAUL KETTL, M.D.

Scenes of school violence have exploded into America's living rooms in the last several years. As we watch adolescents run out of their high schools with hands on their heads, or emergency personnel carry the bodies of children from a grade school, we all wonder how such a thing can happen. What could cause a child or adolescent to take a gun and shoot a fellow classmate?

This is a simple question, but one with a complex answer. It is generally agreed today that psychological factors may be the most important cause of violent behavior, but we are a long way from a full understanding of the causes of violence. Clearly, something is wrong with these children and adolescents who perpetrate violence, but what? Unfortunately, research into the causes of violence remains in its infancy. We have many more theories about violence than data to support them. However, solid data about the causes of violence are beginning to emerge, and in this chapter I examine the biological and social causes of violent behavior.

Violence is a complex behavior, an interaction of psychological, biological, and social factors that can lead a human being to a violent act that we may then witness on our televisions. Most thinkers on this subject believe that psychological influences are the most important factors leading to violent behavior. Among these psychological influences, the most important seems to be a personal experience of violence. If you have experienced violence yourself, or witnessed it while growing up, you are at a greater risk for behaving in a violent way. Violence, in this context, is a learned part of your behavioral repertoire, ready to be called on in the future.

Although it is true that many people who act in a violent way have been victims of violence themselves, it is far from clear exactly how being a victim of violence causes a person to become violent. Moreover, while most thinkers on the subject today feel that psychological causes are predominant in causing violent behavior, few data support the idea that psychological causes are more important than biological causes, mainly because of the dearth of information about biological causes of violence.

BIOLOGICAL CAUSES OF VIOLENCE

So, what *do* we know about the biological causes of violence? While we do not know enough, tantalizing bits of information are beginning to emerge that lead us to the beginning of the story of the causes of violence in children, adolescents, and adults.

Male Sex

To begin, the most clear biological cause of violence is male sex. While we can debate whether the sex differences that cause an increase in violence in men are biological, cultural, or social, there can be little debate that men are more likely to perpetrate violence than are women (see Chapters 1 and 2, this volume). To understand why this difference exists, researchers have examined two of the biological factors that separate the sexes: chromosomal makeup and hormonal differences.

Once chromosomal analysis became possible, scientists discovered that some individuals did not have the typical 46-XY karyotype. Some individuals had more than 46 chromosomes, and some men had more than one Y chromosome. Some individuals who had the karyotype XYY had been arrested for violent offenses. This led some to wonder if the extra Y chromosome led these individuals to act in a more violent way, in essence, getting twice the male "dose" from the Y chromosome. The problem with this idea is that few individuals actually have had their chromosome karyotype checked. Even studies that have examined the karyotype of males, comparing XY males to XYY males, have not uniformly seen increases of aggression in XYY males. Some studies have suggested that XYY males may be more impulsive than other males, which could lead to aggressive behavior (Burrowes et al. 1988). But for now, the XYY male theory has little evidence to support it.

Another feature that biologically separates men from women is the higher level of testosterone circulating in men. While some joke that men suffer from "testosterone poisoning," one wonders whether higher levels of testosterone could lead to violence.

In mice, variations in attacks seem to be related to variations not only in the baseline plasma testosterone level but also in responsiveness to testosterone induced before puberty (Van Oortmerssen et al. 1987). Variations in attack latency were related to baseline testosterone level and to the variations in responsiveness to testosterone that were induced in the mice before puberty.

In humans the effects of testosterone are harder to measure, and in children their measurement is even more difficult. However, a study of healthy adolescent males revealed that high levels of circulating testosterone led to "an increased readiness to respond vigorously and assertively to provocations and threats" (Olweus et al. 1988). This study also suggested that high levels of testosterone made the boys more impatient and irritable. Another study of testosterone was done in boys, ages 4 to 10, who exhibited violent or unmanageable behavior severe enough to require that the boys be admitted to a state hospital. All the children met the diagnostic criteria for conduct disorder and scored higher than the 98th percentile on the aggression subscale of the Child Behavior Checklist. Serum levels of testosterone, sex hormone binding globulin, dehydroepiandrosterone (DHEA), and dehydroepiandrosterone sulfate (DHEAS) were measured as part of the study. None of these hormonal levels were significantly different from normal, leading the researchers to conclude that testosterone does not seem to be a useful biological marker for aggression in childhood (Constantino et al. 1993).

So, while it is clear that male sex is a risk factor for aggression and violence, the reason for this risk remains unclear. To be fair, it is still not evident that the reason for the differential levels of violence in males and females is biological versus psychological or social.

Serotonin Dysregulation

The link between serotonin dysregulation and violent behavior rests on more substantial evidence. In most of these studies, serotonin dysregulation is linked with aggressive behavior independently of the psychiatric diagnosis(es). Findings from these studies have been rather consistent and represent perhaps the strongest evidence linking a biological factor (low levels of circulating serotonin) to aggression. However, a few studies showed higher levels of circulating serotonin in aggressive children, adolescents, and young adults.

A series of studies demonstrated that adult patients who are suicidal are more likely to have low levels of serotonin or of 5-hydroxyindoleacetic acid (5-HIAA), a serotonin metabolite (Banki et al. 1984; Burrowes et al. 1988; Mann et al. 1992), in their cerebrospinal fluid. Moreover, the different levels of circulating serotonin are thought to be related not to a specific disease but rather to aggression or impulsivity independent of the psychiatric diagnosis(es) (Apter et al. 1990; van Praag et al. 1990).

In addition to these basic studies documenting the link between low serotonin levels and aggression in adults, there have been several studies of serotonin in aggressive children. In a 2-year prospective follow-up study of 29 children, 5-HIAA concentration significantly predicted severity of aggression at follow-up. Lower 5-HIAA concentrations and lower autonomic activity were correlated with poorer outcome (Kruesi et al. 1992). In another study of 43 male adolescents (ages 13–17) incarcerated at a facility for juvenile offenders, measures of platelet serotonin function were obtained. In these adolescents, whole-blood serotonin was higher in those with conduct disorder, childhood type, than in those with conduct disorder, adolescent type. In addition, whole-blood serotonin levels were positively correlated with the severity of violence for which the individuals were arrested as well as staff ratings of social skills impairment. In this study, the higher the whole-blood serotonin level, the more violent the offense (Unis et al. 1997).

Another study of children (Halperin et al. 1997) examined serotonergic function and family history of aggression. In this study of 41 boys, all of whom had attention-deficit/hyperactivity disorder, the investigators examined prolactin response to fenfluramine challenge to assess central serotonergic function. Fenfluramine primarily releases central stores of serotonin and blocks its reuptake. Administration of fenfluramine causes a dose-dependent increase in plasma prolactin. The magnitude of the prolactin response to fenfluramine is believed to reflect overall serotonergic function in the hypothalamic-pituitary axis. Aggressive boys who had parents with a history of aggression had a significantly lower prolactin response to fenfluramine than did aggressive boys whose parents had no history of aggression (Halperin et al. 1997). The findings from this study suggest that not only aggression itself but a positive family history of aggression may be linked to abnormal serotonin function. Although the authors were careful to point out that family history of aggression could be transmitted both genetically and environmentally, the finding of a family link is interesting.

Violence against oneself is also linked to low serotonin activity. Patients who engaged in self-mutilating behavior were also found to have low serotonergic activity, as inferred from the blunted prolactin response to D-fenfluramine (Herpetz et al. 1995).

Another study, of 781 21-year-old men and women, measured whole-blood serotonin and assessed each youth for history of violence on the basis of cumulative court conviction records as well as the individual's self-report. Whole-blood serotonin levels were related to violence in men but not in women. In violent men, whole-blood serotonin levels were approximately half a standard deviation above the mean—a finding specific to violence, not to general crime (Moffitt et al. 1998).

It has been suggested, as we discussed earlier, that the best predictor for violent behavior later in life is the personal experience of violence earlier in life. Could serotonin dysregulation play a role in how these factors are mediated in the body? In one study (J. Kaufman et al. 1998), L-5-hydroxytryptophan was administered intravenously to 10 depressed and abused children, 10 depressed nonabused children, and 10 control (nondepressed and nonabused) children. The children who were depressed and abused secreted significantly more prolactin after administration of L-5-hydroxytryptophan than the children in the other two groups. Moreover, clinical ratings of aggressive behavior were significantly correlated with total prolactin levels after administration of L-5-hydroxytryptophan. The authors concluded that dysregulation in the serotonergic system in abused children seems to be related to experience as well as to familial factors (J. Kaufman et al. 1998).

In conclusion, serotonin dysregulation has been consistently linked to aggression. Although our knowledge of brain regulation, and of dysregulation in violence, is clearly in its infancy, the results described here are tantalizing. They suggest that the biology of the serotonergic system may play a role in the genesis of violence and that the experience of violence may contribute to this difference.

Other Neurotransmitters

Other neurotransmitters have been studied to look for links between neurotransmitter abnormalities and aggression. Some studies have shown a positive correlation between norepinephrine and aggression—a finding that has strengthened the arguments for using beta-blockers as antiaggression agents (Eichelman 1992). Other studies cited by Eichelman (1992) have investigated dopamine and γ-aminobutyric acid (GABA) for their role in aggression. Investigation of cortisol in aggression is ongoing as well. These studies, while interesting, have not provided the robust evidence for a role of these neurotransmitters in aggression found in the studies on serotonin. Certainly, our knowledge of the neurochemistry of the brain is just emerging, and the future should bring more promising information.

Brain Structure

Another way to explore the brain is to look for a "violence center," or structure in the brain that may mediate violent behavior. Brain imaging studies or anatomic examinations of brains that have been injured through trauma or tumors have been used to provide these gross pathology data.

Agitation and aggression can often follow traumatic head injury. However, most traumatic head injury occurs in motor vehicle accidents, in which the brain can suffer diffuse coup and contra-coup injury. In their review of the neurobiology of impulsive aggression, Kavoussi et al. (1997) argued that individuals who sustain head injury may not be a random population. Individuals who get into situations such as fights or speeding car crashes may have preexisting problems with impulsivity. However, these authors cited some data showing that patients with frontal lobe injuries may be more likely to show aggression (Garza-Trevino 1994). Garza-Trevino (1994) suggested lesions in the limbic structure, in the temporal lobes, and in the frontal lobes as possible sites for abnormalities in aggressive individuals. Bremner and Narayan (1998) wondered if trauma may result in reduced volume of the hippocampus as measured by magnetic resonance imaging. They also speculated that hippocampal atrophy may be associated with learning or memory problems later in life.

Possible associations between violence and differences or alterations in the "structure" of the brain are currently the focus of investigation, but the data are still young, and the studies are marked by small sample sizes. To examine frontal lobe performance, Westby and Ferraro (1999) administered the Wisconsin Card Sorting Test, the Stroop Color-Word Test, and the Trails B tests to 38 perpetrators of domestic violence and 38 control subjects. Although those who perpetrated violence did perform more poorly on these frontal lobe tests than the control subjects, the difference explained only about 7% of the variance.

Another way of looking at brain injury or brain pathology is to examine violence rates in epilepsy. Violence in persons with temporal lobe epilepsy has been examined, and, at times, temporal lobe epilepsy has even been used as a defense in court. While in a postictal delirium, individuals with epilepsy may strike out or flail their arms at those who come close, but goal-directed violence does not seem to occur. In one study of patients with temporal lobe epilepsy, well-directed violent and self-destructive behavior was not a feature of the epileptic psychosis, occurring instead more specifically in postictal psychosis (Kanemoto et al. 1999).

Thus, pathology studies of the brain through neuroimaging or direct pathological examination have not been consistently successful in identifying a "violence center" in the brain. Nor is such a center likely to be found in the future.

Violence and Psychiatric Disorders

Years ago, charges that persons with serious psychiatric disorder(s) are violent were dismissed by some mental health clinicians, including myself. The stigma surrounding mental illness has been so great, I feared that this allegation was a result of the stigma against mental illness itself. However, over the last several years, data have emerged making it clear that individuals with major psychiatric disorders such as schizophrenia, bipolar disorder, and major depression are more likely to commit violence (Eronen et al. 1998; Tehrani et al. 1998).

Certainly, most individuals with these disorders are not violent, but the rates of violence are higher in those who cope with these disorders (see Chapter 5, this volume). In fact, men with major mental disorders (schizophrenia or a major affective disorder) are more than twice as likely to be arrested for a criminal offense, and four times as likely to be arrested for a violent offense, than men without these disorders (Hodgins 1992). Men are more likely overall to commit an offense, especially a violent offense. If a woman commits a violent offense, one is more likely to suspect a psychiatric disorder as a contributing cause. Women with major psychiatric disorders are five times more likely to commit an offense, and a remarkable 27 times more likely to commit a violent offense, than women without a major psychiatric disorder (Hodgins 1992). The reasons for this greater likelihood are unclear. For some individuals, violence occurs in response to hallucinations that direct them to act violently. In others, violence is connected with their delusional system. Some authors propose that genetic factors in psychiatric disorder(s) may be linked to violence (Tehrani et al. 1998).

Higher rates of violence are seen in both males and females with mental illness. In the general population, men are more likely to be violent. However, when major mental illness enters the picture, these sex differences melt away. An examination of violence in men and women in the 4 months before psychiatric hospitalization for their mental illness found no sex difference in the number of threats and fights. However, men with psychiatric disorder(s) were more likely to use weapons and engage in "more serious violence" (Hiday et al. 1998).

Clearly, other psychiatric disorder(s) are linked with violence. Antisocial personality disorder, almost by definition, is often linked with violent behavior. In addition, substance abuse is often associated with violent behavior (Eronen et al. 1998). Disinhibition of behavior that is associated with intoxication is just a step away from violence or criminal behavior. The U.S. Department of Justice reports that 40% of persons in local or state jails or on probation used alcohol at the time of their offense. Drug use is also often linked with violence. Violent behavior may result not only from intoxication but also from the "business" of dealing drugs. Territories for sales are staked out by those who have made selling drugs their business. Encroachment into this territory is protected for economic reasons—and leads to shootings.

Psychiatric disorder(s) in children and adolescents is also linked to violent behavior. It has long been recognized that children with attention-deficit disorder are more likely to engage in antisocial behavior. This was dramatically demonstrated in a review of 1,956 children, ages 6-17, who were adjudicated delinquents in Cook County, Illinois (Zagar et al. 1989). Their mean age was 14, and 80% were male. Forty-six of these youth had attention-deficit disorder without hyperactivity, and 9% had attention-deficit disorder with hyperactivity. Fifteen percent had mental retardation. Thus, the vernacular statements that "something is wrong" with these children are clearly correct. The fact that so many children have a treatable psychiatric condition also leads to the hope that early intervention and treatment may change the course of some of these lives (see Chapter 5, this volume).

Summary of Biological Factors

Clearly, our understanding of the biology of violence is in its infancy. However, available data demonstrate risk factors that may, in the broadest use of the term, be considered "biological." Male sex, altered serotonin function, attention-deficit disorder in children, and major mental illness in adults all have been rather consistently linked to violent behavior. In addition, antisocial personality disorder, alcoholism, and other drug abuse can be clearly linked to violent behavior. While there is no "typical" violent offender, the factors discussed above should be considered in the assessment of individuals at risk of violent behavior. So far, neuroimaging studies or neurochemical measurements cannot identify violent individuals. The best data in the neurosciences, at the moment, rest with the relation between dysregulation of the serotonergic system and violent behavior.

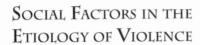

SOCIAL FACTORS IN THE ETIOLOGY OF VIOLENCE

Violent behavior is a complex phenomenon that cannot be explained on the basis of only one set of variables. Biological factors are clearly important in the genesis of violent behavior, but social factors must also be examined to have a fuller explanation of the genesis of violence.

Gangs

In examining social factors in school violence, it is clear that gangs have had an increasing presence over the years. The presence of gangs almost doubled from 1989 to 1995, according to the U.S. Departments of Justice and of Education (P. Kaufman et al. 1999). Some of these gangs are composed of those that immediately come to mind: namely, urban youths who band together, often engaging in drug use or other illegal activity. Some comprise youths who cluster together in less formally organized groups. These groups may stake out territories in school corridors, harass other students, or make other trouble in the school. One of the social factors contributing to violence in the school is the growth of gangs.

Television

In the average American home, television brings stories and messages into the living room approximately 7 hours per day. Children from age 2 years onward watch more than 3 hours per day (Neilsen Media Research 1993). Many children spend more time watching television than doing any other waking activity. While debates about the content of television are still raging, there can be little doubt that the sheer volume of television viewing steals time from growing up.

Effects of Television

The effects of television stem not only from its content—which all too often is not wholesome—but also from the enormous presence of television in the daily life of children. The mere act of watching television removes children from social, intellectual, and physical growth through play, group activities, creative work, reading, and sports. Although television can bring wonderful entertainment into the home, and literally dumps the world into the living room, it also steals time from all other parts of growing up.

Unfortunately, the content of television is not benign. By the time a child graduates from elementary school, he or she will have witnessed more than 100,000 acts of violence and 8,000 entertaining murders from his or her living room (Kroll 1993). An 18-hour survey of 10 channels conducted by *TV Guide* showed 1,846 acts of violence in 175 scenes of television drama (Hickey 1992). If the personal experience of violence is the most important psychological precipitant of violence, then we have exposed two generations of American children to wide-ranging and frequent, if vicarious, experiences of violence in their living rooms.

While it is clear the real experience of violence through assault or family abuse is far more severe than that experienced through the media, it is evident that the sheer volume of violent entertainment consumed by America's children is not beneficial. Children learn from what they experience—even on television. Studies have consistently shown that just as the experience of violence in person may lead to violent behavior, so too can the experience of violence on television. Reviews on the subject have been quite consistent. The American Psychiatric Association (1993), American Academy of Pediatrics (1990), American Medical Association (Kroll 1993), National Institute of Mental Health (1982), and Surgeon General's Scientific Advisory Committee (1972) all come to the same conclusion: Experiencing violence on television can lead to violent behavior in our children. Although not all, especially those in the broadcast industry (Stipp and Milavsky 1998), agree that television causes violent behavior, the bulk of reviewers, including those cited above, feel that television is one cause of violent or aggressive behavior.

That is not to say that television causes all children to be violent. As stated numerous times in this chapter, violence is a complex behavior, with many causes that come together in a susceptible individual, resulting in a violent act. In those who are predisposed to violent behavior for whatever biological or psychological reasons, violent entertainment can make these impulses flare. Exposing children already predisposed to violence to violent entertainment is like pouring kerosene on a fire.

Violent entertainment on television leads some children to act in a violent fashion, but it has an effect on all children. Clearly, it would be silly to presume that a presence so universal in children's lives such as television, one that consumes at least 3 hours of every waking day, would have no effect. Those children predisposed to acting violently have this tendency flared by television. Children who are not likely to act in a violent manner also are affected by television violence. They view the world as a "mean and scary" place (Singer 1985) and may be less likely to explore the world because of this experience.

Parents can intervene to try to limit the harmful effects of television violence (Kettl 1995). The detrimental effects of television viewing are reduced if parents discuss television viewing with their children (Venbrux et al. 1994). Moreover, parents can limit the amount of television their children experience. The American Academy of Pediatrics (1990) recommends that children watch no more than 1–2 hours of television per day. The American Academy of Pediatrics also recommended that children 2 years and under not watch television. This not only limits the amount of violence they experience on television but also allows them to more fully experience the world through other activities.

Television Viewing History in Clinical Practice

Television dominates our society. That fact is a source of worry as we seek to rear our children, but it leads to an area of clinical exploration. Because many children spend more time watching television than doing any other waking activity, an exploration of television viewing provides the clinician an opportunity to better understand and explore the child's life. Ignoring television viewing in the child's clinical evaluation is literally ignoring the largest part of a child's waking life.

Taking a television viewing history can be an important part of any child psychiatry and pediatric evaluation. Getting information about television viewing will tell the evaluating clinician a fair amount about the ecology of the child's household. A television viewing history should include questions on how many hours a day a child watches television and who watches television with the child. Children who view excessive amounts of television may be more at risk for problems with depression and anxiety (Singer et al. 1998). If television viewing is not limited at all, it leads to suspicions that there are few limits in the household. If the parents are never present when the child watches television, it again gives the clinician an idea of a lack of parental involvement.

Television also can be the "freeway to the unconscious." Children are often reluctant to respond to questions about their feelings, hopes, and fears, especially in the initial clinical interaction. However, questions asked about television usually will be answered freely by children, and this process can lead to important clinical information. Because television is ubiquitous, virtually all children have some exposure to the stories on television. Hence, they can select their favorites, and the shows that children select as their favorites tell a lot about them. The clinician might ask, "What is your favorite show?" and "Who is your favorite TV character?" A child's stated preference for watching reruns of the *Cosby Show,* because everybody on that show seemed to care for each other, will tell volumes about her current home and worries. On the other hand, a child's saying that his favorite show is pro wrestling, because "those guys always beat somebody up," also leads to a number of clinical hypotheses. Children will talk readily about television, and ignoring that part of the interview is ignoring the largest part of their waking life.

Television News: Contagion of Threats of Violence

The massacre at Columbine High School in Colorado captured America's attention (see Chapter 7, this volume). The scene of hundreds of high school students streaming out of their school with their hands over their heads after being threatened by fellow students with guns seared its way into America's consciousness. This image was hard to forget. Would an image this dramatic lead some susceptible students to "copy" the event to imitate some of the drama? The Pennsylvania Emergency Management Agency reported that before the tragedy at Columbine High School, it would typically respond to one or two bomb threats per week. However, in the 2½ weeks after the event, more than 200 bomb threats were reported from Pennsylvania schools (Donnelly and Murphy 1999).

Is this just an isolated event, or can "contagion" occur with a widely broadcast tragedy, encouraging other susceptible young people to commit similar acts? Can exposure to an act of violence be a cause of another act of violence? If so, who is most at risk for imitation, and how long does the period of imitation last?

Unfortunately, few data are available to guide us in the answer to these questions. Television research does provide us with some answers in the imitation of violent acts. Gould and Shaffer (1986) noted an increase in suicide attempts reported to New York City area emergency rooms in the 2 weeks following airing of a television drama with a fictionalized suicide by one of the show's characters. However, a review of the event by other investigators examining broader data failed to replicate this finding (Phillips and Paight 1987). Berman (1988), in his review of the subject, also found no increase in overall suicide rates after airing of a television drama showing a fictional suicide, but there was some copying of the suicide method used in the story. The data overall do not support the notion that fictional television suicides lead to an increase in suicides. But enough questions about the subject have been raised that the major television networks now most often do not include themes of suicide in television drama programming because of the concern over "copycat suicides."

However, the events viewed across America in the Columbine High School massacre were, unfortunately, not fiction. They were real events, with repeated analysis and focus by television news shows, commentaries, and talk shows. Is there imitation after real events?

Following the death of Marilyn Monroe, a series of copycat suicides were reported. The concept of imitation suicides following a news story was investigated by a number of researchers, most notably David Phillips at the University of California in San Diego. He found that teen suicides increased in the week following airing of television news stories about suicide. The more notoriety given the stories by television news organizations, the greater the increase in suicides (Phillips and Carstensen 1986). These increases occurred in the week following the news events, and the suicides occurred among teenagers. However, after the State Auditor General of Pennsylvania committed suicide subsequent to being convicted of taking money as a kickback, there was an increase in suicides among middle-age adults, with the increase still evident 8 weeks after the suicide (Kettl et al. 1992).

These data suggest that television coverage of suicides does lead to imitation suicides, with the number following such suicides in excess of the number of suicides that would naturally occur in the population. Television news organizations have debated their responsibility at times, but most have no clear standards to guide them in covering news events that may spur imitation. They rely on the judgment of editors to guide decisions. However, it is clear that imitation suicides occur after a suicide that is covered by the news media. The tragedy at Columbine High School raises the question, Do dramatic violent events lead to perpetration of other violent events or threats of events by susceptible individuals? (See Chapter 7, this volume.)

News organizations need to recognize the power they have over the culture. While no one would suggest that freedom of the press be abrogated in any way, news editors must recognize their power and inherent responsibility in serving the public. They need to recognize that their decisions not only inform people but also may affect their behavior. More data on contagion of social violence are clearly needed to determine how much contagion is a social cause of violence.

Video Games and the Internet

Television is not the only mass medium receiving increased attention as a cause of school violence. The growing use of video games and the Internet have also been proposed as potential suspects in the cause of youth violence.

Video games have been a part of America's youth since the onset of "Pong" in the early 1970s. Over the last three decades, video games have become more complex, interactive, and exciting and more reliant on violence to grab the attention of our youth. Today's games enable children and adolescents with clear 3-D graphics to practice shooting guns or to chase down women in simulated violent action. The action in the games is so dramatic, and so lifelike, that it leads some to wonder whether these video games may be a cause of youth violence. Thus far, this theory remains a hypothesis. Clear evidence for this hypothesis is not yet available. In one study of 278 seventh- and eighth-grade children in the Netherlands, no significant relation was found between video game use and aggressive behavior. However, in the same study, a negative relation was found between video game playing and "prosocial" behavior (Wiegman and van Schie 1998). But, a rhetorical question remains. Is it good for children and adolescents to practice violence as entertainment? Although the answer seems obvious, the effects of video games on our youth need to be clarified with systematic studies on the subject (Emes 1997).

Likewise, the Internet brings a library of information into each computer terminal and has the potential to bring this information to the fingertips of every child and adolescent. However, the Internet is not edited, and violent and sexually violent images, along with pornography, are also available at one's fingertips. Information on bomb making and the use of firearms is freely available at the click of a mouse. The Internet brings into the home "chat rooms," where one can converse privately with others who may also be considering violence. These chat rooms can become support groups that may encourage children and adolescents to act out fantasies of violence.

Some have wondered whether the use of the Internet may lead to decreased "real" or face-to-face communication. One study of 169 people in 73 households showed that greater use of the Internet was associated with declines in the subject's communication with family members in the household and a decline in the number of people in their social circle. Subjects who used the Internet more seemed to experience increased depression and loneliness (Kraut et al. 1998).

As with video games, however, no studies have clearly demonstrated that the Internet is systematically linked to violence in children and adolescents. Although the hypothesis is reasonable, and there exist clear cases in which children have obtained information on bomb making from or have displayed their violent thoughts on the Internet, systematic studies are not yet available. More research is needed to find out the effects of video games and the Internet on children and adolescents.

Guns

It is impossible to examine social causes of violence without at least a brief look at the prevalence of guns in our society. Schools reflect the social circumstances of the community in which they are situated. Unfortunately, the American community is one where guns are prevalent and all too often used. Gunshot wounds are the leading cause of death among teenage boys in America. The homicide rate in the United States (10 per 100,000 people) is double that in the developed country with the next highest rate, Bulgaria (4 per 100,000) (Conway 1996). This extraordinarily high presence of guns in homes not only increases the chances that our children will be killed but also drives up the cost of health care in America. The General Accounting Office estimates that the cumulative lifetime cost for patients who sustain firearm injuries is more than $14 billion for their direct medical care alone (Conway 1996).

Firearm deaths and injuries among America's schoolchildren are epidemic. From 1962 to 1993, the total number of firearm deaths increased by 137%; this rate included a rise in firearm-related homicides and suicides (Ikeda et al. 1997). Today, in America's middle schools and high schools, guns are a constant presence. A survey of more than 2,000 middle-school students revealed that 3% of the students ever carried a gun to school (see Chapter 2, this volume). Moreover, those middle-school students who began substance abuse early and used substances more frequently were more likely to carry guns or other weapons to school, even after the data were adjusted for age, sex, and ethnicity (DuRant et al. 1999).

Fights among adolescent boys have always been a feature of middle school and high school life. However, the presence of guns in school changes the dynamics of that social situation. A survey of 289 middle-school students in 1991 showed that weapons were present in 43% of the fights (Malek et al. 1998a). In a study of 567 seventh-grade students (Malek et al. 1998b), 34% had been involved in a fight at least once. However, those students who more often fought and observed fights were more likely to carry a weapon, leading the authors of the study to conclude, "Those students who actually carry weapons are much more likely to fight" (Malek et al. 1998b, p. 94). This same conclusion was reached in a study of 289 seventh-grade students (Malek et al. 1998a) and a study of more than 10,000 adolescents ages 12 to 21 (Lowry et al. 1998). Of course, violence affects more people than those who perpetrate it (see Chapter 8, this volume). In one study, over a 1-month period, 5% of seventh-grade students skipped school because of the fear of violence (Malek et al. 1998b).

The presence of guns and other weapons not only may encourage students to fight but also may lead to more serious injuries. Students who carry a weapon, including those who carry a handgun, suffer more severe injuries (Lowry et al. 1998; Malek et al. 1998a).

Gun violence is a factor not only in assaults but also in suicides (see Chapter 5, this volume). Gunshot-related suicides occur at epidemic rates. From 1968 through 1985, the rates of suicide by all methods other than gunshot wounds were constant, but the rate of suicide by firearms increased by 36% (Lowry et al. 1998). The rate of suicide by firearms doubled for adolescents and young adults during the same period (Lowry et al. 1998). A study of suicides in Shelby County, Tennessee, and King County, Washington, showed that the presence of one or more guns in the home was associated with an increased risk of suicide (Kellerman et al. 1992). Examining violence in our schools involves not only violence committed by students against each other but also violence against themselves.

Surveys show that Americans strongly support controls such as child-proofing of guns or installation of devices that permit the gun to be fired only by an authorized person (Teret et al. 1998). However, these aspects of gun use are now only hopes. The gun lobby has been effective in blocking these ideas and others that would make gun use safer in this country and would help to safeguard against the epidemic of gun use by our youths. The presence of guns in our society is a lethal social risk factor that spreads to our schools and impacts America's children.

CONCLUSION

Violence has many etiologies. In this chapter, I have examined biological and social factors that, we should keep in mind, are also intertwined with psychological factors.

Perry and Pollard (1998) point out that all experiences change the brain. However, experiences early in life, while the brain is still developing, have more influence on brain homeostasis. Environmental influences also impact the developing brain. For example, Alaska Natives and residents of the Yukon who are born at times of more light are more at risk of suicide than those born at other periods (Kettl et al. 1998).

Biological and social factors of youth violence affect each other. Childhood trauma must be viewed from a neurodevelopmental perspective, in which it is recognized that any trauma a child experiences "can result in the persistence of fear-related neurophysiologic patterns affecting emotional, behavioral and social functioning" (Perry and Pollard 1998, p. 33).

School violence is a public health problem affecting all children and all communities (Winett 1998). Psychiatrists, mental health professionals, and health professionals are in a unique position to provide both secondary prevention of school violence by treating the victims and perpetrators and primary prevention by conducting research on the social and biological causes of youth violence and disseminating the knowledge gained through public education.

REFERENCES

American Academy of Pediatrics, Committee on Communications: Children, Adolescents and Television. Elk Grove Village, IL, American Academy of Pediatrics, 1990

American Psychiatric Association, Board of Trustees: American Psychiatric Association Position Statement on TV Violence. Washington, DC, American Psychiatric Association, 1993

Apter A, van Praag HM, Plutchik R, et al: Interrelationships among anxiety, aggression, impulsivity and mood: a serotonergically linked cluster? Psychiatry Res 32:191–199, 1990

Banki CM, Arato M, Papp Z, et al: Biochemical markers in suicidal patients. Investigations with cerebrospinal fluid amine metabolites and neuroendocrine tests. J Affect Disord 6:341–350, 1984

Berman AL: Fictional depiction of suicide in television films and imitation effects. Am J Psychiatry 145:982–986, 1988

Bremner JD, Narayan M: The effects of stress on memory and the hippocampus throughout the life cycle: implications for childhood development and aging. Development and Psychopathology 10:871–885, 1998

Burrowes KL, Hales RE, Arrington E: Research on the biologic aspects of violence. Psychiatr Clin North Am 11:499–509, 1988

Constantino JN, Grosz D, Saenger P, et al: Testosterone and aggression in children. J Am Acad Child Adolesc Psychiatry 32:1217–1222, 1993

Conway T: The internist's role in addressing violence. Arch Intern Med 156:951–956, 1996

Donnelly F, Murphy J: Schools/midstate officials and parents express relief year's over. Harrisburg Patriot News, June 6, 1999, A9

DuRant RH, Krowchuk DP, Kreiter S, et al: Weapon carrying on school property among middle school students. Arch Pediatr Adolesc Med 153:21–26, 1999

Eichelman B: Aggressive behavior: from laboratory to clinic: quo vadit? Arch Gen Psychiatry 49:488–492, 1992

Emes CE: Is Mr. Pac Man eating our children? A review of the effect of video games on children. Can J Psychiatry 42:409–414, 1997

Eronen M, Angermeyer MC, Schulze B: The psychiatric epidemiology of violent behaviour. Soc Psychiatry Psychiatr Epidemiol 33 (suppl 1):S13–S23, 1998

Garza-Trevino ES: Neurobiological factors in aggressive behavior. Hospital and Community Psychiatry 45:690–699, 1994

Gould MS, Shaffer D: The impact of suicide in television movies: evidence of imitation. N Engl J Med 315:690–694, 1986

Halperin JM, Newcom JH, Kopstein I, et al: Serotonin, aggression and parental psychopathology in children with attention-deficit hyperactivity disorder. J Am Acad Child Adolesc Psychiatry 36:1391–1398, 1997

Herpetz S, Steinmeyer SM, Marx D, et al: The significance of aggression and impulsivity for self-mutilative behavior. Pharmacopsychiatry 28 (suppl 2):64–72, 1995

Hickey N: How much violence? What we found in an eye-opening study. TV Guide, August 22–28, 1992, p 10

Hiday VA, Swartz MS, Swanson JW, et al: Male-female differences in the setting and construction of violence among people with severe mental illness. Soc Psychiatry Psychiatr Epidemiol 33 (suppl 1):S68–S74, 1998

Hodgins S: Mental disorder, intellectual deficiency, and crime: evidence from a birth cohort. Arch Gen Psychiatry 49:476–483, 1992

Ikeda RM, Gorwitz R, James SP, et al: Trends in fatal firearm-related injuries, United States, 1962–1993. Am J Prev Med 13:396–400, 1997

Kanemoto K, Kawasaki J, Mori E: Violence and epilepsy: a close relation between violence and post-ictal psychosis. Epilepsia 40:107–109, 1999

Kaufman J, Birmaher B, Perel J, et al: Serotonergic functioning in depressed abused children: clinical and familial correlates. Biol Psychiatry 44:973–981, 1998

Kaufman P, Chen X, Choy SP, et al: Indicators of school crime and safety, 1998 (NCES 98-251/NCJ-172215). Washington, DC, U.S. Departments of Education and Justice, 1999

Kavoussi R, Armstead P, Coccaro E: The neurobiology of impulsive aggession. Psychiatr Clin N Am 20:395–403, 1997

Kellerman AL, Rivara FP, Somes G, et al: Suicide in the home in relation to gun ownership. N Engl J Med 327:467–472, 1992

Kettl P: The power of "Power Rangers." J Pediatr Health Care 9:101–102, 1995

Kettl PA, Christ MJ, Bixler EO: Imitation suicides after a live televised suicide. Paper presented at the 145th annual meeting of the American Psychiatric Association, Washington, DC, May 2–7, 1992

Kettl PA, Collins T, Sredy M, et al: Seasonal differences in suicidal birth rate in Alaska Natives compared to other populations. American Indian and Alaska Native Mental Health Research 8:1–10, 1998

Kraut R, Patterson M, Lundmark V, et al: Internet paradox. A social technology that reduces social involvement and psychological well being? Am Psychol 53:1017–1031, 1998

Kroll L: Television violence (Resident forum–resident physicians section). JAMA 270:2870, 1993

Kruesi MJ, Hibbs ED, Zahn TP, et al: A 2-year prospective follow-up study of children and adolescents with disruptive behavior disorders: prediction by cerebrospinal fluid 5-hydroxyindoleacetic acid, homovanillic acid, and autonomic measures? Arch Gen Psychiatry 49:429–435, 1992

Lowry R, Powell KE, Kann L, et al: Weapon-carrying, physical fighting, and fight-related injury among U.S. adolescents. Am J Prev Med 14:122–129, 1998

Malek MK, Chang BH, Davis TC: Fighting and weapon carrying among seventh-grade students in Massachusetts and Louisiana. J Adolesc Health 23:94–102, 1998a

Malek MK, Chang BH, Davis TC: Self-reported characterization of seventh-grade students' fights. J Adolesc Health 23:103–109, 1998b

Mann JJ, McBride PA, Brown RP, et al: Relationship between central and peripheral serotonin indexes in depressed and suicidal psychiatric inpatients. Arch Gen Psychiatry 49:442–446, 1992

Moffitt TE, Brammer GL, Caspi A, et al: Whole blood serotonin relates to violence in an epidemiologic study. Biol Psychiatry 43:446–457, 1998

National Institute of Mental Health: Television and Behavior: Ten Years of Scientific Progress and Implications for the Eighties. Rockville, MD, U.S. Department of Health and Human Services, 1982

Neilsen Media Research: Report on Television. New York, Neilsen Media Research, 1993

Olweus D, Mattsson A, Schalling D, et al: Circulating testosterone levels and aggression in adolescent males: a causal analysis. Psychosom Med 50:261–272, 1988

Perry BD, Pollard R: Homeostasis, stress, trauma, and adaptation: a neurodevelopmental view of childhood trauma. Child Adolesc Psychiatr Clin N Am 7:33–51, 1998

Phillips DP, Paight DJ: The impact of televised movies about suicide. N Engl J Med 317:809–811, 1987

Phillips DP, Carstensen LL: Clustering of teenage suicides after television news stories about suicide. N Engl J Med 315:685–689, 1986

Singer DG: Does violent television produce aggressive children? Pediatr Ann 14:804–810, 1985

Singer MI, Slovak K, Frierson T, et al: Viewing preferences, symptoms of psychological trauma, and violent behaviors among children who watch television. J Am Acad Child Adolesc Psychiatry 37:1041–1048, 1998

Stipp H, Milavsky JR: U.S. television programming's effects on aggressive behavior of children and adolescents. Current Psychology: Research and Reviews 7:76–92, 1988

Surgeon General's Scientific Advisory Committee on Television and Social Behavior: Television and Growing Up: The Impact of Televised Violence. Washington, DC, U.S. Government Printing Office, 1972

Tehrani JA, Brennan PA, Hodgins S, et al: Mental illness and criminal violence. Soc Psychiatry Psychiatr Epidemiol 33 (suppl 1):S81–S85, 1998

Teret SP, Webster DW, Vernick JS, et al: Support for new policies to regulate fire-arms: results of two national surveys. N Engl J Med 339:813–818, 1998

Unis AS, Cook EH, Vincent JG, et al: Platelet serotonin measures in adolescents with conduct disorder. Biol Psychiatry 42:553–559, 1997

Van Oortmerssen GA, Jijk DJ, Schuurman T: Studies in wild mice, II: testosterone and aggression. Horm Behav 21:139–152, 1987

van Praag HM, Asnis GM, Kahn RS, et al: Monoamines and abnormal behaviour. A multi-aminergic perspective. Br J Psychiatry 157:723–734, 1990

Venbrux N, Kettl PA, Bixler EO, et al: The role of discussion on television's effects on children (NR120), in 1994 New Research Program and Abstracts, American Psychiatric Association 147th Annual Meeting, Philadelphia, PA, May 21–26, 1994, p 85

Westby MD, Ferraro FR: Frontal lobe deficits in domestic violence offenders. Genet Soc Gen Psychol Monogr 125:71–102, 1999

Wiegman O, van Schie EG: Video game playing and its relations with aggressive and prosocial behavior. Br J Soc Psychol 37:367–378, 1998

Winett LB: Constructing violence as a public health problem. Public Health Reports 113:498–507, 1998

Zagar R, Arbit J, Hughes JR, et al: Developmental and disruptive behavior disorders among delinquents. J Am Acad Child Adolesc Psychiatry 28:437–440, 1989

4

Trends in School Violence

Are Our Schools Safe?

KATHLEEN M. FISHER, PH.D., C.R.N.P.
PAUL KETTL, M.D.

At present, 50 million students in the United States attend 108,000 public schools, and there are a number of students in religious and private schools. However, data on school violence are available only for public schools. The Center for the Study and Prevention of School Violence (1999a) reports that crimes occur all too commonly in America's schools. Each school day, 16,000 crimes are committed, one crime every 6 seconds that schools are in session. These crimes, however, are not simply restricted to children and adolescents. Every school day, 6,250 teachers are threatened with injury, and 260 teachers suffer an assault (see Chapters 2 and 3, this volume).

Our culture has witnessed an increased number of teen parents, resulting in children raising children. Fewer parents are at home when their children return from school—a situation that leaves children and adolescents time and opportunity to engage in inappropriate behavior, including crime. The highest frequency of crime occurs immediately after school: from 2:30 P.M. to 8:30 P.M. (Center for the Study and Prevention of School Violence 1999b). Other social effects, such as gang involvement, drug use, and alcohol use, are all too common in schools and in the surrounding school environment (see Chapters 1 and 2, this volume).

As these social effects swirl around our schools, they impact the education delivered in school. The presence of violence—but more impor-

TABLE 4–1.   School crime rates, by type of crime, among youths ages
              12–19 years: United States, 1989 and 1995

| | Proportion of schools reporting the crime, % | |
Type of crime	1989	1995
Victim of violent or property crime	14.5	14.6
Victim of violent crime	3.4	4.2
Male victim of violent crime	5.0	5.0
Female victim of violent crime	2.0	3.3
Street gangs in school	15.0	28.0
Drugs available in school	63.2	65.3

Source.   Data from Kaufman et al. 1998.

tantly the *fear* of violence—affects the attendance of students and their ability to focus while they are in school. In like manner, crime at school affects the retention rate for teachers.

How is the crime rate now different from what it was in the past? Table 4–1 presents data from the Bureau of Justice Statistics (1998) and the U.S. Departments of Justice and of Education (Kaufman et al. 1998) on school crime rates for 1989 and 1995. These data clearly show that while crime rates as a whole are stable, there has been a slight increase in persons who have been victims of a violent crime. However, this increase in the violent crime rate was explained solely by the increase in violent crime against females in school. The rates of violent crime against males remained exactly the same. Although there was no difference in the rate of drug availability at school, the presence of street gangs in schools almost doubled from 1989 to 1995. By 1995, 28% of schools had reported the presence of street gangs in their hallways and classrooms (see Chapters 2 and 3, this volume).

The National Center for Education Statistics of the U.S. Department of Education conducted a nationwide survey of public school principals (Heaviside et al. 1998). Each was asked to report on the number and description of crimes that occurred in their schools during the 1996–1997 school year. Each event had to be significant enough to have been reported to police or law enforcement officials. This survey of 1,234 public schools noted 190,000 fights without weapons and 115,000 thefts. In addition, there were 98,000 acts of vandalism. The bulk of school crimes in schools continue to be simple fights without weapons, theft, and vandalism. However, in these 1,234 schools, there were 11,000 attacks or fights with weapons,

TABLE 4–2.   Violence and discipline problems in public schools
(N = 1,234): United States, 1996–1997

Incident	No. reported
Fight without weapons	190,000
Theft	115,000
Vandalism	98,000
Physical attack or fight with weapon	11,000
Robbery	7,000
Rape/sexual battery	4,000

Source.   Data from Heaviside et al. 1998.

7,000 robberies, and 4,000 rapes or instances of sexual battering (Table 4–2). In this sample, no murders were reported. So, while school crime most often involves fistfights or acts of theft or vandalism, unfortunately, physical attacks with weapons, robberies, and rape occur all too frequently.

TYPES OF CRIMES IN SCHOOLS

Although crimes are common in schools, it is reassuring that the vast majority of these crimes are minor. In fact, according to the National Center for Education Statistics survey (Heaviside et al. 1998), 43% of the nation's schools reported no crime at all in the 1996–1997 school year. Still, the frequency of crimes is significant enough that almost all schools (78%) have in place some kind of violence prevention or violence reduction effort (Kaufman et al. 1998).

Violence occurs within schools. Although such violence most commonly includes fistfights and property crime, our students and our teachers are nevertheless subject to attack. Schools are an integral part of American society—one that is all too often a violent one. Although violence does occur in schools, our nation's children and adolescents are safer in school than they are on the streets or in many homes (see Chapter 2, this volume).

While the extent of school crime is unfortunate, the rates of school crime pale in comparison to the rates of crime outside of school. Data from the National Center for Education Statistics and the Bureau of Justice Statistics demonstrate that most murders and suicides among young people occur while they are away from school. During the 1992 and 1993 calendar in all locations, 7,357 were murdered and 4,366 committed suicide (Kaufman et al. 1998). When children leave school, between the hours of 3:00 and 8:00 P.M., juvenile crime rates triple. Every week, 40 teens are murdered, and, as FBI reports note, at least 70% of the time the victims are killed with handguns (Hennes 1998). Homicide is now the second leading cause of death among young adults ages 15 to 24 and the leading cause in young African American males (Conway 1996). While America reels from news of gunshots killings and wounds inside the school building, we have become calloused to the fact that dozens of teens are shot to death each week in this country.

YOUTH—A RISK FACTOR FOR VIOLENCE

Teens are more likely to be both perpetrators and victims of violence than are individuals in other age groups. In 1996, approximately one-third of all victims of violent crime were between the ages of 12 and 19 years. Moreover, almost half of all victims of crime were 25 years or younger (Bureau of Justice Statistics 1998). The availability of weapons and the growing presence of street gangs create a dangerous combination. Sadly, gunshot wounds are now the leading cause of death among teenage boys (Conway 1996).

Murder rates in general have been decreasing over the last several years, and after reaching a peak in 1996, teen murder rates have also been dropping. However, the drop in homicide rates among teens occurred after an astonishing rise in violence in the early 1990s. Between 1985 and 1993, for example, the number of adults committing murder decreased by 20%. For this same time period, however, homicides among 18- to 24-year-old males increased by 65%, and those committed by 14- to 17-year-old males increased 165% (Bergman 1996). A high proportion of these crimes and subsequent deaths involving minority youths were associated with drug trafficking (Bergman 1996). Thus, victimization rates for children and adolescents, as well as their involvement in crime, continue to increase despite the overall decrease in violent crimes in this country.

This sea of violence affects not only the victims and perpetrators of crime but all of America's youth. This fear of violence continues to affect children both inside and outside of school. This violence, which occurs primarily outside of school, certainly has an effect on students during school hours. The National Center for Injury Prevention and Control of the Centers for Disease Control and Prevention, the Departments of Justice and of Education, and the National School Safety Center have examined homicides and suicides associated with schools to identify common features of school-related violent deaths. In 1997, they surveyed 16,262 students from 151 of our nation's public schools. This study examined events occurring to and from school, as well as on both public or private school property or during attendance of a school-sponsored event. Their survey, the Youth Risk Behavior Surveillance Survey (YRBSS), reported that 4% of students nationwide had missed one or more days of school during the 30 days preceding the survey because they felt unsafe at school or while traveling to or from school (Kann et al. 1998). It is reasonable to assume that children who attend school but fear becoming a victim of a crime are unable to concentrate, are easily distracted, and are experiencing stress. Future research needs to examine the impact of crime on children's participation while at school and their ability to learn (see Chapters 3 and 8, this volume).

PREVALENCE OF WEAPON CARRYING AT SCHOOL

Arria et al. (1995) conducted a longitudinal analysis of data on weapon carrying and interpersonal aggression among children attending mid-Atlantic urban public schools between 1989 and 1993. In 1989, 1,714 children participated in the study; by 1993 that number had decreased to 1,515. The researchers found that involvement in weapons-related behavior started early, well before the middle-school years. They noted that knife- and gun-carrying activities increased with age, whereas stick carrying decreased. Gun carrying increased over time, and by 1993, 9.9% of boys and 1.4% of girls reported that they had carried a gun in the previous year. Bringing a weapon to school for protection was more commonly reported than for hurting or threatening someone (Arria et al. 1995).

A YRBSS survey conducted in 1996 found that 20% of high school students carried a weapon (e.g., gun, knife, or club) to school in the 30 days preceding the survey. This represents a decrease of 26.1% from 1991, when a similar survey was carried out (Kann et al. 1998). A further decline in the percentage of male high school seniors who reported having carried a weapon to school at least once in the previous 30 days was reported by the National Center for Education Statistics and the Bureau of Justice Statistics. A decrease from 14% in the 1993 school year to 9% in 1996 was observed (Kann et al. 1996). As encouraging as these trends are, it is hard to accept the fact that *any* children feel the need to arm themselves in their schools or in their neighborhoods.

School Homicides

Headlines of horrible tragedies in schools have captured the attention of the nation. At Columbine High School in Littleton, Colorado, two students killed 15 people, including themselves, while live television cameras were reporting the images to the country and while live telephone reports from inside the school were released to the public (see Chapter 7, this volume). One month later, in Georgia, another multiple shooting occurred while President Clinton was in Colorado to comfort the students affected by the prior shooting. These events were superimposed on four other similar events in the previous 18 months. In March 1998, in Jonesboro, Arkansas, four females and a teacher were slain by their young male classmates. The following month in rural Edinboro, Pennsylvania, a teacher was slain at a school event. In May 1998, other school shootings in Fayetteville, Tennessee, and Springfield, Oregon, left three students dead. These series of events seared the problem of school violence into the consciousness of America.

Still, school homicides are relatively infrequent events. The YRBSS reported that fewer than 1% of all homicides among children and adolescents ages 5–19 in 1995 occurred in or around school grounds or on the way to and from school (Kann et al. 1996).

Examining the recent school and school-related shootings does lead to some commonalties. Each shooting was perpetrated by a male(s) with a firearm. Each perpetrator seemed to carry a long-standing grievance that simmered for months before the event. It is suspected that each one was suffering from an emotional disorder, but the data on this are less clear.

Despite the recent notoriety, school-related shooting deaths are not a new phenomenon. The Center on Juvenile and Criminal Justice surveyed school shooting deaths from the 1992–1993 school year through the 1997–1998 school year. These data show clearly that school shooting deaths occur with some regularity. Between 20 and 55 children are killed each year in schools. While this tragedy cannot be underestimated, we must remember that 40 teens are shot to death each week in the streets (Alter 1999).

Prevalence of School-Associated Violent Deaths

Table 4–3 shows the number of school-associated violent deaths since the 1992–1993 school year. The school year 1998–1999, with a total of 29 school shooting deaths, had the third lowest incidence of school shooting deaths since 1992–1993. However, with the Columbine tragedy and its high toll of victims, the 1998–1999 school year will long be remembered as the most shocking and horrific school year to date.

TABLE 4–3.   School homicides: United States, 1992–1993 to 1998–1999
              school years

School year	Deaths
1992–1993	54
1993–1994	51
1994–1995	20
1995–1996	35
1996–1997	25
1997–1998	43
1998–1999	29

Source.   National School Safety Center 1999.

The highest incidence of school shooting deaths occurred during the two academic years between 1992 and 1994. An analysis of these events (Kachur et al. 1996) revealed the following: of a total of 105 deaths, 76 were of students, including 63 homicides and 13 suicides. These deaths occurred in 101 different schools in 25 different states. The majority (71%; $n=74$) of deaths occurred in high schools. The majority (60%; $n=63$) of deaths involved individuals in urban schools. In 77% of the incidents ($n=81$), firearms were the weapons of choice. Knives were used in 17% of deaths, and in 5 of the deaths a rope was used for hanging or strangulation (Kachur et al. 1996).

Victims of School Homicides

An understanding is emerging about who is likely to be a victim of school homicide and where the attacks are likely to occur. The YRBSS survey found that 65% of victims of school-associated violent deaths were students. An additional 11% of victims were teachers or members of the school staff. However, a remarkable 23% of school homicide victims were members of the community who were killed in these incidents (Kann et al. 1998). This last number further emphasizes the point that school homicides occur in a societal context in the midst of a local community. Essentially, we are all potential victims, since our schools exist in the midst of communities.

School violence—even school-related homicide—is not an event that occurs simply within the school building. A surprisingly large number of school homicides occur off campus in school-related activities. The YRBSS identified 35% of school homicides as occurring off campus. Although 28%

of school homicides happened inside school buildings, the majority (36%) of the victims were killed on school property but outside the school building (Kann et al. 1998).

School-Associated Isolated Deaths and Multiple-Victim Deaths

The National Center for Injury Prevention and Control and its previously mentioned partners updated and expanded the original YRBSS study of school-associated violent deaths between July 1994 and June 1998 (Kann et al. 1998). They identified 173 incidents, the majority being homicides that involved the use of firearms. Although the total number of events decreased steadily since the 1992–1993 school year, from 1995 through 1998 an average of five multiple-victim events occurred each school year. They observed for 1992 through 1998 that whereas the total number of school-associated violent deaths decreased, the total number of multiple-victim events appears to have increased (Kann et al. 1998). Data were collected prior to the Columbine massacre, which to date had the largest number of victims of a school shooting (Drummond 1999).

Violence at Different Levels of the Educational System

The National Center for Education Statistics has examined violence rates in elementary schools, middle schools, and high schools. No system of education, even with young children, is free of school violence. Forty-five percent of elementary schools have experienced one or more violent incidents. However, rates of violence begin to grow after elementary school, and violence rates for middle schools and high schools are quite similar. Seventy-four percent of middle schools and 79% of high schools have experienced one or more violent incidents (Heaviside et al. 1998).

IMITATION OF SCHOOL VIOLENCE

Live television coverage showed children streaming out of Columbine High School in Littleton, Colorado. This dramatic scene was followed by innumerable retrospective looks at the event in the media, accompanied by endless analyses. The event, with youngsters running out of their school in fright, hands over their heads, with SWAT teams at the ready, captured the imagination of America and focused attention on this terrible incident.

Among the American public viewing the event, however, were scores of children and adolescents who were attracted to the drama, the excitement, or perhaps the sheer emotion of the event. "Copycat" bomb threats occurred throughout the country (see Chapter 7, this volume). Although, thankfully, few of these bomb threats in schools proved to be real, the consequences of the threats dramatically swept the country. In Pennsylvania, where typically schools would experience one to two bomb threats a week, 200 bomb scares and threats of violence were made in the 2½ weeks following the Columbine High School tragedy (Donnelly and Murphy 1999). An analysis in *Education Week* showed that in the 4 weeks after Columbine, more than 350 students were arrested on charges related to threats against schools, school officials, or their peers (Drummond 1999). The authors noted that in hundreds of other cases schools were shut down or evacuated and students were sent home. This epidemic of threats further led to a heightened level of fear and tension in schools.

Not all of these events were simply threats. In Port Huron, Michigan, a janitor discovered a bomb in a school planted by two 14-year-olds, who were assisted by a 12-year-old and a 13-year-old. No one was hurt in this incident, but the event further raises the question of how much violence results from imitation.

Unfortunately, good data on imitation of violence in school are not available. Data presented earlier in this chapter show that school homicide has occurred with some variability within a relatively narrow range, at least since 1992. The lack of data substantiating clear imitation in school homicide, however, does little to influence the fear and concern of America's parents. This fear is fueled by the hundreds of bomb threats and threats of violence that occurred in the weeks following the Littleton tragedy. These threats occurred with sufficient frequency to make concern about one's own child's safety a prime topic for dinner-table conversation or for quiet discussions at the soccer fields with other parents. These threats laid to rest assurances that "it could never happen here" (see Chapter 1, this volume).

CONCLUSION:
EXPLORING PERCEPTIONS AND REALITY

Concern about school violence, resulting from the tragic events of children and adolescents shooting their peers or their teachers, has enveloped the American consciousness. In the past, parents worried about car accidents or bullies at school. Now, parents also worry about whether their child will be a shooting victim at school. These concerns heighten the tensions in our schools and communities and create the perception that our schools are unsafe. The epidemic of bomb threats and violent acts experienced at our schools following the Columbine tragedy further contributes to these fears. These threats encouraged the dismissal and closing of many schools, as administrators, anxious for the 1998–1999 school year to end, found it impossible to separate real from imagined threats of violence.

However, the data presented in this chapter clearly show that America's children are far safer in school than on the streets or in many homes. Sadly, our "culture of violence" envelops our children and teens, as is demonstrated by the increasing rate at which they are becoming victims of violent crime, despite the overall decreasing murder rates in this country.

Although one can never absolutely guarantee the safety of any child, or any person, in any social situation, school homicides occur relatively infrequently. As noted previously, before Columbine, fewer than 1% of schools across the country experienced a violent death on their campus in the previous 7 years. School homicides, when they occur, present themselves in the context of a greater community, involving events in the home and the community that the school serves. Further, these events are shocking and horrific and shatter the safety zone that was felt to surround our nation's schools.

A death of any child, no matter what the circumstances, is a tragedy. The senseless death of a child in school-related violence has a violent impact on children, adolescents, and the community. The trends in school violence reported here suggest that school homicides are not on the increase. The availability of guns, however, raises concerns that firearms are replacing fists in the settling of disputes among our young people. Unfortunately, rates of violence against females and the presence of gangs in schools are also on the increase. The total number of events of school-associated deaths has decreased since 1991, but the total number of multiple-victim events has recently increased. The death of any child is a tragedy; prevention efforts are imperative. Although school violence is not increasing, these data suggest that a focus on gang violence and violence against females would be an appropriate next step.

REFERENCES

Alter J: On the cusp of a crusade. Newsweek, May 10, 1999, p 59

Arria A, Wood N, Anthony J: Prevalence of carrying a weapon and related behaviors in urban schoolchildren, 1989 to 1993. Arch Pediatr Adolesc Med 149: 1345–1350, 1995

Bergman A: Our society is not more violent. Pediatrics 98:1198–1120, 1996

Bureau of Justice Statistics: Victim Characteristics. Washington, DC, U.S. Department of Justice, 1998

Center for the Study and Prevention of Violence: Safe school planning. 1999a Available at http://www.colorado.edu/cspv/factsheets/factsheet4.html. Accessed October 24, 1999

Center for the Study and Prevention of Violence: Urban after-school programs. 1999b Available at http://www.colorado.edu/cspv/factsheets/factsheet-11.html. Accessed October 24, 1999

Conway T: The internist's role in addressing violence. Arch Intern Med 156:951–956, 1996

Donnelly F, Murphy J: Schools/midstate officials and parents express relief year's over. Patriot News, June 6, 1999, A1, A9

Drummond S: Arrests top 350 in threats, bomb scares. Education Week on the Web, May 26, 1999. Available at http://familyeducation.com/article/0,1120,1-7051,00.html

Heaviside S, Rowand C, Williams C, et al: Violence and discipline problems in U.S. public schools: 1996–97 (NCES 98-030). Washington, DC, U.S. Department of Education, 1998

Hennes H: A review of violence statistics among children and adolescents in the United States. Pediatr Clin North Am 45:269–280, 1998

Kachur SP, Stennies GM, Powell KE, et al: School-associated violent deaths in the United States, 1992 to 1994. JAMA 275:1729–1733, 1996

Kann L, Warren C, Harris W, et al: Youth risk behavior surveillance—United States, 1995. MMWR Morb Mortal Wkly Rep 45(11), 1996

Kann L, Kinchen S, Villiams B, et al.: Youth risk behavior surveillance—United States, 1997. MMWR Morb Mortal Wkly Rep 47(SS-3), 1998. Available at: http://www.cdc.gov/nccdphp/dash/MMWRFile/ss4703.htm. Accessed July 10, 1999

Kaufman R, Chen X, Choy SP, et al: Indicators of school crime and safety, 1998 (NCES 98-251/NCJ-172215). Washington, DC, U.S. Departments of Education and Justice, 1998

National School Safety Center: School-associated violent deaths report. Westlake Village, CA, National School Safety Center 1999. Available at http://www.nssc1.org/home.htm. Accessed June 8, 2000

II

ASSESSMENT AND MANAGEMENT

Diagnostic Assessment, Management, and Treatment of Children and Adolescents With Potential for School Violence

MOHAMMAD SHAFII, M.D.
SHARON LEE SHAFII, R.N., B.S.N.

Mental health professionals, including psychiatrists, have a difficult time assessing and treating potentially violent individuals. This is particularly true with children and adolescents. Will a child or adolescent who talks about committing an act of violence really do it? What parameters can a clinician use to make this assessment?

At present, our knowledge of assessing, treating, and, in particular, predicting violent acts by youths is in an embryonic phase. One is reminded of the 1960s and 1970s when our state of knowledge of depressive disorders in children and adolescents was in its infancy and the clinician had great difficulty predicting the potential for suicidal behavior and suicide. Extensive clinical research efforts in the 1970s and 1980s resulted in the development of a data-based foundation for the "study, documentation, classification, and development of behavioral scales and psychoneuroendocrinological measurements for [the diagnosis and treatment of] depression in children and adolescents" (Shafii and Shafii 1992, p. 8). The pioneer research clinicians in this area were Annel (1972), Anthony (1970, 1978), Anthony and Scott (1960), Brumback and Weinberg (1977), Cantwell and Carlson (1979), Cytryn and McKnew (1974, 1979), Glaser (1967), Kashani et al. (1983, 1986, 1987), Kovacs (1980–1981), Poznanski (1980), Poznanski et al. (1982, 1985), Puig-Antich et al. (1984a, 1984b, 1984c, 1984d, 1985), Ryan et al. (1987), Sandler and Joffe (1965), Shafii and Shafii (1982a, 1982c), Weller et al. (1984, 1986), and Welner et al. (1979).

In this chapter, the comorbidity of violence and the potential for violent behavior, suicidal behavior, and depressive behavior are explored within the context of psychological autopsy. Practical issues regarding diagnostic assessment of potentially violent youth are discussed. These issues include first-aid, duty to warn and protect, comprehensive evaluation from a developmental perspective, and management and treatment, with emphasis on individual and family psychotherapy and pharmacotherapy.

PSYCHOLOGICAL AUTOPSY OF SUICIDE IN CHILDREN AND ADOLESCENTS

The threefold increase in the suicide rate among children and adolescents during the 1960s and 1970s, as compared with the 1950s, created national concern, as there is now for school violence. In the late 1970s and early 1980s, extensive research efforts were undertaken to study suicidal behavior and completed suicide in children and adolescents.

The clinical ethos in the 1960s and 1970s was that children and adolescents who talked about, threatened, or attempted suicide did not actually commit suicide—the thinking was that if they were serious about it, they would have done it. The research question arose: Is there any relationship between children and adolescents who talk about, threaten, and/or attempt suicide and those who commit suicide?

In the early 1980s, in an attempt to address questions related to suicide, we decided to use the method of psychological autopsy to explore the behavior, attitudes, and feelings of children and adolescents who had committed suicide by interviewing the families, friends, peers, teachers, counselors, neighbors, physicians, clergy, and any other person who had had contact with the deceased (Shafii et al. 1984, 1985). A matched pair control group was included in the study for comparison. We found that 85% of the children and adolescents who committed suicide had verbalized suicidal ideas at least once during the previous year, as opposed to 18% of the control group. Some of the findings from this study are summa-

TABLE 5–1. Relation between suicidal behavior or risk factor and completed suicide in children and adolescents in a psychological autopsy study

	Prevalence of suicidal behavior, %	
	Suicide victims	Control subjects
Verbalized suicidal idea(s)	85	18
Suicide threat(s)	55	12
Suicide attempt(s)	40	6
Exposure to suicide or suicidal behavior in other(s)	60	12
History of neglect and/or abuse	55	29

rized in Table 5–1. Our findings, which were substantiated by Brent et al. (1988), Shaffer (1988), and others, dispelled the myth that children and adolescents who talk about, threaten, or attempt suicide do not commit suicide. Most certainly they do!

At the time, another myth about children and adolescents who commit suicide was also prevalent. Many people, including clinicians, thought that children and adolescents who committed suicide did so in a moment of impulse and were otherwise "healthy." However, in postmortem psychiatric diagnosis based on DSM-III criteria, we found that 95% of suicide victims had a diagnosable psychiatric disorder(s), compared with 48% of the control subjects (Shafii et al. 1988). Of the suicide victims, 76% had major depressive disorder and/or dysthymia, usually associated with conduct disorder and/or alcohol and drug abuse, whereas only 29% of the control subjects had these disorders. Later, studies by Brent et al. (1988) and Shaffer (1988) confirmed our findings. These research efforts changed the clinician's and the public's perception of depression, suicidal behavior, and completed suicide in children and adolescents. Similar research efforts on school violence can help to discover whether or not the youth who contemplates, talks about, or commits school violence has any major psychiatric disorder.

Another surprise was that the suicide victim's closest friends and peers knew more about his or her behavior and psychological condition than anyone else. Our clinical impression is that, compared with the 1960s and 1970s, friends and peers are more willing to share information with significant adults when their friends talk about, threaten, or attempt suicide. There is less hiding of suicidal ideas and less romanticizing of the suicidal act. More often than not, friends and peers now see suicidal ideas and behavior as signs of an emotional or psychiatric disorder. They feel responsible for getting their friend some help. Some teens even come with their friend to the emergency room to share their concern with the clinician.

Also, in the 1960s and 1970s, children and adolescents with inhibited and depressive tendencies were seen as clinically different from those with impulsive and aggressive tendencies (i.e., internalizers vs. externalizers). However, our research showed that children and adolescents who committed suicide more often manifested both inhibited behaviors (e.g., isolation, withdrawal, quietness, depressive symptoms) and antisocial behaviors (e.g., breaking and entering, theft, vandalism, violent behavior toward others) than did the control group (76% vs. 24%). These findings, and later others, substantiated that, in addition to major depressive disorders and/or other mood disorders, children and adolescents who committed suicide often had conduct disorder, oppositional defiant disorder, and/or attention-deficit/hyperactivity disorder (ADHD). Comorbid diagnoses were prevalent (Shafii et al. 1985, 1988). In summary, *violence against the self and violence toward others are opposite sides of the same coin.*

PSYCHOLOGICAL AUTOPSY OF SCHOOL VIOLENCE

Our knowledge about violent behavior in children and youth, particularly in schools, needs careful, systematic, data-based research. An approach similar to the psychological autopsy of suicide could be used in cases of school violence to decipher early signs, contributing factors, and underlying psychopathology.

In the case of school violence, however, a major obstacle is the issue of confidentiality. Fear of litigation and of the possible use of confidential research materials against the perpetrator and his or her family often blocks communication and careful data collection. The first step for doing sound research on school violence should be granting researchers and their research materials immunity from subpoena. Trust between the researchers, perpetrators, victims, families, friends, peers, school personnel, and others is the most important aspect of clinical research in this area. It is true, even now, that some reports about the perpetrators of violence and their families are published in news media and available in court proceedings, but most of this information is of a limited nature because of the issues of confidentiality and objectivity, along with the fear of liability and litigation.

PSYCHIATRIC ASSESSMENT OF
POTENTIALLY VIOLENT YOUTHS

Because data-based research on school violence is limited, the senior author, as an experienced child and adolescent psychiatrist, uses an approach similar to that used in evaluating suicidal or depressed children or adolescents and their families. In assessing the potentially violent child or adolescent, the guidelines that we have been using in assessing suicidal or depressed children or adolescents, as presented in this section, are helpful (Shafii and Shafii 1982c [pp. 177–179], 1992; Mokros and Poznanski 1992). Other clinicians might use a different approach or follow other guidelines.

First Aid for Potentially Violent
Children and Adolescents

Children and adolescents occasionally think about hurting or killing others or themselves. However, when they verbally express their thoughts or directly or indirectly show violent or self-destructive behavior, it becomes a extremely serious situation.

The following first-aid guidelines are essential:

1. Adults must recognize and accept the reality that children and adolescents can physically hurt others and themselves and that they do commit homicide and suicide.
2. All violent, homicidal, and suicidal messages and behavior should be taken seriously.
3. People working with children and adolescents need to examine their own internal feelings about violence, homicide, and suicide honestly in order to increase their sensitivity and receptivity toward subtle destructive or self-destructive cues.
4. All adults, and especially clinicians, need to be aware of their tendencies to deny, to minimize, or not to recognize violent, homicidal and/or suicidal clues.
5. A thorough psychiatric examination of the child or adolescent and the family is essential if there is any evidence or suspicion of destructive or self-destructive behavior.
6. If the clinician does not have the time, knowledge, or interest in providing a thorough psychiatric evaluation, immediate referral to a child and adolescent psychiatrist, general psychiatrist, or qualified allied mental health professional is necessary.

7. A potentially violent, homicidal, and/or suicidal child or adolescent and the family should be seen immediately.
8. The parents or responsible adult should be instructed that, until the child or adolescent is seen, one of them must be with the child or adolescent at all times—never out of sight.
9. All potentially hazardous objects and/or materials such as guns, ammunition, explosives, combustibles, prescribed and nonprescribed drugs, knives, razors, ropes, and the youth's belts and shoelaces should be removed from the home or, at the very least, be kept under lock and key.
10. Even with careful precautions, an actively violent, homicidal, and/or suicidal youth is at high risk and needs to be continuously attended until psychiatric assessment is completed.
11. If the youth is unmanageable and/or defiant or poses an immediate risk to others and/or to themselves, police and emergency services need to be notified immediately.

Duty to Warn and Protect

From the very beginning of evaluation and treatment, it is important to make clear to both the youth and the parents that confidentiality is not absolute. When the youth's, the parents', or someone else's life is in danger or the possibility for physical harm exists, the clinician has an ethical, professional, and legal obligation to break confidentiality and take any measures necessary to prevent violence against others or the youth (see Chapters 9 and 10, this volume).

In cases of the threat of violence, as Perlin (1999) notes, if the clinician determines that the youth

> presents a serious danger of violence to another,...[the clinician] incurs an obligation to use reasonable care to protect the intended victim[s] against such danger. The discharge of this duty may require the therapist to take one or more of various steps, depending upon the nature of the case. Thus it may call for...[the clinician] to warn the intended victim[s] or others likely to apprise the victim[s] of the danger, to notify the police, or to take whatever other steps are reasonably necessary under the circumstances. (p. 20)

Psychiatric Assessment

In assessing the potentially violent, homicidal and/or suicidal child or adolescent, the following guidelines are useful:

1. In a psychiatric assessment, the clinician should spend as much time as necessary to see the patient and other members of the family. Shortcuts can be costly. It is not uncommon for skillful clinicians to spend 3–4 hours in the initial contact for assessment.
2. In interviewing the young person and the family, it is appropriate to show concern but maintain neutrality. The clinician must listen to all sides of the story, both on a one-to-one basis and with the family as a group. He or she should avoid making value judgments or attaching blame.
3. Clinicians must remember that their first responsibility is to save lives. Everything else is secondary; no consideration should compromise this responsibility.
4. At the time of crisis, frequently it is difficult to assess the intensity and lethality of violent, homicidal, and/or suicidal behavior and ideas. When the intensity and lethality are in doubt, it is prudent to admit the young person to the hospital, preferably to a child or adolescent psychiatric setting.
5. In interviews with a child or adolescent and the family, the clinician should explore violent, homicidal, and/or suicidal ideas openly and thoroughly.
6. If it is discovered that the youth has a plan for a violent, homicidal, and/or suicidal act, or clues are found accidentally, the violent behavior is more serious.
7. The clinician needs to take a careful and thorough history regarding the availability of and access to guns, ammunition, explosives, combustibles, and other dangerous objects or materials.
8. Changes in behavior such as isolation from the family; alienation from peers; early use of cigarettes, alcohol, marijuana, and other drugs; secretiveness; and increased time away from home are important cues.
9. Verbalization of violent, homicidal, suicidal, and death wishes should be taken seriously. Examples of such verbalizations are "I would like to take a gun and blow his head off"; "I'd like to blow up the school"; "I wish I wasn't around"; "I hope I'll sleep forever and never wake up"; or "Soon I'll be out of your way."
10. Violent, homicidal, and/or suicidal behavior does not know any age, race, or socioeconomic class.
11. Failure in human contact is the most significant contributing factor to the development of violent, homicidal, and/or suicidal behavior.
12. The risk of violence, homicide, and/or suicide increases significantly when one or more of the following are present:

Preoccupation With Violence and Death

- A previous act of violence or a suicide attempt
- Frequent talk of committing violence or suicide
- Fascination with or carrying gun, knives, and clubs on their person and to school
- Association with gangs and violent groups
- Excessive preoccupation with violence via video games, computer games, and electronic media
- Preoccupation with death and dying

Alcohol and Drug Abuse

- History of alcohol or drug abuse
- History of alcohol or drug abuse by any other family member

Personality Profile

- Lack of empathy
- Explosive anger or chronic hatred
- Rigidity, perfectionistic tendency; overexpectation by the self or by the family
- Extreme overreaction and/or withdrawal at the time of failure
- Impulsive and/or destructive behavior such as lack of regard for danger; cruelty toward siblings, peers, and animals; fire setting; and antisocial behavior
- Racism, prejudiced ideas and behavior, homophobia, and lack of tolerance for diversity

Psychiatric and Neurological Disorders

- Presence of psychiatric disorders such as conduct disorder, depressive disorders, bipolar disorders, ADHD, or schizophrenia and other psychotic disorders
- Presence of central nervous system (CNS) disorders such as grand mal seizures and absence seizures
- History or insult to the CNS such as trauma, head injuries, and infection

Family Characteristics

- Witnessing violence
- Physical or sexual abuse or neglect

- Availability of guns, ammunition, and explosives
- Violent death from homicide or suicide of a family member, relative, idol, or other significant person
- Major loss during early childhood, such as of a parent or another meaningful person

Structured Diagnostic Instruments and Rating Scales

Structured and semistructured diagnostic instruments and rating scales used for the last decade or two for research purposes are now being utilized in daily practice for comprehensive clinical assessment of children and adolescents. Some third-party payers actually now inquire whether these instruments have been used for assessment.

Structured Checklists and Rating Scales

The following structured checklists and rating scales can be used, in addition to the extensive clinical interview, to obtain information about symptoms and behavior in order to enhance systematic diagnostic assessment. These instruments decrease the subjectivity of a clinical impression and help in making a more comprehensive diagnosis and assessment of the intensity and severity of the symptoms.

Child Behavior Checklist (CBCL; Achenbach and Edelbrock 1982, 1984). The CBCL is a 160-item questionnaire that assesses social competence and behavior problems during the preceding 2–6 months. The questionnaire, designed for children and adolescents ages 4–16 years, is completed by parents or teachers. This instrument is easy to administer and takes only 15–20 minutes to complete. The CBCL is the most commonly used instrument in research and clinical practice. Behavior problems are factored into distinct groups on the basis of age and sex. For example, for 12- to 16-year-old boys, the factors include "somatic complaints, schizoid, uncommunicative, immature, obsessive-compulsive, hostile-withdrawn, delinquent, aggressive, and hyperactive" (Mokros and Poznanski 1992, p. 142).

In assessing violence potential in children and adolescents, most research clinicians use the CBCL to assess tendency toward aggressivity and violence. Clinicians particularly look at the following "externalizing" factors: hostile-withdrawn, delinquent, aggressive, hyperactive, sex problems, and cruelty.

Conners Parent Rating Scale—Revised and Conners Teacher Rating Scale—Revised (Conners 1997a, 1997b). If there is a question about the presence of attention-deficit disorders, the Conners rating scales, which have been used for a number of years, are very helpful (Conners 1997a, 1997b; Loney and Milich 1982). Both long and short versions are available; the long version covers not only attention-deficit disorder but also oppositional defiant disorder and conduct disorder.

The parents' version, an 80-item scale, and the teacher's version, a 59-item scale, cover "common problems" the child or adolescent might have had during the preceding month at home or in school. The Conners rating scales are easy to administer and take only about 15 minutes to complete.

Children's Aggression Scale (CAS; Halperin et al. 1997).   Finding a specific scale for assessing aggressive behavior in children and adolescents is difficult. The Children's Aggression Scale is a welcome addition in this area. Both parent (CAS-P) and teacher (CAS-T) versions are available. As Donovan et al. (1999) noted, "These scales assess the frequency of aggressive acts of varying severity and generate five scores each including: Verbal Aggression, Aggression Against Objects and Animals, Provoked Physical Aggression, Initiated Physical Aggression, and Use of Weapons" (p. 87). The scales are weighted to reflect the severity and the intensity of the behavior. The parents' version covers the youth's behavior at home and outside the home during the past year. The teacher's version covers the youth's behavior in school for the previous 2–10 months.

Children's Depression Inventory (CDI; Kovacs 1985).   In assessing a violent youth, it is very important to determine whether the youth is also depressed. Although the diagnosis of depression is made clinically, the depressive rating scales can help the clinician assess the severity and the intensity of the depression.

The CDI, based on the Beck Depression Inventory (BDI; Beck 1976), is one of the first self-report instruments for assessing the severity of depression in children ages 6–12 years. We have found that the CDI or the BDI also can be used with adolescents ages 12–18 years. The CDI, which takes only 8–10 minutes to administer, includes 27 items "evaluating dysphoria, pessimism, self-esteem, anhedonia, morbid concerns, suicidality, self-deprecation, social withdrawal, tendencies to ruminate, school performance, social conduct, and vegetative symptoms such as appetite and sleep disturbances, tiredness, and somatic complaints" (Mokros and Poznanski 1992, p. 143).

Depression Self-Rating Scale (DSRS; Birleson 1981).   The DSRS was developed for use with children and adolescents by modifying the Zung Depression Scale for Adults (Zung 1965). The DSRS, which "consists of 18 items that assess the range of symptoms associated with depression in children" (Mokros and Poznanski 1992, p. 144), has more specificity than the CDI regarding depression and complements the latter instrument. The DSRS takes 5–8 minutes to administer.

Structured Diagnostic Interviews

During the last two decades, a number of comprehensive structured diagnostic interviews have been developed to systematically assess child and adolescent psychiatric disorders. Clinical and epidemiological research has been the impetus for these efforts.

In our recent research on the neurobiology of depression in children and adolescents, we used checklists and rating scales—CBCL, CDI, and DSRS—and the structured diagnostic interview instrument Diagnostic Interview for Children and Adolescents (discussed below) (Shafii and Shafii 1998; Shafii et al. 1990, 1996). In daily clinical practice, we have found that this combination of checklists, rating scales, and structured diagnostic interview instrument, as an addition to the clinical interview, is very helpful for making a comprehensive assessment and diagnosis.

The following structured diagnostic interview instruments could be used both in a comprehensive assessment of violent children and adolescents and in daily clinical practice.

Diagnostic Interview for Children and Adolescents (DICA; Herjanic and Reich 1982; Welner et al. 1987).   The DICA, now called Missouri Assessment of Genetics Interview for Children (MAGIC; Reich and Todd 1999a, 1999b), is a structured interview instrument administered by a trained clinician that covers all major DSM-III-R (American Psychiatric Association 1987) and DSM-IV (American Psychiatric Association 1994) criteria for psychiatric disorders in children and adolescents, including relationships at home and with peers, homicidal and suicidal behavior, and school and social adjustment. The DICA (or MAGIC) has child, adolescent, and parent versions (Herjanic and Reich 1982; Reich and Todd 1999; Welner et al. 1987). Initially, the DICA (or MAGIC) takes 2½–3 hours to administer for each version, but as the clinician becomes more experienced, the interview can be administered in 1½–2 hours. We have found that the DICA (or MAGIC) is very easy to administer and is helpful not only for thoroughly exploring symptoms in determining the primary diagnosis but also for detecting comorbid diagnoses.

Diagnostic Interview Schedule for Children (DISC; A.J. Costello and M.K. Dulcan, "DISC: Diagnostic Interview for Children," unpublished manuscript, 1985; Shaffer et al. 1989).   The DISC is a structured diagnostic interview instrument designed to be administered by nonclinicians for epidemiological studies, although it is also used by clinicians for research purposes. A child's version (A.J. Costello and M.K. Dulcan, "DISC: Diagnostic Interview for Children," unpublished manuscript, 1985) and a parent version (Shaffer et al. 1989) are available.

Children's Interview for Psychiatric Syndromes (CHIPS; Weller et al. 1999). CHIPS is a structured interview instrument, designed to be administered by clinicians and researchers, that covers all DSM-IV criteria for major psychiatric disorders in children and adolescents. CHIPS is easy to administer. A parent version, called P-CHIPS, is also available (Weller et al. 1999).

Semistructured Diagnostic Instruments and Rating Scales

Schedule for Affective Disorders and Schizophrenia—Child's Version (K-SADS; Puig-Antich et al. 1983). K-SADS is based on the adult Schedule for Affective Disorders and Schizophrenia (SADS). Both a present episode (P) version and an epidemiological (E) version, including present and lifetime episodes, are available (Orvaschel and Puig-Antich 1986; Orvaschel et al. 1982). K-SADS is a semistructured, comprehensive diagnostic interview instrument administered by a trained clinician; it takes 2½–3 hours to complete. K-SADS is used extensively for clinical research.

Children's Depression Rating Scale—Revised (CDRS-R; Poznanski et al. 1979, 1985). CDRS-R, based on the Hamilton Rating Scale for Depression for adults, is "a semi-structured, clinician-rated instrument designed for use with children between the ages of 6 and 12 years, although it has been used effectively with adolescents" (Mokros and Poznanski 1992, p. 147). The CDRS-R takes 20–30 minutes to administer and score. The items cover "school work, capacity to have fun, social withdrawal, appetite or eating patterns, excessive fatigue, physical complaints, irritability, guilt, self-esteem, depressed feelings, morbid ideations, suicidal ideation, and weeping" (Mokros and Poznanski 1992, p. 147).

CDRS-R can be given to both children and parents. Unlike self-report depressive rating scales such as the CDI and the DSRS, CDRS-R depends on the clinician's impressions and ratings based on specific questions and the clinician's unstructured probing. CDRS-R covers the youth's behavior and feelings over the past 6 months.

In our research and clinical practice, we have found CDRS-R to be a highly sensitive and specific instrument in assessing the severity of depression and in monitoring changes in depressive symptoms over time.

Interviews With Siblings, Peers, and School Personnel

With the permission of the patient and the family, and depending on the nature and intensity of the threat of violence, it would be helpful for the clinician to interview the patient's siblings, close friends, peers, and school personnel. At times these interviews yield valuable information that is not available from other sources.

Developmental History

In addition to a thorough exploration of the child's or adolescent's developmental history, the clinician needs to pay specific attention to the following (Shafii and Shafii 1982b, pp. 10–43):

Prenatal Period

1. Nature of conception and pregnancy
2. Parental use of drugs and alcohol from conception through pregnancy
3. Physical or psychological distress throughout pregnancy and delivery

Infancy and Toddlerhood: Ages 0 to 3 Years

1. Difficult temperament
2. Regulatory disorders (disturbances in sleep, appetite, rest, and wakefulness, "colicky baby")
3. Hyperreactivity to touching and holding
4. Disturbances in separation-individuation and object relations such as eye contact from birth, social smile (2 months), recognition smile (4 months), stranger anxiety (6–7 months), separation anxiety (8 months), "becoming dare devil" (10–17 months), rapprochement (17–25 months), and internalization of maternal image or object constancy (25–36 months) (Mahler 1971; Mahler and Furer 1972; Shafii and Shafii 1982b, pp. 14–24, 33–35)

Preschool Years: Ages 3 to 6 Years

1. Difficulty in getting along with or playing with other children (e.g., physically fighting, hurting others, or withdrawing)
2. Frequent temper tantrums
3. Short attention span and hyperactivity
4. Delay in symbolic thought process or overwhelming preoccupation with the world of fantasy at the expense of relating to others
5. Lack of empathy

6. Lack of shame or overwhelming shame
7. Uninhibited and very impulsive or overwhelmingly inhibited and fearful behavior

Early School Years: Ages 6 to 12 Years

1. Lack of development of moral feelings or conscience (superego)
2. Rigid or unbending sense of righteousness
3. All-or-none quality in thinking
4. Difficulty in relating to peers (e.g., exploiting, manipulating, or following sheepishly)
5. Hyperactivity, explosiveness, inattentiveness
6. Cruelty to animals, peers, and/or others
7. Preoccupation with violence
8. Preoccupation with sexual themes or behavior
9. Use of drugs or alcohol
10. Pseudomaturity or immaturity
11. Lying and secretiveness
12. Deep resentment of authority

Adolescence: Ages 12 to 18 Years

Human Relations

1. Lack of empathy
2. Difficulty relating to parents and authority figures
3. Difficulty relating to peers (e.g., being a loner or having an intense relationship with one or two peers or small group)

Thought Processes

1. Delayed or difficulty in the development of abstract thought processes
2. Preoccupation with violence and violent fantasy
3. Seeing solution of problems and conflicts through violent acts
4. Preoccupation with having and using guns, knives, explosives, combustibles
5. Difficulty in integrative thinking such as perceiving good and bad qualities in the same person
6. Extreme negativism and nihilism
7. Inability to anticipate the consequences of one's behavior
8. Difficulty in perceiving the future
9. All-or-none quality in thinking
10. Intolerance for diversity, preoccupation with racism, homophobia

Behavior, Morality, and Conscience

1. Use of drugs and alcohol
2. Poor performance in school (e.g., because of hyperactivity, inattentiveness, disinterest)
3. Overachieving in school but feeling slighted or unappreciated for efforts
4. Lack of development of conscience or having big holes in conscience

Perception of the Self

1. Extreme concern about physical development (e.g., height, weight, muscular development, and physical strength)
2. Extreme or shocking forms of attire, hair color and cuts, body jewelry, or tattooing
3. Difficulty in development of identity (e.g., overvaluing or undervaluing the self)
4. Feelings of superiority, disdain, and contempt toward others

Family History

A thorough assessment of the family constellation and history is needed, with emphasis on the following:

1. Marital relationship (current and past, if applicable)
2. Relationships with parents, siblings, and relatives
3. Drug and alcohol abuse
4. Legal entanglements
5. Work history
6. Physical and emotional violence and abuse
7. Sexual abuse
8. Psychiatric and neurological disorders
9. Availability of hazardous materials and dangerous objects such as guns and ammunition, knives, explosives, combustibles
10. Homicidal or suicidal behavior, homicide, suicide
11. Availability of support systems and other role models

Physical Assessment

A comprehensive psychiatric assessment includes a complete physical assessment. With today's specialization and subspecialization, many children and youth have received fragmented and/or narrow physical assessment with some areas missing. This piecemeal approach has become more prevalent in the era of managed care, with clinicians having to fight to receive prior approval for each and every test and referral. The psychiatrist needs to function as a primary care physician, initiating and coordinating various tests and referrals and integrating them into a comprehensive whole.

In the case of a potentially violent or violent youth, the psychiatrist needs to be especially vigilant. A thorough physical assessment is needed for a comprehensive diagnosis and for possible use of medication. This physical assessment should include the following:

1. Thorough, recent physical examination, including exploration of history of seizure disorder, head injuries, and CNS insult
2. Laboratory studies for baseline data, including complete blood count (CBC) and differential; liver function tests, including alanine transaminase (ALT; formerly SGPT); and γ-glutamyltransferase (GGT)
3. Thyroid function tests, including thyroid-stimulating hormone (TSH), triiodothyronine (T_3), and thyroxine (T_4)
4. Comprehensive serum chemistry panel
5. Urinalysis plus a 24-hour urine creatinine clearance test if lithium is being considered
6. Urine drug screen if drug abuse is suspected
7. Electrocardiogram
8. Electroencephalogram—sleep-deprived to rule out grand mal seizures, absence seizures, and other CNS abnormalities

Psychodiagnostic Assessment

Although increasing numbers of third-party payers refuse to allow comprehensive psychological testing, we insist on having this done. In most cases, the third-party payers eventually acquiesce, or the family, if they can manage, or another source(s) pays for it.

Some potentially violent youths have a long history of learning difficulties, cognitive dysfunction, attention-deficit disorder, thought disorders, or pessimistic, paranoid ideation that, at times, expresses itself more clearly in projective and cognitive testing. Close consultation and communication with an experienced child and adolescent psychologist can help in the assessment of intellectual functioning, psychoeducational level, and the inner world of these youths. Such consultation can strengthen the psychiatric clinician's position regarding the treatment plan and recommendations to the family, school, and/or legal authorities. The psychological consultation also allows the clinician to gain a broader, deeper perspective and more objectivity in the clinical assessment. In many cases, the psychological consultation confirms and validates the psychiatrist's clinical impression. If there is a discrepancy between the two, the consultation can help identify what factors need further exploration and evaluation.

Contact With School

With the permission of the youth and the parents, the clinician needs to contact the school counselors and teachers to inquire about the youth's academic performance, behavior, attitude, peer choices, and relationships. In addition, the clinician needs to explore past history of conflicts in school, including verbal or physical threats or acts of violence, suspicion of drug and alcohol abuse, and other potentially dangerous behavior. In some cases, a school visit might be indicated. If the school appears to be a psychotoxic environment for a particular youth, immediate measures should be taken to find an alternative school or other placement.

Interviewing Siblings and Peers

In most cases, siblings and particularly peers have more information about the youth's attitude, behavior, and plans than anyone else. If the youth and/or the parents do not have enough information, or if they have not shared certain information with the clinician, interviewing peers and siblings in privacy can be very helpful.

It goes without saying that the clinician must have prior permission from the youth and his or her family to initiate and conduct such interviews. If either the youth or the family refuses permission, the clinician may need to get the court's permission.

MANAGEMENT AND TREATMENT

Clinicians' past experiences and internal attitudes toward violence and homicidal behavior influence, both directly and indirectly, the evaluation, management, and treatment of potentially violent and violent youths. Violence toward the self or others strikes a deep chord within any human being, including clinicians. The clinician can easily lose objectivity or minimize the potential for an act of violence.

The clinician should function as a good detective does. Listen to what is said and, even more importantly, what is *not* said, remembering that at least two-thirds of human behavior is nonverbal. Nonverbal cues and body language, because they are closer to the preconscious and the unconscious, can be more revealing. Every message—every communication—from the patient, the family, and others needs to be taken seriously. Overlooking a message might cost a life.

Establishing Rapport

Establishing rapport and showing genuine concern for a violent, homicidal, and/or suicidal youth and the family are essential. Frequently, a clinician has empathy for a depressed or suicidal youth. However, for a violent or homicidal youth, the clinician may feel quiet disdain. A clinician needs to be constantly aware of these feelings in managing and treating violent youth. Lack of awareness of his or her own feelings may result in the clinician's missing clues and in overidentifying with or overdistancing from the patient and the family. This lack of awareness will hamper the clinician's subjective objectivity and interfere with establishing meaningful rapport.

From a psychodynamic and developmental point of view, the youth who exhibits violent behavior, whether directed toward the self or others, has difficulty in establishing and maintaining human relationships. Genuine human contact with a clinician might be the youth's last chance to reconnect with another caring human being. The clinician needs to remember that the troubled, violent youth has had many failures in human relationships. He or she is wary and mistrustful and is hypersensitive to oversolicitous or callous behavior. The youth senses immediately whether the clinician is genuine, honest, and "leveling" with him or her. A meaningful relationship with a concerned clinician may be the last lifeline for the violent youth.

The sooner the clinician puts all the cards on the table and in plain, straightforward, and frank language explains the process and procedure of evaluation and treatment, the better the treatment will be. "Beating around the bush," or not answering the patient's and the family's questions straightforwardly, is the "kiss of death" for rapport. The clinician must avoid professional jargon, euphemisms, and platitudes. Exaggerating or minimizing the issues undermines the rapport. Vivid and graphic language carefully chosen with appropriate affect will have a powerful effect on the management and treatment process.

Short-Term Psychiatric Hospitalization

Frequently, short-term psychiatric hospitalization is indicated for violent, homicidal, or suicidal youths. If one is in doubt or concerned about whether or not a youth might act out against others or the self, it is prudent to hospitalize the youth immediately. It is not uncommon for the family and the patient to resist hospitalization because of the fear of "stigma." The patient and the family should be directly confronted to make it clear that there might not be a next time. If the youth or the parents refuse hospitalization and the clinician cannot convince them to change their minds, legal action is required. However, if one has established a good rapport with the patient and the family, emergency legal action is rarely needed.

Hospitalization temporarily removes the youth from the psychotoxic environment and emphasizes both to the young person and to the family the seriousness of the behavior. Hospitalization often mobilizes resources within the youth and the family and makes them more receptive to therapeutic input and change. It also provides the opportunity for a more comprehensive psychiatric and physical assessment of the patient on a 24-hour basis. The patient's behavior, attitude, and response to authority, structure, and peers can also be observed more closely. The patient's style of responding to stress and conflict can be observed more thoroughly. Alternatives to violent thoughts or behaviors can be suggested by the staff and therapists.

Most youths who are referred for assessment of violent behavior or potential for violence are taking a plethora of prescribed psychostimulants, antidepressants, neuroleptics, and mood stabilizers with no or limited success. Hospitalization provides an opportunity to decrease and discontinue these medications and to observe the patient free from any drugs. Later, the clinician can judiciously prescribe appropriate medication if indicated.

Involvement in intensive individual, group, and family therapy, along with participation in school and recreational activities, can help the clinician and treatment staff to further observe, understand, and treat the young person and the family.

Long-Term Residential Placement

In some cases, the violent youth can benefit from long-term residential placement immediately after initial evaluation or, more likely, after short-term psychiatric hospitalization. Indications for long-term residential placement are

1. Chronic use of drugs and alcohol
2. Association with gangs or peers with a history of drug and alcohol abuse or violent and antisocial behavior
3. Continued isolation of the self at home

4. Incorrigible behavior at home or in school
5. Continuous threat of violence at home or in school
6. Homicidal or suicidal preoccupations
7. Ineffective parenting or severely dysfunctional family

We have found that for a number of violent youth, especially those threatening to commit violent acts at school, placement in a long-term residential setting with emphasis on wilderness experiences can be very helpful. Some of these facilities integrate sound developmental and psychiatric principles with a modified Alcoholics Anonymous step approach. Peer group accountability and the honor system often are used to encourage violent youths to become more introspective, to control behavior, and to become more honest with themselves and others. These programs emphasize personal responsibility and accountability and discourage the use of projection and blaming others. They encourage the youth to find effective ways of verbal communication for conflict resolution, rather than automatically thinking of relying on acts of physical violence. Some youths might need to be in such a setting for an entire school year or longer.

After discharge from this type of setting, regular outpatient follow-up and involvement in Alcoholics Anonymous or a similar self-help group are essential.

Individual Psychotherapy

Individual psychotherapy is recommended for almost all violent, homicidal, and/or suicidal youths whether it be on an inpatient or an outpatient basis. The young person needs to reestablish healthy, meaningful human contact in the privacy of a dyadic relationship. No matter how old the youth is, role-playing, games, play, and the creative arts, such as drawing, painting, clay modeling, writing, and music, can significantly enhance this therapeutic connectedness. The therapist can help the patient become aware of feelings of caring and empathy toward others. Part of the therapeutic work with violent patients is helping them to put themselves in the other person's place and to understand and to experience the other person's thoughts and feelings. Role-playing, at times, can be effective in helping the patient experience this process and gain skills in this area.

As we know, many violent, homicidal, and/or suicidal youths have been or are being traumatized. Traumatized youths frequently dissociate themselves from traumatic experiences, becoming numb to their own feelings and others' feelings and indifferent to their own and others' pain and suffering (see Chapter 8, this volume). They view having feelings as being a "sissy or coward." Clinicians must be sensitive to these defensive postures and emphasize that it is actually a sign of courage, "guts," and "manhood" to experience sadness, disappointment, tearfulness, and caring for others. Violent youths need to realize that because they feel that other people did not care for them, it does not mean that they should not care for others and for themselves. Frequently, for violent youths, reestablishment of self-respect and self-worth begins with caring for others.

Helping the traumatized youth become aware of, verbalize, and reexperience previous traumas in measured doses facilitates mastery. This approach can decrease psychological and physical overreaction to affronts and stresses. Eventually, the patient may be able to work through anger, hatred, and resentment and find internal peace and forgiveness.

There will be many setbacks—false starts, disappointments, and premature hopes—in this dyadic relationship. The therapist can help the patient experience feelings of guilt, shame, and embarrassment in the therapeutic process. As long as the violent youth keeps the promise of not acting violently toward others or self, there is great hope for recovery.

With use of Martin Buber's idea of the "I–Thou" relationship in individual therapy, not only in verbal exchanges but also in silent and nonverbal exchanges, human connectedness begins to grow and flourish again. This human connectedness or human bond is the antidote to the destructive poison of violence against others and the self.

One of the early signs that a violent youth is beginning to repair fragile bonds is that the youth begins either to show interest in having a pet or to take better care of the family pet. The pet may symbolically represent the patient, the therapeutic relationship, and/or other meaningful people in the patient's life. The therapist could encourage the patient to bring his or her pet to the office. Choosing unusual pets such as boa constrictors or other snakes, ferrets, rats, and tarantulas is not uncommon, although some youths do choose dogs, cats, hamsters, or mice. The patient often describes the pet's feeding behavior with glee. Taming aggressive behavior frequently begins with developing a relationship with a domesticated or wild animal.

The youth needs to become more aware of his or her assets and liabilities in order to shore up shattered self-esteem or to modify "macho tendencies" and overestimation of the self. Accepting and experiencing affront and failure without extreme reaction is an important part of the therapeutic process (see Chapter 1, this volume). In an inhibited and depressed young person, verbal expression of hostile and aggressive feelings is encouraged. In an aggressive, callous, or delinquent youth, containment of anger, impulsive behavior, and hostile verbal expressions is encouraged.

Frequently, the violent youth has comorbid diagnoses of both depression and conduct disorder. In this situation, a delicate balance is needed between appropriately healthy verbal expression and containment of explosive verbalization and impulsive behavior. A major theme of therapy will be dealing with these two sides of the same coin.

Establishing human contact is the most important part of the therapeutic process. A violent youth might resist coming to treatment, storm out of the office, sit for hours in pouty silence, become belligerent, or call the therapist all names imaginable. Consistent presence of a caring human being who is not intimidated by the patient's hostility or deluded by the patient's pleasantries may save not only other peoples' lives but also the patient's. A caring therapeutic relationship may help the patient become a happier, more productive citizen relatively free from intrapsychic and interactional conflicts.

Psychopharmacotherapy

Depending on the underlying psychiatric or physical disorder, judicious use of medication may be necessary. With the availability of serotonin reuptake inhibitors (SRIs) and new antiepileptic agents, mood stabilizers, and novel antipsychotics, the pharmacotherapeutic armamentarium for treating violent youths has been expanded.

As far as we know, only psychostimulants for the treatment of ADHD and some of the SRIs such as fluoxetine, sertraline, and paroxetine have been found in double-blind crossover studies to be effective in the treatment of major depression and obsessive-compulsive disorder in children and youth. Other drugs found to be effective in adults can be useful in treating underlying disorders of violent youths, some of which will be discussed below.

Medication cannot be a substitute for or replace individual, group, and family therapies. But medication can be a useful adjunct. Third-party insurance providers and health maintenance organizations (HMOs), for the sake of cutting costs and increasing profits, frequently push the psychiatrist to use only medication and just provide "med check" services for these troubled youths. They frequently decline authorization for a qualified psychiatrist to provide an integrative therapeutic approach of both psychotherapy and pharmacotherapy. If they reluctantly agree to psychotherapy, they allow only a few sessions. It is hoped that with the recent public and professional protests, along with efforts by the United States Congress and other branches of the federal government, this dangerous, short-sighted practice will be short-lived.

The following information is based on clinical experience and communication with other experienced clinical colleagues concerning the treatment of potentially violent or violent youths. Some medications have a disinhibiting effect on violent youths with underlying CNS dysfunction and/or borderline personality traits. Instead of calming irritability and violence, the medication intensifies symptoms further. The clinician needs to find, by trial and error, the appropriate medication and optimal dose. The optimal dose is usually in the low- to moderate-range level. Children and youths metabolize medication faster and, consequently, need more frequent daily doses.

The clinician should keep in mind that pubescent youths, because of an avalanche of hormonal secretion, might show an increase in side effects and probably will be less tolerant to the same amount of medication that they were taking at a younger age. This usually happens for males between ages 12 and 14 years and for females between ages 11 and 13 years.

Before any medication is prescribed, as suggested earlier, it is essential for the patient to have a complete physical examination and appropriate laboratory studies for baseline values. Also, the side effects of prescribed medications should be clearly and thoroughly explained to the patient and the family. Follow-up visits should include exploration of possible side effects, along with dose adjustment, monitoring of serum levels, and appropriate laboratory studies as indicated.

Also, the clinician needs to explain and discuss the possibilities and dangers, including sudden death, of some of the medications' cross-reactivity when used with other medications or "drugs" such as antihistamines, acne medications, antifungals, erythromycin, and others. The clinician should emphasize, on more than one occasion, to both the patient and the family that no additional medications should be taken without checking with or calling the clinician.

If in doubt about cross-reactivity of a particular medication, the clinician should call a qualified clinical pharmacist in a medical center for consultation. In most medical centers, clinical pharmacists receive monthly or even more frequent updated information on various medications.

On the basis of clinical experience, the following medications and dose ranges are suggested in mild to moderate cases of youth violence, depending on the patient's underlying psychopathology. In severe and more complex cases, the following recommendations may not be effective. Then, the clinician may need psychopharmacological consultation, since extensive polypharmacy and significant increases in dosage may be indicated.

1. For a youth with underlying major depression or dysthymia associated with signs of anxiety, agitation, irritability, and anger, a small to mod-

erate dose of sertraline (25–50 mg) daily in two divided doses can help reduce symptoms significantly.

2. For a youth who is depressed but preoccupied with violent thoughts against others or the self and shows some of the symptoms of obsessive-compulsive disorder, fluoxetine in a dose range of 10 to 40 mg daily in two divided doses is indicated.

3. If the youth is depressed, withdrawn, and quiet, and lacks energy, paroxetine, an activating agent, can be helpful in the dose range of 10 to 40 mg daily in two divided doses.

4. For a youth with rapid-cycling bipolar disorder, or bipolar II disorder and/or cyclothymia, divalproex sodium, a derivative of valproic acid, is the drug of first choice, in the range of 250 to 1,000 mg daily in two or three divided doses to reach a plasma concentration of 50–125 µg/mL. In females, there is a rare possibility of the development of polycystic ovarian disease. Divalproex sodium is not recommended for children 6 years or younger and should be used with caution for children between ages 6 and 10 years because of the possibility of fatty degeneration of the liver. In the 6- to 10-year-old age group, frequent liver function tests are recommended.

5. For a youth with bipolar I disorder or aggressive bipolar II disorder who has not responded well to valproic acid derivatives such as divalproex sodium, lithium in the dosage range of 600 to 1,200 mg or higher daily in two to three divided doses for a serum level of 0.8 mEq to 1.4 mEq can be effective.

6. For a youth with a mood disorder and/or a seizure disorder, gabapentin in the dosage range of 600 mg to 1800 mg or more daily in two or three divided doses can be extremely effective for absence seizures (complex partial seizures), nocturnal seizures, mood disorders, anger outbursts, and oppositional behavior. At present, gabapentin is the drug of choice. For patients with seizure disorders, pharmacotherapy should be done in consultation with a pediatric neurologist.

7. For a youth with absence and mood disorders, if gabapentin has not been effective, carbamazepine in the dosage range of 600 mg to 1,200 mg daily in two divided doses can be effective. Sertraline 25–50 mg daily in two divided doses may be added for stabilization of mood and irritability.

8. For a youth with the symptoms of ADHD and violent behavior, in addition to psychostimulants such as methylphenidate 20–60 mg daily in two or three divided doses or a new combination of dextroamphetamines and amphetamines 10–40 mg daily in two divided doses, a SRI such as sertraline 25–50 mg daily in two divided doses can be very helpful.

9. In some cases, if none of the above medications are helpful, one can add or substitute neuroleptics such as thioridazine 200–400 mg daily in two divided doses.
10. New antipsychotic medications such as risperidone 1–6 mg daily in two divided doses, olanzapine 2.5–7.5 mg daily in two divided doses, or quetiapine fumarate 25–200 mg daily in two divided doses may be helpful, especially for a youth with underlying borderline personality disorder, schizoaffective disorder, or schizophrenia or another psychotic disorder.

Family Therapy

After the initial interviews, seeing the potentially violent or violent youth and the family together when first beginning therapy may be explosive and counterproductive. The therapist can see the parents separately on a regular basis to educate and to help them to understand and to deal more effectively with their troubled youth. If there is evidence of serious marital disharmony or psychiatric disorders in one or both of the parents, the experienced therapist might treat them independently or refer them to a qualified colleague. If a parent(s) is referred to another therapist, communication between the therapists is essential.

Group Therapy

In addition to individual psychotherapy and family therapy, some youths can benefit from group therapy. If the youth has underlying borderline traits, avoidance personality, schizoid personality, or psychotic features, group therapy may be counterproductive (see Chapter 8, this volume).

Follow-Up

After discharge from the hospital, continuous outpatient psychotherapeutic work with the young person and the family is necessary. Inpatient hospitalization is the beginning of treatment rather than the end. At least 2 years of outpatient treatment and follow-up is recommended. We know that most youths who complete suicide do so within 2 years of the previous suicide attempt (Otto 1972). No data are available about the subsequent behavior of potentially violent or violent youths after hospital discharge, but the possibility exists that they, too, may act out violently and therefore need close supervision and active follow-up for a long time.

Occasionally, rehospitalization is indicated. The youth and the family should be helped to see that rehospitalization does not mean failure; rather, it is a preventive measure for helping the patient and the family to regroup their psychological resources in order to deal with a stressful situation.

Conclusion

Assessing, predicting, and treating violent or potentially violent individuals, particularly children and adolescents, is not an easy task. Parents, educators, and even clinicians have a tendency to deny, overlook, or minimize the potential for youth violence. The first step in the diagnostic assessment and treatment of potentially violent youth is for clinicians to be aware of these tendencies.

Comprehensive assessment begins with practical and effective first-aid management. Specific guidelines are provided for psychiatric evaluation, including individual and family characteristics that may increase the risk of violence. In addition to comprehensive clinical interviews of the youth and the family, the use of structured diagnostic instruments and rating scales is discussed. Psychiatric assessment is conceptualized within a developmental perspective.

Establishing and maintaining a consistent human relationship or human contact with a potentially violent youth and his or her family is the foundation of effective management and treatment. The indications for short-term psychiatric hospitalization and long-term residential placement are discussed. The essential aspects of individual psychotherapy and pharmacotherapy, in addition to family therapy, group therapy, and follow-up, are examined.

References

Achenbach TM, Edelbrock C: Manual for the Child Behavioral Checklist and Revised Child Behavior Profile. Burlington, University of Vermont, 1982

Achenbach TM, Edelbrock C: Psychopathology of childhood. Annu Rev Psychol 35:227–256, 1984

American Psychiatric Association: Diagnostic and Statistical Manual of Mental Disorders, 3rd Edition, Revised. Washington, DC, American Psychiatric Association, 1987

American Psychiatric Association: Diagnostic and Statistical Manual of Mental Disorders, 4th Edition. Washington, DC, American Psychiatric Association, 1994

Annel AL: Depressive States in Children and Adolescents. New York, Halstead Press, 1972

Anthony E: Two contrasting types of adolescent depression and their treatment. J Am Psychoanal Assoc 18:841–859, 1970

Anthony EJ: Affective disorders in children and adolescents, with special emphasis on depression, in Depression: Biology, Psychodynamics and Treatment. Edited by Cole J, Schatzberg A, Frazier S. New York, Plenum, 1978, pp 173–184

Anthony EJ, Scott P: Manic-depressive psychosis in childhood. J Child Psychol Psychiatry 1:53–72, 1960

Beck AT: Depression: Clinical, Experimental, and Theoretical Aspects. New York, Harper & Row, 1967

Birleson P: The validity of depressive disorder in childhood and the development of a self-rating scale: a research report. J Child Psychol Psychiatry 22:73–88, 1981

Brent DA, Perper JA, Goldstein CE, et al: Risk factors for adolescent suicide: a comparison of adolescent suicide victims with suicidal inpatients. Arch Gen Psychiatry 45:581–588, 1988

Brumback RA, Weinberg WA: Childhood depression: an exploration of a behavior disorder of children. Percept Mot Skills 44:911–916, 1977

Cantwell D, Carlson G: Problems and prospects in the study of childhood depression. J Nerv Ment Dis 167:522–529, 1979

Conners CK: Conners Parent Rating Scale—Revised (L). North Tonawanda, NY, Multi-Health Systems, 1997a

Conners CK: Conners Teacher Rating Scale—Revised (L). North Tonawanda, NY, Multi-Health Systems, 1997b

Cytryn L, McKnew D: Factors influencing the changing clinical expression of the depressive process in children. Am J Psychiatry 131:879–881, 1974

Cytryn L, McKnew DH: Affective disorders, in Basic Handbook of Child Psychiatry (Noshpitz JD, Series Editor), Vol 2. New York, Basic Books, 1979, pp 321–341

Donovan AM, Halperin JM, Newcorn JH, et al: Thermal response to serotonergic challenge and aggression in attention deficit hyperactivity disorder children. J Child Adolesc Psychopharmacology 9(2):85–91, 1999

Glaser K: Masked depression in children and adolescents. Am J Psychother 21:565–574, 1967

Herjanic B, Reich W: Development of a structured psychiatric interview for children: agreement between child and parent on individual symptoms. J Abnorm Child Psychol 10:307–324, 1982

Halperin JM, Newcorn JH, Schwartz ST, et al: Age-related changes in the association between serotonergic function and aggression in boys with ADHD. Biol Psychiatry 41:682–689, 1997

Kashani JH, McGee RO, Clarkson SE, et al: Depression in a sample of 9-year-old children: prevalence and associated characteristics. Arch Gen Psychiatry 40:1217–1223, 1983

Kashani JH, Holcomb WR, Orvaschel H: Depression and depressive symptoms in preschool children from the general population. Am J Psychiatry 143:1138–1143, 1986

Kashani JH, Carlson GA, Beck NC, et al: Depression, depressive symptoms, and depressed mood among a community sample of adolescents. Am J Psychiatry 144:931–934, 1987

Kovacs M: Rating scales to assess depression in school-aged children. Acta Paedopsychiatrica 46:305–315, 1980–1981

Kovacs M: The Children's Depression Inventory (CDI). Psychopharmacol Bull 21:995–998, 1985

Loney J, Milich R: Hyperactivity, inattention and aggression in clinical practice. Advances in Developmental Behavioral Pediatrics 3:113–147, 1982

Mahler MS: A study of the separation-individuation process and its possible application to borderline phenomena in the psychoanalytic situation. Psychoanal Study Child 26:403–424, 1971

Mahler MS, Furer M: Child psychosis: a theoretical statement and its implications. Journal of Autism and Childhood Schizophrenia 2:213–218, 1972

Mokros HB, Poznanski EO: Standardized approaches to clinical assessment of depression, in Clinical Guide to Depression in Children and Adolescents. Edited by Shafii M, Shafii SL. Washington, DC, American Psychiatric Press, 1992, pp 129–155

Orvaschel J, Puig-Antich J: Schedule for Affective Disorder and Schizophrenia for School-Age Children, Epidemiological Version, 4th Edition. Pittsburgh, PA, Western Psychiatric Institute and Clinic, 1986

Orvaschel J, Puig-Antich J, Chambers W, et al: Restrospective assessment of prepubertal major depression with the Kiddie-SADS-E. Journal of the American Academy of Child Psychiatry 17:49–59, 1982

Otto U: Suicidal acts by children and adolescents. Acta Psychiatr Scand Suppl 233:7–123, 1972

Perlin ML: Tarasoff at the millennium: New directions, new defendants, new dangers, new dilemmas. Psychiatric Times 16(11):20, 1999

Poznanski E: Childhood depression: the outcome. Acta Paedopsychiatrica 46:297–304, 1980

Poznanski EO, Cook SC, Carroll BJ: A depression rating scale for children. Pediatrics 64:442–450, 1979

Poznanski EO, Carroll BJ, Banegas MC, et al: The dexamethasone suppression test in prepubertal depressed children. Am J Psychiatry 139:321–324, 1982

Poznanski EO, Freeman LN, Mokros HB: Children's Depression Rating Scale revisited. Psychopharmacol Bull 21:979–989, 1985

Puig-Antich J, Chambers WJ, Tabrizi M: The clinical assessment of current depressive episodes in children and adolescents: interviews with parents and children, in Affective Disorders in Childhood and Adolescents: An Update. Edited by Cantwell DP, Carlson GA. New York, Spectrum, 1983, pp 157–159

Puig-Antich J, Geotz RM, Davies M, et al: Growth hormone secretion in prepubertal children with major depression, II: sleep-related plasma concentrations during a depressive episode. Arch Gen Psychiatry 41:463–466, 1984a

Puig-Antich J, Geotz RM, Davies M, et al: Growth hormone secretion in prepubertal children with major depression, IV: sleep-related plasma concentrations in a drug-free, fully recovered clinical state. Arch Gen Psychiatry 41:479–483, 1984b

Puig-Antich J, Novacenko H, Davies M, et al: Growth hormone secretion in prepubertal children with major depression, I: final report on response. Arch Gen Psychiatry 41:455–460, 1984c

Puig-Antich J, Novacenko H, Davies M, et al: Growth hormone secretion in prepubertal children with major depression, III: response to insulin-induced hypoglycemia after recovery from a depressive episode and in a drug-free state. Arch Gen Psychiatry 41:471–475, 1984d

Puig-Antich J, Lukens E, Davies M, et al: Psychosocial functioning in prepubertal major depressive disorders. Arch Gen Psychiatry 42:511–517, 1985

Reich W, Todd R: Missouri Assessment for Genetics Interview for Children (Magic-C, Child Version). St Louis, MO, Washington University, 1999a

Reich W, Todd R: Missouri Assessment for Genetics Interview for Children (Magic-P, Parent Version). St Louis, MO, Washington University, 1999b

Reich W, Herjanic B, Welner Z, et al: Development of a structured psychiatric interview for children: agreement on diagnosis comparing child and parent interviews. J Abnorm Child Psychol 10:325–336, 1982

Ryan ND, Puig-Antich J, Ambrosini P, et al: The clinical picture of major depression in children and adolescents. Arch Gen Psychiatry 44:854–861, 1987

Sandler J, Joffe W: Notes on obsessional manifestations in children. Psychoanal Study Child 20:425–438, 1965

Shaffer D: The epidemiology of teen suicide: an examination of risk factors. J Clin Psychol 49:36–41, 1988

Shaffer D, Fisher P, Piacentini J, et al: Diagnostic Interview Schedule for Children (DISC-2.1P)—Parent Version. New York, New York State Psychiatric Institute, 1989

Shafii M, Shafii SL: Depression in infancy, childhood, and adolescence: failure in human contact, sadness, and withdrawal, in Pathways of Human Development: Normal Growth and Emotional Disorders in Infancy, Childhood and Adolescence. New York, Thieme-Stratton, 1982a, pp 77–95

Shafii M, Shafii SL: Pathways of Human Development: Normal Growth and Emotional Disorders in Infancy, Childhood and Adolescence. New York, Thieme-Stratton, 1982b

Shafii M, Shafii SL: Self-destructive, suicidal behavior, and completed suicide, in Pathways of Human Development: Normal Growth and Emotional Disorders in Infancy, Childhood and Adolescence. New York, Thieme-Stratton, 1982c, pp 164–180

Shafii M, Shafii SL: Clinical manifestations and developmental psychopathology of depression, in Clinical Guide to Depression in Children and Adolescents. Edited by Shafii M, Shafii SL. Washington, DC, American Psychiatric Press, 1992, pp 3–42

Shafii M, Shafii SL: Melatonin in healthy and depressed children and adolescents, in Melatonin in Psychiatric and Neoplastic Disorders. Edited by Shafii M, Shafii SL. Washington, DC, American Psychiatric Press, 1998, pp 149–167

Shafii M, Whittinghill JR, Dolen DC, et al: Psychological reconstruction of completed suicide in childhood and adolescence, in Suicide in the Young. Edited by Sudak H, Ford AB, Rushforth NB. Boston, MA, John Wright PSG, 1984, pp 271–294

Shafii M, Carrigan SP, Whittinghill JR, et al: Psychological autopsy of completed suicide in children and adolescents. Am J Psychiatry 142:1061–1064, 1985

Shafii M, Steltz-Lenarsky J, Derrick AM, et al: Comorbidity of mental disorders in the postmortem diagnosis of completed suicide in children and adolescents. J Affect Disord 15:227–233, 1988

Shafii M, Foster MB, Greenberg RA, et al: Pineal gland and depressive disorders in children and adolescents, in Biological Rhythms, Mood Disorders, Light Therapy, and the Pineal Gland. Edited by Shafii M, Shafii SL. Washington, DC, American Psychiatric Press, 1990, pp 97–116

Shafii M, MacMillan DR, Key MP, et al: Nocturnal serum melatonin profile in major depression in children and adolescents. Arch Gen Psychiatry 53:1009–1013, 1996

Weller EB, Weller RA, Fristad MA, et al: The dexamethasone suppression test in hospitalized prepubertal depressed children. Am J Psychiatry 141:290–291, 1984

Weller EB, Weller RA, Fristad MA, et al: Dexamethasone suppression test and clinical outcome. Am J Psychiatry 143:1469–1470, 1986

Weller EB, Weller RA, Fristad MA, et al (eds): ChIPS—Children's Interview for Psychiatric Symptoms. Washington, DC, American Psychiatric Press, 1999

Welner A, Welner Z, Fishman R: Psychiatry adolescent inpatients: eight- to ten-year follow-up. Arch Gen Psychiatry 36:698–700, 1979

Welner A, Reich W, Herjanic B, et al: Reliability, validity, and parent-child agreement studies of the Diagnostic Interview for Children and Adolescents (DICA). J Am Acad Child Adolesc Psychiatry 26:649–643, 1987

Zung WWK: A self-rating depression scale. Arch Gen Psychiatry 12:63–70, 1965

6

Coping With School Violence

An Eyewitness Account

BECKY ROWAN, M.ED.

It is hard for me to remember what my life was like before October 1, 1997. Sometimes I wonder how it must have felt not to have the memories of that day.

WEDNESDAY, OCTOBER 1, 1997

The day began as any other day for me, a high-school counselor in Pearl, Mississippi. I remember being anxious—not because I anticipated the un-imaginable event that transpired, but because of statewide standardized testing for approximately 300 ninth-graders at Pearl High School. I re-member thinking as I drove to school that I hoped everyone would be there that day—both faculty and students—and that, if an auditor from the State Department of Education were to come by, everything would go smoothly, along with numerous other things associated with the testing process. The first bell rings at 8:20 A.M., but I arrived that morning at about 7:30 A.M.

As I walked across the commons, a large, open area where our stu-dents gather before school and that also serves as a cafeteria at lunch, a few

117

students were already there. Lydia always stood or sat close to the door of the counseling office. I remember that on that morning, as on many others, we spoke to each other. Lydia was very excited that day because class rings were going to be delivered and she wanted to know what time the representatives would be there. For the next 30 minutes or so, Ernest Larry, the other counselor at Pearl High School, and I were busy counting out test booklets and getting ready for teachers to come in and check out materials so we would be ready to begin testing promptly. Several parents were going to come about 8:15 A.M. to help us monitor testing. I remember a student and his father in the office that morning waiting to see John Craven, our assistant principal.

At approximately 5 minutes after 8:00 A.M., I was standing at the door of the office talking with a friend. We heard a pop that sounded like a firecracker. My friend and I started toward the door. I almost had my hand on the door to push it open when I heard a second pop. Someone screamed, "It's a gun!" People scattered, running to take cover in the several offices and rooms in the counseling office. Mr. Larry and I and three others ran into the vault where records are kept. As we stood there, other shots were fired, and suddenly I remembered that my son and Mr. Larry's son might be in the commons. I said, "Oh, Mr. Larry, Matthew and Scott may be out there! We have to get out of here!"

I was standing by the door with my hand on the doorknob. Nobody in the room thought to get on the floor or anything like that. We were just standing there horrified. I remember cracking the door and someone yelling, "Close the door. He's still out there!" Another teacher in the room with us said that it was Luke Woodham. She had actually seen him shoot. He was a student of hers. I remember thinking, "No, not Luke—not a student." I had assumed it was someone other than anyone we might know. Someone finally yelled, "He's gone."

We came out. I walked out of the counselor's office and saw several bodies on the floor. Book bags were everywhere. It was deathly quiet. I walked over to a teacher who had already gotten to that area and asked if one of those on the floor was Scott, my son. He said, "No." I was too horrified to look, afraid of what I might see.

Then, along with several other faculty, I tried to help the wounded and dying. The first student I got to was Lydia, lying on the floor by my office door. We talked to her, not realizing how seriously wounded she was, and told her that it would be okay and help was on the way. At this time, I remember crouching beside her on the floor along with two other teachers, constantly looking over my shoulder, asking, "Is he gone?" and screaming for the paramedics to hurry.

I left Lydia with those two teachers and walked over to Christine, Luke's former girlfriend, whom he had shot at point-blank range in the neck with a .30.30 hunting rifle. Two teachers were there trying to stop the bleeding, but it was hopeless. I remember that her hands and her face were already blue. Pools of blood. I walked to Alan Westbook, who, as he tried to run from Luke, was shot in the back as he grabbed another girl to shield her from the bullet. Water . . . bone fragments—I didn't think Alan would make it. Across the commons, two others. At this point, teachers were with them.

Back over to Lydia—still not knowing where the killer or my son were. After what seemed an eternity but was only a span of a couple of minutes, paramedics arrived. It still did not seem real to me. I kept saying to myself, "They'll be okay—there's help here now. They'll be okay. Where's Scott? I need to call my mother. Where are the other students?" Thousands of questions—all in the span of a minute or two. Back in my office, I was lucky enough to get a phoneline out to call my mom, who I was afraid would hear this on the news, to tell her Scott and I were okay, athough I still had no clue about Scott.

By that time, we were trying to get outside to help other students who had fled the building. I remember stepping on gun shells. Police and paramedics were everywhere as we ran outside. I saw a fire truck and an ambulance down at the band hall. I thought, "Oh, no, Scott is down there and the shooter has been there, too." I ran out, but, as I later found out, two of the wounded students had run out of the commons to the band hall and paramedics were on the scene there helping them. Still no sign of Scott. Over and over I am thinking, "Where is Scott?" Students everywhere— huddled, crying—some had run up into a wooded area. Highway patrolmen everywhere. One officer asked if I would come out to the driveway of the parking lot where parents were in cars to try to assure them that their children were probably okay. I tried to be as calm as possible and reassure the parents as best I could. All the time inside I was going crazy wondering about my own son.

One of the most vivid memories of that day was Lydia's mother arriving at the scene. I did not know until after I was outside the building that Lydia had died. I remember Joel Myrick, our other assistant principal, who had subdued Luke as he had tried to drive away, walking with Lydia's mom across the lawn. Big tears were streaming down Joel's face, as he knew what news was about to be shared with this mother. Joel—the big, husky, military guy, the loveable guy, the guy who you would think would be the last person you would see afraid or crying. My heart broke. I realized that this nightmare was not a dream. It was real.

Our athletic director was gathering faculty together. The police wanted all of us to board a school bus and ride to the police station where we would give statements. As we loaded that bus, I saw my friend who had been with me with Lydia. She did not know that Lydia was dead. As I ran to her sobbing and telling her about Lydia, I remember her saying over and over, "No, no, no." I remember saying, "We didn't know—we didn't know." As I looked out the window of the bus, I saw parents, students, and cars lining the streets. We were quiet, trying, I think, to let it all sink in.

As the faculty sat in a room together in the police station, stunned and horrified, we held hands and prayed. The police chaplain, a minister in our community, talked with us. At one point, the door opened and I caught a glimpse of Christina's stepmother. Then I heard her anguished cry as she was told of her daughter's death. There is no way to describe the emotion of that moment.

I later found out that Scott had left home but had forgotten something and had gone back home to get it. He was turning into the street leading to the school when the shots rang out. I am so thankful he did not witness or experience what so many did. Mr. Larry's son was in the commons during the shooting, but he was close to a door and escaped safely.

Those who actually witnessed the shooting stayed at the police station to give statements. I had not actually seen Luke. As I reflect on that, I wondered so many times how I did not see him. He was only a few feet away and the office has glass windows. Had I looked to my right instead of straight across the commons, he would have been there.

As we were driving home from the police station, we passed by Lydia's home, and I saw her mom and several others standing in the front yard. I told Brian, my husband, to stop and let me say something to her. As I hugged her, I remember telling her that I thought as a parent she would want to know that Lydia was not alone. That some of us were there. That I was sorry. We only spoke briefly that day . . . but I am glad I had the opportunity to talk with her.

I was home by about 11:00 A.M. that morning. It seemed like a lifetime since I had left home a few hours before. How my life had changed, and I still had no clue just how much. I only remember sketches of that afternoon and night—people calling, watching the news, my insides shaking—that afternoon and night are blurry to me. We got word that the faculty would meet the next morning at 10:00 A.M. in our central office complex.

THURSDAY, OCTOBER 2, 1997

The faculty gathered for a debriefing session. Our principal, Roy Balentine, spoke to us tearfully and told us how grateful he was for how we had responded and how sorry he was. He updated us about injured students. Alan Westbrook was in critical condition at that time. He stayed in the hospital for several weeks and had several surgeries.

The faculty and staff were divided into small groups. We shared. I remember people crying, feeling guilty, saying, "If I had walked across the commons, then it would have been me and not these children who died." Our ROTC commander, crying, told of being the first to get to Christina and trying to keep her from dying, knowing she was already gone. Our band director spoke of seeing Luke going down a hall after he had shot seven students and reloading and then turning and coming back up the hall and thinking, he's going to kill all of us. A teacher telling of students huddled behind the columns in the commons—being still—hoping Luke would not shoot them. A teacher who had been absent that day telling of the guilt she felt for not being there. A distraught, heartbroken faculty.

The administration had planned for us to have school open Friday for those students and parents who wanted to come and have a brief memorial service. Faculty members wanted to go back into the building before the students arrived; they allowed us to go that Thursday. I'll never forget us walking back into the commons area. We gathered in a circle around the place close to my office where Lydia and Christina had died. We held hands, we prayed, we cried. I remember after that going over and standing by the door of my office and sobbing. We didn't stay long that day, but it was one of the best things we did as far as helping our students the next day. We needed to have time for ourselves before we could give time to them. No media . . . just us.

That night, visits to two funeral homes to offer support and love to grieving parents.

FRIDAY, OCTOBER 3, 1997

As I drove into the parking lot that morning, I could not believe the media. Big satellites, trucks—national news, local news. Everywhere. It was amazing to me. I never thought about what a factor the media would be in what we would deal with, and are still dealing with, in the aftermath of the shooting. A team of school counselors, mental health professionals, and pastors met early that morning. We discussed what needed to be done: helping students get into the building, conducting small-group counseling sessions with students, and being available for parents and faculty to share their concerns.

Students and parents began to arrive. Many were scared to come into the commons area. We held hands and walked through the doors together. One wounded student came, and as his parents walked into the commons with him, I was overcome with emotion. Faculty, students, parents, administrators, policemen, city officials—we supported each other through the most difficult time of our lives.

After a brief memorial service, students were asked to attend small-group sharing sessions. They could meet in their homeroom or in any room as long as they felt comfortable. We went through questions such as the following: What happened? Where were you? What thoughts have you had? How did you react? What impact has this had on you? How has this affected your family? Each session was closed by reminding students of strengths, reassuring them that it would take time to heal and that someone would be available to share with them in the days ahead. Although only about half our student body was there that day, sharing with each other made us a little stronger for what lay ahead. And we had no idea the events that would unfold in the next few days would make things harder than ever.

That afternoon I attended two funerals. I ached all over. I felt as if my insides were fragmented. Would we ever be back to normal? I wasn't sure.

MONDAY, OCTOBER 6, 1997— FIVE DAYS AFTER THE SHOOTING

Over the weekend, a counseling team composed of school counselors and mental health counselors was assembled to help students and faculty as we returned to school for a full day. We had an enrollment of about 1,000 students, and that first day back, about 900 students were present. Counselors were assigned to each classroom to help teachers in talking with students. A counselor was assigned to follow the schedules for the deceased, as well as the schedule of Luke Woodham. Students shared feelings and told their stories. We wondered why and how any of this could have happened in a community like ours.

The Friday night football game had been rescheduled for this night. We were playing a rival team at their field a few miles from our school. The pregame atmosphere was subdued. I remember being scared as I saw the crowd. Since I grew up in this community, I knew almost all the people around me in the stadium. But I had a nagging fear. I kept looking over my shoulder into the faces of people I didn't know. Was there another Luke somewhere here that might open fire on us? Anxious. An extended moment of silence for the victims was observed. One cheerleader, one who had witnessed Luke shoot Christina, wept. One football player, as the team came out, came with them on crutches. He had been shot, and Luke had looked him in the eye after he shot him and said, "Man, I'm sorry. I didn't know that was you." That boy's mother, a teacher, was standing a few feet away in the commons that morning, watching her son as Luke shot. That young man said that night, "I hope I can play again soon . . . I wish I could play tonight . . . Maybe next week." Our student body president, the head cheerleader, said, "The game is a welcome break from the worry and pain. It gives us something else to think about. It helps you forget at least a little." After Pearl High School won that game, the same pretty cheerleader said, with sad, watery eyes, "It's always there. I don't think any of us will ever forget. What happened is always going to be there." I was reminded of that again recently as I read what a Columbine student said: "Sometimes you forget for 30 seconds, and every 30 seconds helps."

TUESDAY, OCTOBER 8, 1997

Maybe today will be more of a normal day, I thought as I drove to school. Hopefully, the worst is over. Little did I know that it would be the most frightening day of my life.

After 9:00 A.M. that morning, my principal came and asked me to find where five students were. He needed that information immediately. Something was very wrong. That morning, police came into our school into classrooms and arrested five students. Police walked into classrooms, asked if certain students were there, and then informed them that they were under arrest for conspiracy to commit murder. They were led out in handcuffs, leaving behind rooms of students, scared and confused. I went to classrooms where these students had been and asked the remaining students to remain calm and not to panic, and stressed, above all else, that they were safe. They were scared, so scared. And so was I.

I went to the room where Scott was. Not knowing anything, I cautioned him about not saying anything to anyone. These students were his classmates, one in his honors classes, one who sang in the youth choir at our church with him, and one whose mother was a teacher in our school district. I cautioned him to trust no one. As I look back on that, it was so strange because we had never had reason to feel this way before.

We had gone to school as usual that day. Word spread about the arrests. I am amazed as I look back on that day that we did not have mass panic. It is truly a commendation to our students and faculty for keeping their composure under the most trying circumstances. Our faculty had no knowledge that these arrests were going to take place. It was a police matter. We simply had to trust our administration, police department, and city officials that they were doing what they thought was best at that time. And I did trust them—I think most everyone did. But it was not easy getting through that day. We had a brief faculty meeting that afternoon, and our superintendent, school board, and school board attorney talked with us about the situation and what we needed to do. Without the support, care, and concern of these people, our faculty and student body could not have carried on as they did. And the media were about to become one of the biggest factors we had to deal with. Our principal, superintendent, school board attorney, and school board president were our spokespersons. I think we were all afraid to speak to anyone at this point. I certainly was.

That night of the arrests, Scott and I were home. My husband was out of town on business. I was absolutely scared to death. I didn't want Scott to leave the house. I called my other son at the University of Mississippi, cautioning him to be careful who he talked with about anything. I was frantic. Who could be trusted? How could this have involved anyone else? I couldn't sleep at all. I was so frightened. What could tomorrow hold?

The Following Weeks and Months

The next days, weeks, and months were filled with sketches. Rumors of cults, hit-lists, bomb threats—all kinds of things that caused fright. Our district, in collaboration with Region 8 mental health, brought in a counselor to help us for the rest of that year. Because I was so directly involved in the incident, it was hard for me to talk to some students. I could not bear to think that anyone would have known anything like this would happen. All I could see at times were Lydia and Christina on the commons floor. Innocent. Dead.

MAY 1998—GRADUATION

We dedicated the program to the memories of Lydia and Christina. The student body president talked about being bound forever by the memories of their senior year. The media were still there, but we asked that they not report on the graduation ceremony. We wanted this to be a happy night. And it was. But the memories were there for all of us.

JUNE 1998—THE TRIAL

Luke Woodham was convicted of murdering his mother. In a second trial, Luke Woodham was convicted of murdering two students. I attended the day of the trial when our students and faculty testified to the events of that day in October. I sat in the balcony of the courtroom with the parents of the two victims. I heard the cheerleader who saw Luke shoot Christina cry as she turned to identify Luke as the shooter. She told me just a few days ago how she thought she was prepared, but when she turned and looked at him, how frightened she was. She said to me, "Mrs. Rowan, I grew up 20 years that day." She also shared with me how supported and loved she has felt. How a student that she had not gotten along with had come to her after the shooting and told her she was sorry for all she had had to see that day. How she believed our student body is more aware of what they say to each other. Yes, there are still cliques, there are still people who do not get along with each other, there are still hurtful remarks made, but, all in all, she believed we are much more conscious of how our actions affect others. How she felt sorry for Luke in the courtroom. "He had no one," she said, "and I had the love and support of friends and parents." How she could not understand how anyone could possibly do anything that horrible.

NINE MONTHS LATER

Even today as I walk across the commons in the morning, I can't help but think of that day. My son is a senior. He will graduate next week. As I have sat in the commons for banquets and proms, I have enjoyed the activities that we have had for our students. But I have never forgotten that I am sitting in the place where two innocent children died.

MEMORIES

Fourth of July—driving in the car, hearing fireworks, remembering standing in that room hearing shots.

Football game—a year later, the visiting team fires a cannon as their team comes onto the field. I cover my head and crouch down. I look down onto the field at a cheerleader who had been standing beside Christina, who had seen Luke shoot her. She grabs the cheerleader next to her and buries her head.

Watching television—gunshots or people screaming; it brings it all back.

Ketchup—sometimes I look at it and see a pool of blood.

A balloon pops in the commons—students become silent with fright.

My hands—I see them holding on to Lydia's.

Yellow crime tape, a news segment—an assistant principal tells me he can't stand to see this tape either: we remember.

Sirens—I hear them that day.

Smells—certain ones remind me of the smell of smoke that day.

Students—telling me how they are afraid to eat lunch in the commons. How much they appreciate a teacher for wiping the blood off their shoes that day. How guilty they feel for not having protected their friends. How they say we are closer and more aware of how precious life is.

LOOKING BACK

Certainly, as I look back over the past year and a half, there are things that I wish we could have done that perhaps we didn't do. But we did do so many things right:

We returned to school as quickly as possible.

We gave students the opportunity to talk through the situation.

We returned to normal scheduled activities as quickly as possible.

Our community worked together, police, city officials, school personnel—everyone—all worked with one goal in mind: to help our children recover from perhaps the most horrible event of their lives.

Our administration kept us informed as much as possible about the events. We took a strong hand with the media, not allowing them to disturb our students after school resumed.

A teacher wrote the following in our yearbook as a tribute to the two victims:

> Their lives were taken . . . senselessly.
> Our lives were changed forever . . . indescribably.
> In our minds the tragedy lives . . . disturbingly.
> In our hearts their memories live forever . . . beautifully.

7

Columbine High School Shootings

Community Response

PHILIPPE WEINTRAUB, M.D.
HARRIET L. HALL, PH.D.
ROBERT S. PYNOOS, M.D., M.P.H.

On April 20, 1999, the worst school shooting in United States history took place at Columbine High School, located just outside of Littleton, Colorado, a suburb of Denver. As of the writing of this chapter, a little more than a year has elapsed since that terrible event. As a result, the full story of what happened is still not known. In addition, it may take many years before the full psychological impact on the victims and community can be fully determined.

In this chapter, we attempt to chronicle how government officials, civic leaders, psychiatrists, and other mental health professionals in the Denver metropolitan area responded to the shootings and their aftermath. The massive outpouring of help and support from the local community, other parts of Colorado, the nation, and the world makes it impossible to know, much less describe, all the interventions provided to alleviate the victims' suffering.

We focus here on several topics. First, the events of April 20 and important background information related to the shootings are summarized. Second, the acute and longer-term psychological impact on the victims and the larger community is described. Third, the interventions that were felt to be helpful and are considered to be the hallmark of a good disaster response are highlighted. Fourth, the lessons learned—lessons that should enhance our knowledge of how to respond to school shootings—are discussed. Fifth, the community's current plan to deal with the long-term sequelae of this event is outlined. Last, unanswered questions that may be a focus of future research into adolescent violence are outlined.

A public health approach is a prerequisite for any successful series of interventions following a psychiatric disaster of this magnitude. Such an approach requires collaboration and coordination among many different agencies in order to first identify and then treat traumatized individuals in need of services. We describe how a collaboration of this type was forged among the school district, government agencies, mental health professionals, and important civic leaders in Jefferson County and the Denver metropolitan area. What local psychiatric leaders learned after this tragedy is that most communities and mental health professionals are not prepared, from previous training and experience, to respond to a psychiatric disaster of this magnitude on a long-term basis without outside consultation from experts in the field. Fortunately, such consultation was sought after this tragedy and led to the type of public health approach necessary to adequately deal with the crisis. It is believed that the development of the infrastructure to successfully implement a coordinated response among major agencies could enable all communities in the United States to optimally respond to psychiatric disasters involving teen violence in the school setting.

COLUMBINE HIGH SCHOOL

Before this incident, there were very few outward signs that Columbine High School was at risk for the violence that occurred within its walls on April 20, 1999. Located near Littleton, Colorado, in an upper-middle-class community of unincorporated Jefferson County, Columbine has a graduation rate of more than 90%, and most of its graduates go on to college. Although reports after the shootings suggested that conflicts between different student groups helped create a tense climate that contributed to the event, the school had not received publicity about the tension between groups prior to April 20. At the time of the shootings, its student body of 1,965 was more than 91% white. Of the remaining students, 16 were black, 112 Hispanic, and 42 Asian.

April 20, 1999, the Day of the Shootings

Eyewitness accounts, media reports, and descriptions from law enforcement agencies revealed a scene of chaos, carnage, and terror for hundreds of students, their families, and teachers and other staff on the day of the shootings. At about 11:20 A.M., around the start of the school lunch hour, two Columbine students, Eric Harris, 18 years old, and Dylan Klebold, 17 years old, arrived at the school clad in black trenchcoats and wearing masks. Heavily armed with rifles, semiautomatic weapons, and homemade pipe bombs, they began firing shots outside on the school grounds and threw pipe bombs onto the school roof. Two students were found dead outside, and others were wounded during this initial round of shots. The assailants then entered the school, where they proceeded to shoot many of the students and one teacher.

After entering the school, Harris and Klebold initially began firing at people in the cafeteria. They then went upstairs to the library, where they killed 10 students before committing suicide with gunshots to the head. During this shooting rampage, the assailants exploded bombs within the school, and these explosions produced fires and smoke in various parts of the building. The fires and smoke set off fire alarms, which rang continuously during the long ordeal for those students trapped in the building before help arrived.

Victims were traumatized in many different ways. A total of 38 individuals sustained injuries, primarily from gunshot wounds: the 12 students and 1 teacher who were killed, the 2 assailants who committed suicide, and an additional 23 individuals, mainly students, who survived their injuries. At least several of the injured were critically wounded, and some have been left with permanent disabilities.

Many students and teachers witnessed the shootings and the subsequent impact on the victims. These experiences were extremely traumatic not only because of the gore and carnage witnessed but also because of the brutal manner in which the acts were committed. For example, it was reported that as they were shooting people, the assailants laughed and verbalized pleasure in what they were doing.

Another major stressor for many students, teachers, family members, law enforcement officers, paramedics, and others involved in the tragedy was the helplessness and fear engendered by the incident. There was a several-hour period when approximately 300 students trapped in the building did not know if they also would be targets of the assailants. With the aid of cellular phones, some students contacted their families during this period and, in a state of terror, expressed fears that they might be killed in the shooting rampage going on around them. These trapped students, while hiding in various rooms, could hear gunshots, bombs exploding, attempts by the assailants to locate them, and the cries of victims.

ACUTE PSYCHOLOGICAL IMPACT OF THE SHOOTINGS

Much of the Denver metropolitan area, with a population of 2 million, was deeply affected by this tragedy for several reasons. There was initially a long period of uncertainty about the magnitude of the disaster and the potential risk to children and adolescents from other parts of the community. For much of the afternoon of April 20, the entire community was deluged with media reports that the gunmen might still be at large within the school. This uncertainty was due to the fact that law enforcement agents elected to not immediately storm the building for fear that such an action might precipitate additional shootings of innocent victims.

It was also not known for a significant period of time whether other schools were being targeted as part of a conspiracy. As a result, many neighboring schools were locked down as a precautionary measure. Concerns that this event might represent part of a broader-based effort to kill students in other schools led to bomb searches of other schools. Jefferson County and Denver County School Districts canceled classes the day after the shootings because of security concerns. In the ensuing days, bomb threats were made against other schools in Jefferson County and the Denver metropolitan area. The net effect of all these experiences was that many children, adolescents, and their parents had their sense of security and safety shattered.

The massive surge in the need for psychiatric services throughout the Denver metropolitan area soon after the event illustrates the widespread nature of the response to the shootings. There were reports of a dramatic increase in the number of local youths needing psychiatric hospitalization after the shootings. During the months of April, May, and June, Jefferson Center for Mental Health (Jefferson Center), which serves the area where Columbine High School is located, had an approximately 20% increase in the number of patients seen compared with the same period a year earlier.

In large part because of frequent speculations in the media about the causes of the shootings, many local citizens' distress about Columbine was exacerbated by the following fears and beliefs about the societal significance of this event and its implications about community safety and the psychological health of children.

Uncertainty About Causes

In the aftermath of the shootings, the uncertainty about how such a terrible event could have occurred contributed to widespread anxiety in the community. Uncertainty about the causes of the massacre fueled fears that many other high schools could be at risk for this type of violence, since Columbine had seemed, prior to the event, such a model school. There was tremendous concern about why the two assailants, Eric Harris and Dylan Kleblod, had not been identified sooner as youth at high risk for dangerous behavior. It was very unsettling to many that two bright students could be capable of committing such a heinous act. For many citizens, these apparent contradictions led to a fear that perhaps there were many more disturbed teens in the community who were not being identified by parents, teachers, and other important adults in their life. If even highly academically achieving youth could be capable of such violence, how could even the most dedicated monitoring efforts identify all teens at risk for this kind of behavior? These anxieties were exacerbated in the immediate aftermath of the shootings when there were approximately 3,000 copycat incidents nationwide, a more than fivefold increase in the average number of such incidents for that period of time.

Perception of Unheeded and Unnoticed Warning Signals

On the basis of other information available in the mass media, however, many people were distressed for the opposite reason: that warning signals that the assailants were at high risk of becoming violent had gone unheeded and unnoticed. Both of the assailants had apparently been meticulously planning this assault for over a year and had an arsenal of weapons and bombs in their homes. There were also reports that they had made threats and hostile comments to other students on numerous occasions and that at least one teacher had been concerned about violent themes in a writing assignment of one of the assailants.

These concerns were heightened by reports that the massacre could have been much worse if Harris and Klebold had succeeded in carrying out all of their plans. Most distressing was the information that they had brought 76 bombs to school and that 30 of them had exploded. In addition, it was sheer good fortune that most of the bombs failed to go off. Had these bombs exploded and the assailants continued shooting students before killing themselves, the death toll could have been much greater.

Another contributor to the perception that there had been a breakdown in the system's ability to identify high-risk youth was the fact that the assailants' previous problems with the law did not result in the identification of their underlying problems. In January 1998, they became involved with the law for the first time, after committing theft. Both Harris and Klebold, however, successfully completed their juvenile diversion program without officials developing any suspicion that either of them might have serious underlying psychiatric problems. People's fears were further exacerbated when it was reported that Eric Harris had actually been taking a psychotropic medication at the time of the shootings. After this report, there were wild speculations by many, including some professionals, that the medication could have caused the assailant to commit these terrible acts.

Fears of Unsafe Schools

Reports that there were tensions among different groups of Columbine students further compounded fears that schools were not as safe as previously believed. Although there were some conflicting reports about the seriousness of this problem, a sufficient number of students identified this as a potential contributor to the shootings that people throughout the community began to develop concerns that schools everywhere might not be safe because of such problems. What was particularly distressing were reports that the assailants were among a group of students perceived as "outsiders" and "different" from the more mainstream groups. It was reported that these outsiders were frequently taunted and excessively harassed. Since it was not clear whether these alleged problems were unique to Columbine or reflected worsening intolerance and student alienation in most American schools, the reports further eroded the confidence of children, adolescents, and adults in the community about the safety of their schools.

Fears of Unsafe Communities

The numerous copycat incidents and speculations about the causes of the shooting led to a fear among many in the community that societal institutions that were supposed to prevent this type of violence were no longer functioning adequately. The frequent speculations in the press by self-proclaimed experts about the causes of the Columbine shootings further exacerbated the fears of many individuals. Whether the blame was placed on the American family, schools, law enforcement, "psychiatric drugs," or the various agencies charged with helping troubled youth, many people of all ages no longer assumed that they could feel safe anywhere.

Anxieties about the role of media violence, violent video games, and access to guns in contributing to the commission of these acts added further to the sense of helplessness and fear that many families felt. Although there have long been concerns nationally that media and video game violence are unhealthy for young people, these issues became more of a focus of concern after the shootings because of reports that the assailants had been obsessed with violence and loved playing video games with violent themes (see Chapter 3, this volume). Regardless of their position on gun control, most local residents were also disturbed that the assailants, as minors, were so easily able to get access to so many destructive weapons. These concerns led many to feel that we live in a society of rampant violence whose unhealthy influence on young people disrupts the most dedicated efforts of good parents, schools, and helping agencies to provide, for children and adolescents, a safe, nurturing environment that promotes healthy psychological development.

ACUTE RESPONSE OF THE COMMUNITY AND LOCAL MENTAL HEALTH PROFESSIONALS

A massive outpouring of support and offers of assistance from all segments of the community occurred following the shootings. Many in the metropolitan area felt personally affected by the tragedy. If an event of this nature could occur at a school like Columbine, then no one could assume that his or her school was safe. One positive outcome of this reaction was that civic leaders, mental health agencies, and citizens from all walks of life came together to provide resources to help the victims and to coordinate their efforts in devising an effective disaster response.

In this section, we focus primarily on three of the many groups that have played a major role in responding to the mental health needs of the victims and larger community after the shootings. We first discuss the efforts of Victim Services and Jefferson Center, the two agencies that have provided the bulk of acute and ongoing services for those affected by the tragedy. We then review the involvement of the local professional psychiatric organizations, which put a tremendous amount of time into providing assistance, education, consultation, and service to the community. Last, we discuss the role of the University of Colorado Department of Psychiatry, which, in a consultant role, helped support the strengthening of the already existing collaboration among local agencies charged with responding to the mental health needs of the victims and larger community. It also provided expertise on treatment and design of research into the tragedy.

The efforts of these groups were made, it should be emphasized, in conjunction with the assistance provided by local and state government. In particular, a task force appointed by the governor in the immediate aftermath of the shootings to oversee the planning for the long-term needs of the community has interfaced with other agencies in activities designed to assist the victims. In addition, many other organizations, such as the Red Cross, whose contributions are not the focus of this chapter, played important roles in the crisis response.

Victim Services

In psychiatric disasters (e.g. violent crimes, traffic accidents) involving law enforcement in the United States, district attorneys and law enforcement victim-witness assistance services play a central role in helping victims of trauma. These organizations are required to inform all victims of their right to obtain funds for funeral costs, loss of income due to interruptions in work from trauma-related injuries, medical costs, and costs of treatment of psychiatric symptoms. The services provided by these organizations play a key role in reducing posttrauma adversities and ensuring proper care for those physically and psychologically injured.

Following the Columbine High School shootings, the Victim Assistance program, which is administered by the Jefferson County Sheriff's Office, served as the lead agency in coordinating the victim assistance response. Victims' advocates from that office, as well as those from other local organizations such as the Jefferson County District Attorney's Office, the Colorado Organization for Victim Assistance, and the advocacy staff and trained volunteers from throughout the metropolitan area, were on the scene almost immediately to provide support and assistance to the victims.

The Jefferson County Sheriff's Victim Services program, which provides services for approximately 2,000 victims in a typical year, became responsible for approximately 2,000 additional victims on the day of the shootings! That number included all students, teachers, administrators, and other employees at Columbine High School. The Victim Services program more than doubled its staff to meet the need. However, because the number of victims overloaded the response capacity of the organization, many victim assistance services, including crisis intervention, referrals, assistance for applying for Victims' Compensation benefits, and information about the status of the investigation, were often provided by volunteers from other areas for a significant period of time in the immediate aftermath of the shootings.

Victim Compensation, administered out of the Jefferson County District Attorney's Office, together with worker's compensation for the staff of the school, was available to fund formal psychiatric services for the victims, their families, and some other members of the Columbine community who required psychiatric help.

Approximately 8,000 individuals were potentially eligible for victim assistance intervention. Under the Victim Assistance Compensation program, there was no charge to patients for services, and every individual had the equivalent of an advocate or case manager to help with getting access to needed treatment. Because of the large number of individuals in need of services, Victim Assistance applied for and received a grant from the federal government for the additional services.

Community Mental Health Response: Jefferson Center for Mental Health

A psychiatric disaster of this magnitude requires a swift but also evolving response until it becomes more clear what level and coordination of services will be required to meet the psychiatric needs of all those traumatized. Although no organization can ever be fully prepared for a crisis affecting an entire community, Jefferson Center was well qualified to respond in several ways. The center has a long tradition of responding to community tragedies and crises, both large and small. In 1992, Jefferson Center started a service called "Trauma Management Consultants" specifically to respond to workplace violence and other critical incidents in the business community. Trauma Management Consultant specialists have trained, over the years, numerous Jefferson Center personnel in critical incident stress debriefing and other crisis management techniques.

The center also has long worked closely and collaboratively with the schools, and as a result, it had well established working relationships with the individuals in charge of the school's crisis response. Jefferson Center not only had strong relationships with key school district staff as a result of community collaborative programming, but also had easy access to top officials in the Jefferson County Sheriff's Department, District Attorney's Office, and other agencies involved in the Columbine response. Because of these strong relationships, the center was able to respond quickly and effectively.

Another factor that prepared Jefferson Center to manage the longer-term crisis response was its experience as the managed care entity responsible for providing all needed behavioral health care to Medicaid recipients in three counties. In this role, it has developed the ability to 1) manage a network of providers, both internal and external, and 2) coordinate, dispatch, and manage service delivery using a wide range of public and private sector providers. Against this background, what follows is the chronology of how Jefferson Center, in cooperation with other agencies, responded to the unprecedented crisis facing the local community after the Columbine shootings.

Acute Response

April 20.   Jefferson Center staff were on site within 2 hours of the shooting, providing crisis response and leadership for the mental health efforts in the days to come. Jefferson Center mobilized teams of crisis counselors that included Jefferson Center clinicians and volunteers from other mental health agencies. That first night after the shooting, Jefferson Center management and professional staff were on site near Columbine High School at Leawood Elementary School, Columbine Public Library, and the Light of the World Church, providing in excess of 165 hours of crisis counseling services to students, family members, and residents of the community.

The types of psychiatric problems for which people sought and/or needed assistance included

- Acute distress and shock in reaction to the shootings
- Anxiety about the whereabouts of loved ones before the dead and wounded were identified
- Acute grief once it was learned that loved ones had been killed or seriously injured
- Fear for one's safety before it was known that there was no longer any threat of further shootings
- Requests from parents about how to 1) talk to their children about what happened and 2) help their children cope with fears for their own safety

April 21.   On the day after the shootings, Jefferson Center staff began to fully realize the enormity of the tragedy and the tasks that lay ahead to help a whole community heal. In anticipation of the large number of individuals who would need services in the upcoming days, Jefferson Center organized a crisis call center, which used 16 staffed phonelines to respond to crisis calls related to the shootings. Many callers were from the local area, but numerous others were previous trauma victims from all over the United States retraumatized by the television coverage, which frequently mentioned the center's emergency phone number. In addition, 56 clinicians provided psychiatric services at Clement Park, right next to Columbine High School, and at two churches. Representatives from Jefferson Center, the school district, Victim Services, and County Emergency began meeting with the Office of Emergency Management.

April 22. Approximately 100 clinicians from Jefferson Center and other agencies provided about 300 hours of psychiatric services to individuals and groups at three churches, one school, and five other community locations. The Columbine Crisis Chat Line was opened on the Jefferson Center Web site to provide support for teenagers who chose not to use counseling or debriefing services. By the end of the first 3 days of the crisis, approximately 1,600 Jefferson Center staff hours were spent attending crisis calls, coordinating volunteers, helping individuals find critical services, and assisting those most directly impacted: the students, families, and staff of Columbine.

April 23–April 30. During this period, Jefferson Center became the central point for organizing debriefings in response to requests for assistance from schools, businesses, churches, community organizations, and individuals. Jefferson Center worked closely with the school district to meet the counseling and support needs of all students and staff impacted by the tragedy. It was during this period that planning began for a facility in the Columbine area to provide counseling and victim services as well as activities and education for students, families, and community members over the summer. Before the students from Columbine High School returned to school at nearby Chatfield High School, mental health staff participated in a parents' meeting that was attended by 3,500 parents; Jefferson Center staff described for the parents how the mental health needs of the students would be met in the upcoming weeks. From the day of the shootings through April 30, more than 3,000 hours of services were provided to the community.

Mental health services were made available to Columbine students after they resumed classes at Chatfield High School. These services consisted primarily of crisis counseling and referral/triage for students and families, consultation to staff, and desensitization (e.g., to fire drills).

A critical part of the Jefferson Center's crisis response was the public information effort to get word out about symptoms to watch for and how to access services. In conjunction with the Mental Health Association of Colorado, Jefferson Center put together a booklet about the crisis for parents. Entitled "A Partner for Parents: A Handbook for Healing," it was mailed to every parent in the school district, approximately 70,000 households. The booklet provided considerable psychoeducation about trauma. Topics included how to talk to one's child about the Columbine incident, identification of signs of stress reactions in children, and warning signs of possible severe psychopathology in youths at risk of suicidal or homicidal behavior (see Chapter 5, this volume). In addition, the booklet emphasized the importance of parents taking care of their own emotional needs in order to be optimally supportive of their children. The last pages of the booklet had a comprehensive list of resources in the Denver metropolitan area for families seeking the aid of a mental health professional. It also included resources for faith-based treatment through churches, since many members of the community preferred a spiritual approach in dealing with this type of traumatic experience.

Columbine Connections

A prime example of the effective coordination of efforts among different agencies responding to the tragedy was the creation of Columbine Connections, a community resource center located near Columbine High School. It was formed to address the enormous needs of a community that had been subjected to an unprecedented, major trauma. Columbine Connections was the result of a collaboration among several groups. These included the Jefferson Center for Mental Health, the Jefferson County Sheriff's Department, First Judicial District Attorney's Office, Foothills Parks and Recreation District, PACCT (Parents and Community Connecting Together, a grassroots community organization), and a 20-member youth advisory board from Columbine High School.

This collaborative effort had several major goals. One goal was to develop within the community a specialized local capability for providing services and compensation to victims. It was felt that such a collaboration would, in addition, provide easy access to a wide array of services, information, and opportunities needed in order for victims to heal in the aftermath of this violent and tragic event. As part of this collaboration, linkages were formed with important community institutions such as churches and other religious groups, health facilities, major employers, recreation providers, and other agencies in a position to identify and aid those in need of support during the recovery process. Columbine Connections has offered victim services; survivor counseling; parent education and support; parent, adolescent, and peer counseling; a teen drop-in center; and community outreach and linkages involving, among others, recreational agencies, athletic leagues, the faith community, arts community, and educational system.

Jefferson Center's treatment and outreach services included three types of programs and interventions. One type focused on the treatment of children, youth, adults, and families at Columbine Connections and in the schools and community. Another focused on the development and dissemination of psychoeducational information on all aspects of trauma recovery for both victims and those providing services for the traumatized. A strong outreach component, based out of Columbine Connections, sought to provide both psychoeducation and treatment to individuals in need who were not actively seeking assistance. The third focused on the development of specialized programming at Columbine Connections for affected youths in order to provide a safe place, both physically and emotionally, for them to process the wide range of emotions the tragedy had evoked.

The teen component of Columbine Connections, SHOUTS (Students Helping Others Unite Together Socially), was actually the first component of Columbine Connections to open. SHOUTS was created to provide additional support for traumatized youths who are potentially at high risk for developing symptoms of depression and/or posttraumatic stress disorder (PTSD). When it became apparent within the first few days after the shootings that youths were finding support through contacts with their peers, it was decided that they needed a nurturing environment where they could feel safe, be together, and have access to the support of adults if such help was needed. A youth advisory board was quickly formed to give life to the concept. Youths on the advisory board were adamant that some type of center for teens needed to be open by the time school ended on May 27. Because of concern that this tragedy took place right before the summer vacation, when many students would have less access to services and support, project organizers agreed with this goal, and SHOUTS opened on May 28.

At SHOUTS, youths participated in a variety of recreational activities and spent time socializing with peers. There was a large open area with couches and chairs, a dance floor, a café fashioned after the set on the TV show *Friends*, an art room, a computer room, a movie room, and a recording studio. Youths also had access to counseling and support groups. In addition to being a teen drop-in center, SHOUTS also provided adult members of the community a place to gather as well. Saturday evenings were community nights when teens and families came together.

Funding for the Community Mental Health Response

One of the challenges facing local leaders, agencies, and mental health professionals after the shootings was how to get the resources and funding to help the potentially large number of traumatized individuals in need of services. Communities experiencing either natural disasters or certain types of terrorist acts, like the Oklahoma City bombing in April 1995, are eligible for Federal Emergency Management Agency (FEMA) funding.

Such funding, administered through the Emergency Services and Disaster Branch of the federal Center for Mental Health Services (CMHS), part of the U.S. Public Health Service, is typically made available only if the president declares the affected location a disaster area. Despite some initial optimism from federal officials that this funding would be made available for the Columbine victims, it was not made available, in part because there was not enough physical damage at the school to meet one of the eligibility criteria for this type of support. Given that federal disaster officials had originally estimated that Columbine-related mental health services could cost $9 million over 3 years, the loss of potential resources to support the treatment of the victims was disappointing.

However, both the U.S. Department of Justice and the State of Colorado did respond with funding. Two weeks after the tragedy, $125,000 was made available to Jefferson Center for Mental Health from the $1 million that Governor Bill Owens allocated to Jefferson County via the state's Emergency Declaration. The U.S Department of Justice, through the Victims of Crime Act, promptly made approximately $250,000 available to Jefferson Center for Mental Health for mental health victim services. It also made counseling dollars available to the Jefferson County School District and Jefferson County Sheriff's Victim Assistance and provided a substantial amount of additional money for the state's Victims' Compensation fund for psychiatric treatment for Columbine victims.

Even with this additional funding, the treatment needs of the victims overwhelmed the resources of Jefferson Center and other agencies that were providing services. Additional funding was provided through The Healing Fund, which had been created by United Way and the McCormick Tribune Foundation days after the Columbine tragedy to support victims, families of victims, and local agencies with youth and violence prevention programs. The fund ended up with over $4.4 million donated by individuals and businesses responding to the Columbine tragedy. The process of deciding how these funds should be spent was not without controversy. Public attention was focused on the 38 identified deceased and injured victims and their families, and many in the community did not understand the psychological victimization of the uninjured students and teachers in the school, as well as others in the community. The Healing Fund Committee ultimately ended up understanding how important the mental health needs of the community were. They provided funding for 1 year for an outreach team with the equivalent of four full-time staff, several school-based counselors, and some of the costs of Columbine Connections and SHOUTS. The total funding for mental health services ended up being about 10% of the $4.4 million.

Acute Response and Role of Local and University Psychiatrists

Local psychiatrists were as deeply affected by this tragedy as any other group and have played a major role in the community response. Most of their efforts have been through participation in task forces created by the state professional organizations and/or the University of Colorado Department of Psychiatry. The major efforts of these groups have revolved around providing consultation, support, expertise, and pro bono services to a community with a large number of traumatized individuals. What follows is a description of the efforts of these groups. We then describe how these local organizations have come together with the school system and frontline clinicians to begin to develop a series of interventions that will address the long-term needs of the victims and community.

Local Psychiatric Professional Organizations

Like most other citizens, local psychiatrists responded quickly to the shootings. The day after the tragedy, the Colorado Psychiatric Society (CPS) held an emergency meeting to explore what role the organization should play in helping the victims and community at large recover from the psychiatric sequelae of the shootings. Local child and adolescent psychiatric leaders from the Colorado Child and Adolescent Psychiatric Society (CCAPS) were invited to provide their expertise on how to deal with a disaster primarily involving young people.

A number of important topics were addressed, and an action plan to respond to the crisis began to be developed. First, the group focused on their own personal reactions to the tragedy. This exercise was important because it illustrated that one of the major challenges in addressing this type of crisis is being able to help the "helpers." This process led to a discussion of how teachers, school administrators, parents, mental health professionals, and other important adults in the community responsible for the care, supervision, education, and welfare of children were themselves traumatized to varying degrees. Such individuals, it was pointed out, would need support and psychoeducation in order to be able to take on the enormous burdens of responding to the emotional needs of the victims.

There was also considerable discussion of how the organization could best help the community respond to the tragedy. Although it was agreed that it would be helpful for members to make themselves available to provide treatment for individual victims, it was decided that the organization could make a major positive contribution if it was part of the coordinated response to the tragedy. Therefore, the organization decided to make itself available to assist state and local agencies charged with providing psychiatric services to the victims. Offering to provide consultation and talks to various lay and professional groups could provide a very useful educational function for the community.

A task force was formed of members interested in responding to the crisis. In addition, both CPS and CCAPS decided to coordinate their efforts by making this a joint task force under the coleadership of their respective presidents. This emergency meeting was followed by a rapid mobilization to action of the two organizations' memberships as well as a variety of outreach efforts to others in the community. Within 72 hours of the shooting, an urgent memo was sent to all members, requesting that they make themselves available to provide services for any individuals in acute need of help. Within 6 days of the shootings, 100 members offered to provide assistance in doing emergency evaluations, conducting debriefings, and providing consultation to schools and front-line clinicians.

One of the major efforts of the task force and the parent organizations was to disseminate important information about trauma and disaster response. The American Psychiatric Association (APA) and the American Academy of Child and Adolescent Psychiatry (AACAP) sent CPS and CCAPS, respectively, didactic materials that were mailed to local providers who might be called on to help the victims and other members of the community affected by the tragedy. For example, the entire memberships of CPS and CCAPS received a mailing of these materials soon after the shootings. Similar types of information about teen violence, trauma, and disaster response were mailed to pediatricians and family practitioners in Colorado. This latter mailing was the result of a joint effort of CCAPS, Denver's Children's Hospital, and the state chapter of the American Academy of Pediatrics. The APA provided financial support for these educational efforts through a grant to CPS from a fund reserved for psychiatric disasters. These funds were used to help pay for the dramatic increase in administrative costs associated with the mailings and increased volume of phone calls.

Another important focus of the task force was addressing the potential adverse impact of the media on the victims and on efforts to respond to the crisis. Concerns were expressed about how the extensive media coverage of the event was retraumatizing individuals with high levels of exposure to the violence as well as exacerbating the symptoms of children and adolescents with preexisting psychiatric illnesses. The membership also was strongly urged to not grant interviews to the media about their diagnostic impressions regarding the psychiatric status of the assailants. It was stressed that commenting to the media on individuals one has not personally evaluated is a violation of the psychiatrist's code of ethics.

The task force also formed linkages with other important groups involved in the community response to the tragedy. For example, a representative from the state disaster management agency briefed the task force on the magnitude of the problems facing the community and how local organizations could be of help in assisting the victims. In addition, one of the task force's co-chairs served on a multidisciplinary local committee that included representatives from the school district; the committee's mission was to help coordinate the response efforts of the various agencies charged with providing services to the Columbine community and others affected by the shootings.

Role of the University of Colorado Department of Psychiatry

Within days of the shooting, a group of faculty came together under the direction of the interim chairman to assess what role the department of psychiatry should play in responding to the crisis. Composed of more senior members of the department who had expressed an interest in helping out and who had expertise in some aspect of the tragedy, the group included researchers, clinician-educators, and two child and adolescent psychiatrists.

The experience following the Oklahoma City bombing established a precedent for a coordinated community response. There, the local mental health agencies, school district leadership, local university medical school, federal and state departments of education, and external consultants who were national experts in the field worked together to help the victims. Within 3 days of the Columbine shootings, Dr. Robert Pynoos of the UCLA Trauma Psychiatry program, who had been a consultant for the Oklahoma City bombing and the Springfield, Oregon, school shooting, was contacted and became an external consultant to the university soon thereafter.

According to Pynoos et al. (1998), while there is a strong, compelling professional need to provide as much immediate crisis support as possible, at some key point it is necessary to make a transition to a more systematic public health approach. Disaster research has shown that the best way to implement such a public health approach is to conduct a systematic screening of the affected students, school personnel, and their families. This assessment should include a determination of the degree of bereavement and traumatic exposure as well as the level of ongoing distress and functional impairment after the event—all risk factors for a poor psychiatric outcome. This type of screening is necessary because crisis services in the immediate aftermath of psychiatric disasters rarely provide a systematic assessment of the presence of these risk factors, the identification of which permits a more comprehensive and successful targeting and treatment of individuals in need of services. Identification of high-risk individuals also provides information that is essential in planning the array of services needed to provide adequate treatment to the affected population.

National and international efforts after wars, disasters, terrorist attacks, and community violence have repeatedly confirmed the advantages of placing mental health efforts within the school setting. The school setting is the best and most efficient site to identify children in need of services and the optimal location to maximize compliance with the interventions provided. In addition, the provision of services at school enhances parental participation and helps reduce the stigma associated with psychiatric illness. All these factors have been found to facilitate an integration of psychological and academic recovery.

The very school personnel on whom parents and students rely to help normalize their return to school are themselves likely to be badly traumatized and grieving. Rather than just providing psychoeducation to teachers about how to assist their students, it is critical first to provide school personnel with adequate support and attention to their own experiences, losses, ongoing distress, and current reactivity to reminders of the trauma. They must have adequate guarantees of confidentiality so that they can take advantage of treatment without having to worry that their teaching careers will be adversely affected by seeking help. It is only within this context that proper psychoeducation about traumatized students can occur. The success of any school-based program relies on the support of the school administrators, and such support often rests on administrators' understanding of their own experiences and prolonged course of recovery.

The importance of recognizing the violence at Columbine High School as a murder–suicide was emphasized to Jefferson Center and school staff. Preventive efforts should therefore be directed at identifying suicidal, depressed adolescents, ensuring their psychiatric care, and educating the public and families about the psychiatric imperative to restrict access to alcohol, guns, and drugs and to address risk-taking behaviors.

Frequently, a major shortcoming of the response of departments of psychiatry is to want to offer assistance and clinical research efforts without first establishing an appropriate alliance with community agencies and school personnel who carry the primary responsibility for the welfare of students, staff, and families in the community. It is therefore imperative to find appropriate channels through which the university can participate in the public mental health planning. The major challenge for the department in beginning to address these issues in regard to the Columbine tragedy was determining how to approach the school and community. It was decided to approach Jefferson Center, which was providing most of the frontline mental health services for the victims, and the state agency responsible for overseeing mental health services, Colorado Mental Health Services (CMHS), to see if those agencies were interested in collaborating with the university.

PLANNING THE LONG-TERM RESPONSE TO THE COLUMBINE TRAGEDY

After 1 month of acutely responding to the shootings, the community had an opportunity to step back, evaluate its efforts, and assess what type of more long-term interventions the victims and others affected by the tragedy would require as part of the recovery from this traumatic experience. This evolution in the response was aided by two events.

The first event took place in the middle of May. At a time when it still appeared that chances for federal disaster funding were good, CMHS arranged for a team of three mental health disaster professionals with expertise in federally funded disaster responses to come to Colorado and conduct a needs assessment the week of May 18th. They were in town for most of the week, and their expertise was quite useful in planning for the long-term response needed to meet the community's mental health needs.

An important piece of feedback from these consultants was their observation that the level of fear throughout the Columbine community, the Denver metropolitan area, and the state of Colorado was higher than had been seen after other disasters. It was felt that a major contributor to this high level of fear was that, because there was no single definitive explanation for why the assailants committed this crime, no one had any answers on how to prevent such events from occurring again.

In their formal report, the consultants estimated that it would cost approximately $3.9 million to provide mental health services for 18 months. It was recommended that after 18 months, an additional needs assessment be done to ascertain how much longer posttrauma intervention would be required. High-risk, medium-risk, and low-risk groups were identified on the basis of the amount of exposure to trauma related to the shootings.

It was estimated that the high-risk group comprised approximately 9,000 individuals, including all Columbine students, employees, and their immediate families as well as the approximately 200 first responders to the scene of the shooting. The site visitors estimated that one-third of this group would receive active outreach and counseling services. They recommended that two outreach teams, each consisting of 6.25 full-time employees, be funded to meet the needs of the high-risk group. The staff on these teams were to include professional mental health counselors, outreach paraprofessionals, and a mental health professional trained in trauma-related interventions, to whom the outreach teams could refer for consultation and supervision.

It was estimated that the moderate-risk group comprised 12,300 individuals, including students in surrounding schools and students in schools that were "locked down" during the incident. The site visitors recommended that an additional outreach team and mental health professional trained in trauma-related interventions be hired to meet the needs of this group.

The low-risk group, whose numbers the task force said were impossible to calculate, included those who learned about the event through media exposure. It was felt that all residents of Colorado were potentially in this group but that the incidence of individuals needing assistance from this group would be low. The team recommended increasing the staffing of all community mental health centers in the state by two full-time employees each to meet the needs of this group. This ended up being the largest dollar amount requested in the needs assessment, which also recommended funding for organizational infrastructure and program evaluation costs.

The second event that helped the community change its focus from crisis intervention to long-term planning and treatment was the visit to Denver of two external consultants hired by the University of Colorado Department of Psychiatry. The two consultants were one of the present authors, Robert Pynoos, M.D., from UCLA, and Betty Pfefferbaum, M.D., chairperson of the University of Oklahoma Department of Psychiatry, who was actively involved in the psychiatric response to the Oklahoma City bombing and who had done extensive research into that event. They were asked to provide consultation on how to assist in the community response to the tragedy, on the types of interventions that should be provided to those requiring psychiatric services, and on the design of research studies.

There were two reasons why it was felt that the consultants should come to Denver as soon as possible. First, concerns were raised that a large number of Columbine students were at high risk of developing PTSD, depression, and other psychiatric complications resulting from the high levels of trauma exposure. Since without treatment many of these students could be at significant risk of developing major functional impairment and/or of becoming suicidal, it was felt that the expertise of the external consultants on how to identify and treat persons in this group should be obtained as soon as possible. In addition, given the psychological need for traumatized people to suppress their memories of what happened and resist further intervention, it was felt that there was a very narrow window of opportunity to begin obtaining the cooperation of the school district and local community in this endeavor. The hope was that the consultation would help the agencies involved acquire the expertise to develop the infrastructure by the beginning of the next school year so that they could identify and treat those Columbine students in need of services.

IMPEDIMENTS TO HELPING THE VICTIMS

The following impediments to helping the victims were identified by the task force, local agencies, and external consultants.

Negative Impact of the Media

Although the media can provide essential information to survivors, community members, and the general public, its coverage can also be excessive and intrusive and can re-evoke traumatic reactions in at-risk traumatized children, adolescents, and adults. The Los Angeles Unified School District, among others in the United States, has developed specific guidelines to contend with media requests in the aftermath of a school disaster. All requests must go through central school administration, thereby freeing school personnel at the affected school to focus their attention on the emotional and practical needs of their students, faculty, and families. In addition, the guidelines regulate media access to school grounds and set parameters for interviews with students and faculty.

It was stressed by the consultants that a traumatized individual is not able to give true informed consent when approached by the media for an interview. Dr. Pfefferbaum also cited her study which showed that following the Oklahoma City bombing, severity of PTSD symptoms in children correlated with the amount of exposure to television coverage of the event (Pfefferbaum et al. 1999).

Flood of Offers for Crisis Services and for Research

In response to the enormous number of calls from mental health professionals throughout the state and nation offering to provide crisis services to the Columbine victims, CMHS began providing credentialing services to the community several days after the tragedy. Because there were concerns that some untrained individuals with their own agenda were trying to become involved in the response, the state checked that those volunteering had crisis training and also ran their names through the Colorado Bureau of Investigation background check. In addition, the large number of individuals from outside the state wanting to do research on this population raised concerns about possible exploitation of the victims and the risk of a lack of coordination in all research efforts.

Inadequate Expertise in Community

Although many local clinicians had some background and experience in treating victims of trauma, this type of psychiatric disaster requires knowledge and skills not possessed by most mental health professionals. Staff at Jefferson Center had significant experience dealing with the immediate crisis needs but had no experience in planning for long-term intervention efforts of the magnitude required by this event.

Greater Risks for PTSD and Depression

Many traumatized adolescents and school personnel were potentially at high risk of significant morbidity if they were not identified soon. Drs. Pynoos and Pfefferbaum reviewed the scientific evidence that individuals with high levels of exposure to the violence were at significant risk of developing PTSD and depression and that those who were close to the slain victims would also be at risk of complicated bereavement and depression. In addition, it was emphasized that students with preexisting psychiatric problems also would be more vulnerable to exacerbations of psychiatric symptoms.

Differentiating Grief From Acute Stress Reactions

After a massive disaster, there is often failure to recognize that not only PTSD but also depression and grief reactions are prevalent. The importance of tailoring interventions for individual victims on the basis of the most prominent of these two clinical syndromes was emphasized. In addition, many victims have combinations of both conditions, which presents a challenge in clinical management, since the treatment for each, to some extent, involves opposite goals. In the treatment of PTSD, one of the goals is to reduce hyperarousal and intrusive recollections of the event, whereas for those who have lost a loved one, one goal of therapy is to facilitate normal bereavement, helping them to reconstitute a nontraumatic mental image of the deceased in order to promote positive reminiscing.

Impact of Shootings on School Officials and the Local Community

Although there was a consensus in the group that schoolwide screening and subsequent school-based, trauma-focused interventions were essential, there were expectable concerns that school officials, parents, and members of the local community might be uncomfortable with such activities. The consultants discussed how to go about dealing with this issue.

1. It is important to address concerns that the public mental health effort would only exacerbate traumatic distress and interfere with a natural course of recovery. By explaining to school officials, students, and parents the ways in which the information would be used to inform and guide essential clinical services, agencies and other mental health personnel can allay some of the hesitancy.
2. Many of the school personnel had only just begun to recover from their own traumatic experiences and would find it difficult to be "burdened" with this task, despite their interest in the recovery of the student body and school community. In addition to providing mental health assistance to school personnel, clarifying information about the practical implementation of the screening could help assuage concerns of school officials that the students would be overwhelmed by this process.
3. Since many students and families will have obtained support and assistance through religious organizations, it is important to include representatives from churches, synagogues, and other religious groups in planning the mental health effort.

The visit from the external consultants proved to be helpful in beginning to address the problems just described. It resulted in the development of a plan of action and an even greater coordination of efforts among the major agencies involved in the response. Two days after the consultation, the governor's task force appointed a committee from CMHS to screen requests to do research related to Columbine. The school district authorized this committee to determine which research would be appropriate. Over time, the membership of this committee was expanded to include a university liaison and representatives from the school district. In addition, Jefferson Center and the University of Colorado Department of Psychiatry formalized their collaboration, which included an agreement for the department of psychiatry to take the lead in designing research protocols.

Screening for High-Risk Youth

Jefferson Center wanted priority to be given to research efforts that also met a service delivery need. Both Jefferson Center and the University of Colorado Department of Psychiatry agreed that the recommended screening would allow for identification of those at Columbine High School who were in greatest need of services. The limited treatment resources available could be better prioritized if the screening was performed. The major goal of the two groups was to enlist the cooperation of the school district and community to allow the screening of all Columbine High School students when the new school year resumed.

The school district was initially reluctant to consent to screenings in the school setting, because some administrators were concerned that a massive screening would dredge up bad memories and disrupt the students' and teachers' ability to get on with their lives. One of the consultants was helpful in gaining support from the school district for the screening concept. When concerns were raised by the school about the screening being nothing more than research that would not address the treatment needs of the students, the consultant explained that the screening is actually the standard way of identifying high-risk youth in need of services. Assessment and identification of high-risk individuals in potential need of services is the standard of care in the methodology used by businesses and industries responding to workplace disasters and traumatic situations. As a result of this clarification, the school district supported the screening concept and authorized the department of psychiatry to be in charge of this project.

Although the school district administration was now in support of the screening concept, some teachers and administrators at Columbine High School continued to be uncomfortable with the concept of screenings. It was felt that because they themselves had been so badly traumatized by this event, it would be important for the screening personnel to be sensitive to the anxiety-provoking effects of the screening process on those who had been through such a difficult experience.

LONGER-TERM PSYCHOLOGICAL IMPACT

As would be predicted from our current knowledge about the psychological effects of trauma, many individuals from Columbine High School and the larger community have developed significant psychiatric symptoms and associated functional impairment. In this section, we describe the types of problems seen in children, adolescents, and adults during the summer of 1999 and over the course of the ensuing school year. In addition, we describe the types of interventions provided to help the growing number of individuals who were identified as needing services.

One of the challenges in addressing the longer-term needs of the victims and community was the time it took to make a needs assessment and to gain the support of the community. In the immediate aftermath of the shootings, one understandable, and at times appropriate, response in the Columbine community was to believe that the best way to recover from this tragedy was to look to the future and not dwell on the past. As a result, concerned mental health professionals had to respect, to some extent, the need for victims to request help on their own when they felt ready to do so. It should be emphasized that this type of response is very typical in communities where people have been traumatized and are trying to reduce psychic pain by avoiding any offer of help that they fear will overwhelm them with painful memories.

As more children, adolescents, and parents developed symptoms, however, more victims and persons in the larger community requested help. This increase in requests led to the development of a growing infrastructure to assess and treat those in need of services.

As far back as the summer, when the resource center opened, Columbine Connections was busy responding to the needs of the victims and community. Later, in the fall, crisis walk-ins of various types became an almost daily occurrence. One day during the last week of October, for example, three Columbine parents, each contemplating suicide because of psychological distress related to the shootings, walked in seeking assistance. In addition, families requested family therapy as they found that the emotional toll of the shootings became too difficult to bear without professional assistance. The requests for support groups for mothers of Columbine students became so numerous that it was necessary to run groups during both days and evenings.

Columbine Connections has received numerous requests from all over Jefferson County to provide both consultation and intervention for those affected by the Columbine shootings. Examples of the types of services provided include intervention for spouses of those who first responded to the tragedy; treatment of children with school phobia directly traceable to Columbine; consultation to teachers from elementary and secondary schools; and support and information for Boy Scout leaders. Columbine Connections provided outreach to these individuals and groups whenever possible. During the fall, the outreach team of the Columbine Connections Resource Center, comprising four individuals, averaged 50 or more contacts per staff person per week.

Many different groups of individuals, in addition to the students and staff at Columbine High School, developed psychiatric symptoms since the shootings. For example, families living on Leawood Drive, which is across the street from Columbine High School, were significantly affected by the shootings. Some of these residents witnessed wounded students running into their homes, covered with blood, immediately after the shootings.

Parents sought help for a variety of psychiatric symptoms that developed in their children and in other family members. Some families reported that all family members were sleeping together at night in order to feel safe. Many parents were concerned about adolescents who were engaging in unhealthy and reckless behaviors. These behaviors included consuming alcohol, driving 100 miles per hour, and "totaling" cars in auto accidents. In addition, some of the students who were high-school seniors at the time of the shooting were having difficulty adjusting to college because of PTSD symptoms. Parents of these youths requested help after learning that their children were doing poorly academically because PTSD symptoms prevented them from studying or focusing effectively on their schoolwork.

THE 1999–2000 SCHOOL YEAR

Since it was anticipated that the return to school for students at Columbine at nearby schools would be stressful, considerable outreach was provided by Jefferson Center during the summer months to prepare families and school officials for the problems that would emerge. The center's school-based team provided a variety of services to Columbine and other area schools, including outreach and collaboration. These services included meetings with school mental health staff and administration in order to set up programs, problem-solve, clarify needs, and provide education about the services of Jefferson Center. In addition, at one elementary and one middle school, weekly drop-in support services for students, parents, and other community members were made available.

SHOUTS, Columbine Connection's teen drop-in center, has served many youth in need of services. During the fall of 1999, 765 teens participated in activities there—an average of more than 25 teens per day.

About a month before school began, Jefferson Center began working with principals from area schools to determine the mental health needs of their particular school and what kind of skills they wanted in their Jefferson Center mental health counselor. There was also coordination with Victim Assistance and Columbine High School staff to provide support services to Columbine students during registration and freshman orientation.

Jefferson Center's school-based team provided 3–4 counselors every day during registration week at Columbine High School. During that time, some students required a variety of interventions or emotional support from counselors or victim's advocates, especially when touring the area close to where the library had been located.

Jefferson Center had nine school-based therapists in Columbine area schools. There were two full-time counselors at Columbine High School (although during the month of September as many as four counselors were there daily as dictated by need and the request of the school). The middle school and five feeder elementary schools each had one full-time counselor, and two nearby high schools shared a full-time counselor.

The demand for school-based services increased greatly following the start of school. Two months into the school year, therapists at Columbine High School had already seen 400 students and/or families. During the school year, Columbine-based therapists led four weekly drop-in groups, aptly named "Remembering, Recovering, Recapturing," which fostered healing from traumatic events. They also provided daily lunch "stress buster" groups to help students deal with day-to-day stresses and cope better at school. Supportive and consultative services were also available to staff on a daily basis.

During a test fire drill, a therapist witnessed how the shootings have impacted the victims. On hearing the fire alarm, two students hid under their desks while others sat frozen in their seats, unable to move even after the alarm was turned off. Also, 47 students developed severe shooting-related PTSD and/or depression and, as a result, required home-based schooling.

At the request of school administration and school mental health staff, Jefferson Center's elementary school–based staff offered a variety of services that ranged from coordinating violence prevention and tolerance programs to providing individual and family therapy. A needs assessment that was mailed to parents established that many individuals did require services. Of the parents who responded (half of those contacted), 75% identified a concern about their child.

In these elementary schools, concerns were voiced about various types of Columbine-related emotional problems in students. For example, one boy repetitively played out the shooting at school and home. In addition, symptoms of preexisting disorders were exacerbated. As a result of this upsurge in symptoms, most of the therapists had each already seen 20–30 students or families for therapy by October.

The counselor based at Ken Caryl Middle School, the feeder school for Columbine, was extremely busy seeing students and families directly impacted by the shootings and experiencing academic problems, depression, anxiety, and increased anger.

Psychiatrists in the community continued to offer their services to help those impacted by the shootings. The joint CPS/CCAPS task force collaborated with the Jefferson County School District to recruit psychiatrists to provide free consultation to teachers and other school officials at schools through the Jefferson County School District. In addition, the University of Colorado Department of Psychiatry recruited faculty to provide services to members of the Columbine community.

CURRENT ISSUES AND CHALLENGES

Development of a Screening Instrument

On December 1, 1999, a screening questionnaire was administered to students at Columbine High School. Its purpose was to identify students with 1) high levels of traumatic exposure and 2) current symptoms of disorders such as PTSD and depression. The screening instrument was developed by the University of Colorado Department of Psychiatry's task force on Columbine. Community input was solicited by having representatives from other agencies participate in the design of the instrument at the weekly meetings of the task force. Participants included individuals from the school district, state mental health, Jefferson Center, Victim Assistance, and other individuals with an interest in the project. Dr. Pynoos and his group at UCLA provided consultation on the development of this instrument. Parents of Columbine students were also allowed to review the instrument and provide feedback. The goal was to develop a screening device that would be comprehensive enough to elicit important data that would identify high-risk youth but yet not so long and intrusive that it would cause undue stress for already vulnerable youths. High-risk and symptomatic youths identified by the screening would then undergo more detailed assessments to determine the level and severity of their psychopathology in order to plan for their treatment.

Group and Individual Therapy

In addition to screening, a wide array of interventions was being offered during the school year at Columbine High School and other schools in the southern portion of the Jefferson County School District near Columbine High School. These services were provided by Jefferson Center, which employed therapists at Columbine and nearby schools. Previous research has shown that group therapy at school is the most effective and practical way to help traumatized youth after a disaster. The therapists were trained in methods of group treatment used by the UCLA Trauma Psychiatry Program in the Los Angeles schools (see Chapter 7, this volume).

Tensions in the Community

Although the community has done a remarkable job pulling together to help the victims, this kind of tragedy creates tensions that can be viewed as a manifestation of the stress response in victims and individuals in the larger community. Also, tensions will develop as a result of the legitimate, competing interests of different groups in the community following major disasters. What follows are some tensions that arose in the community after the Columbine tragedy.

Debate on Resource Allocation

There has been extensive debate about whether resources should be allocated to preventing teen violence or providing treatment for the victims. This debate was in part precipitated by the reality that there are never adequate resources to address all the psychiatric problems that arise after this type of disaster. Since the Columbine shootings, the community has shown a tremendous desire to develop efforts to prevent this type of violence. This is an understandable and legitimate goal, in part fueled by fear of recurrence. Initially, as a result, it seemed more difficult to get support for treating the mental health needs of the victims than for violence prevention.

Respect for Privacy Versus Media Coverage

There is a delicate balance between the need to respect the privacy of the victims and the need of society to learn from this tragedy through media coverage of the event and research into what happened. As was mentioned earlier, in the discussion of the development of an alliance between the school system and agencies charged with helping the victims, it has been and will continue to be a challenge to strike a balance that addresses these competing but equally legitimate interests. As the shock of Columbine begins to subside for the larger community, ongoing media coverage of the event can play a positive role in reminding people that the victims of this tragedy continue to need help in recovering from their traumatic experiences. Yet this very coverage runs the risk of exacerbating the victims' symptoms through traumatic reminders of what happened if the information is not presented in a careful and sensitive manner.

In addition, the media's and the nation's continuing interest in Columbine has at times infringed on students' privacy. For example, it has been reported that tourists, more than once, have visited Columbine High School since the shootings and asked students if they could have their pictures taken with them. Students have also been asked by the media to take video cameras into school. In addition, representatives of the media have followed students home. Because of this scrutiny, many students and teachers have stopped identifying themselves as being from Columbine when outside of school because they have not wanted to be asked about the tragedy. Of particular concern has been that the frequent, obsessive retelling, to the media, by students of their experience on the day of the shootings, without proper emotional support, has served to exacerbate their symptoms of PTSD.

Traumatic Reminders of the Shootings

A major impediment to the healing process has been the numerous traumatic reminders of the shootings. The return to school was very difficult for many students. Even though the library was walled off and its former entrance covered by a bank of lockers, no one forgot where it was. Its absence was a frequent reminder to students of the terrible events that occurred there.

FURTHER TRAGEDIES AND RETRAUMATIZATIONS

In October, two very disturbing events related to Columbine retraumatized much of the community. The day before the 6-month anniversary of the tragedy, a Columbine student was arrested for allegedly threatening to "finish the job" started by the shooters. Two days after this anniversary, tragically, the mother of one of the surviving shooting victims died from a self-inflicted gunshot wound.

The massive increase in distress in the Columbine community following these events is not surprising and serves to illustrate how vulnerable the victims are to symptom exacerbation with further traumatic reminders. In addition, the events themselves were traumatic and caused students and parents to fear that their school continues to be an unsafe place and that adults, because of their own psychological distress, are unable to provide emotional support to the students.

Throughout the remainder of the fall and winter, retraumatizing events continued. They included the publication by *Time* magazine of a graphic account of the tragedy, a threat made over the Internet to a Columbine student, the murder of two Columbine students at a nearby sandwich shop, the release of graphic tapes of the shootings by the Jefferson County Sheriff's department, and the suicide of a Columbine student. Each of these events was followed by significant increases in requests for services from Columbine Connections.

These ongoing events made it clear to even the most skeptical that many in the Columbine community were still suffering psychologically and would need help and support for a long time. The one positive outcome from these events was that many more patients and students began to seek professional help for psychological problems. In fact, not only was there a greater acceptance in the community of the need for such services, but parents began to demand that services be made available.

CONCLUSION

The Columbine High School shootings represent, without question, the largest psychiatric disaster to ever befall the Denver metropolitan area. What has been remarkable in the face of such a tragedy is the tremendous response of the community in addressing the mental health needs of those traumatized by this event. Thus far, there has been an excellent coming together of the agencies with the resources to identify, treat, and develop long-term interventions for those in need of services. A highly educated surrounding community, the involvement of numerous churches and community organizations, and the willingness of local citizens to organize and work hard to meet the needs of traumatized youths and families have enhanced the effectiveness of services.

A variety of intervention strategies have proven useful in meeting ongoing treatment needs. Many victims have received psychotherapy and medication for treatment of PTSD and depression. In addition, certain experiential interventions, such as relaxation and movement groups, have been very popular with Columbine students, including those who have refused all other types of treatment. EMDR (Eye Movement Desensitization Reprocessing), used as an adjunctive intervention, has been helpful in facilitating effective and efficient treatment.

Clinicians who provided Columbine-related treatment received considerable training from experts in trauma, much of it donated or provided at a reduced cost. Psychoeducation has also been a key component of successful intervention so far, with information related to the impact of trauma on academic achievement being particularly appreciated by parents and teachers.

Although many in the community are still experiencing serious effects of the trauma of April 20, 1999, much healing has gone on. The 1-year observance, on April 20, 2000, while it created anxieties and brought back difficult memories, was a peaceful and meaningful day for the community. Internal school commemoration, districtwide activities, and public community observances were thoughtfully planned by committees with broad representation, including victims, family members, school officials, and community representatives, with strong mental health representation. School-related accomplishments during the year included the first state football championship and prizes in band competition and debate. Sixteen students graduated with a 4.0 grade point average, one with a National Merit Scholarship, and 125 graduated with other types of scholarships.

If the success of the initial efforts can be maintained, there could be an opportunity to begin answering some important research questions posed by this event that affected primarily an older adolescent student population.

Among some of the many questions to be answered include the following:

- What is the incidence of PTSD, depression, and other psychopathology in youths with high levels of exposure to this type of trauma?
- Are there risk factors and protective factors that help predict the outcome in traumatized youth?
- What is the impact of exposure to media coverage on outcome in at-risk youths?
- What are the long-term effects of the traumatic event and aftermath on development and personality formation?
- What types of interventions are best in helping traumatized youths and adults after this type of school shooting?

The students at Columbine are beginning the transition to adulthood, and it is not known how this experience will affect their academic performance, ability to form intimate relationships, and adult functioning. Certainly an event of this type is capable of shaking a young person's confidence in the capacity of adult institutions to provide him or her with a safe, nurturing environment in which to grow and develop. More needs to be learned about how this type of event affects the trajectory of normal development, since significant functional impairment from a traumatic experience could have a pronounced effect on adolescents' preparation for college or vocational training and choice of an occupation.

For the Columbine community and the Denver metropolitan area, the challenge for the future is to continue to build the infrastructure to help those in need and to help prevent future tragedies of this kind. The success of such an effort will depend on the ability of the major players to harmoniously work together and to respect the vulnerability of a traumatized community that will need time to heal from its wounds.

REFERENCES

Pfefferbaum B, Nixon SJ, Krug RS, et al: Clinical needs assessment of middle and high school students following the 1995 Oklahoma City bombing. Am J Psychiatry 156:1067–1074, 1999

Pynoos RS, Goenjian AK, Steinberg AM: A public mental health approach to the postdisaster treatment of children and adolescents. Child Adolesc Clin N Am 7:195–210, 1998

8

Wounded Adolescence

*School-Based Group Psychotherapy
for Adolescents Who Sustained or
Witnessed Violent Injury*

CHRISTOPHER M. LAYNE, PH.D.
ROBERT S. PYNOOS, M.D., M.P.H.
JOSE CARDENAS, PSY.D.

In this chapter, we describe the design, implementation, and qualitative evaluation of a school-based pilot group psychotherapy program for adolescents who directly sustained violent injury or who witnessed the violent injury or death of a close friend or family member. *Wounded adolescence* refers to the profound developmental impact of violent traumatization among adolescents—an impact that extends beyond the diagnostic classification of posttraumatic stress disorder (PTSD) and related disorders (Pynoos et al. 1995). The adolescent group members in this pilot program were quite articulate about the significant developmentally linked disruptions that grew out of their violent exposures, including disturbances in peer relationships, in close friendships, and in motivation and aspirations for school and the future. Most notably, they described a disturbing restric-

The authors gratefully acknowledge support for this work from the Robert Ellis Simon Foundation, the Bing Fund, and the Irene Foundation for Mental Health.

tion in their capacity for intimacy in close relationships. Of concern, this restriction is occurring during a key developmental period—namely, transition to young adulthood.

The epidemiological literature on adolescent exposure to violence is just emerging (Bell et al. 1988; Boney-McCoy and Finkelhor 1995; Fitzpatrick and Boldizar 1993; Kilpatrick et al. 1995). Findings from one nationally representative survey indicate that U.S. youths are directly victimized at alarmingly high rates. Using a sample of 1,245 12- to 17-year-old adolescents, Kilpatrick et al. (1995) found that 26.7% reported no history of violence exposure, 48.1% reported exposure to violence via witnessing only, 2% reported having been physically assaulted only, and 23.1% reported having been physically assaulted *and* having witnessed the violent victimization of others. From this sample, Kilpatrick and his colleagues estimated that 15.8 million American adolescents have witnessed some form of violent assault.

On the basis of their results, Kilpatrick et al. (1995) estimate that 1.8 million U.S. adolescents have met the DSM-IV diagnostic criteria for PTSD (American Psychiatric Association 1994) at some point during their lifetime, and that 1.07 million experienced PTSD within the past 6 months. In addition, they reported that sexual assault, physical assault, and witnessing violence were each associated with past-year substance use, and that current PTSD increased the risk of substance abuse above that associated with victimization alone (Kilpatrick et al. 2000). Of special concern, Kilpatrick et al. found strong evidence of marked synergistic effects of both direct exposure to violence and witnessing of violence on rates of PTSD, illustrated by a lifetime PTSD prevalence rate of 0.6% for those reporting no exposure to violence, 7.7% for those reporting witnessing violence only, 12% for those reporting direct assault only, and 20.5% for those reporting both direct assault and witnessing violence. These findings underscore the importance of our selecting a pilot group of adolescents who had both sustained direct violent injury and witnessed the serious injury or death of a close friend or family member.

DESIGN OF THE THERAPEUTIC PROGRAM

The pilot program had two primary goals: 1) to develop a battery of instruments that could be used in a high school health clinic setting to screen students for exposure, distress, and developmental impact, to provide more in-depth evaluation of identified students, and to monitor course of recovery; and 2) to develop and pilot a structured yet flexible, time-limited, school-based group psychotherapy intervention for adolescent victims of violence that focuses on trauma and grief. Importantly, we developed procedures to assess serial traumatic and loss exposures. These procedures build on a pilot school-based group intervention program for elementary school students exposed to violence and traumatic loss (Murphy et al. 1998).

Each treatment session was designed to address the five therapeutic foci of the UCLA Trauma Psychiatry Program (Pynoos et al. 1998): 1) traumatic experiences and posttraumatic stress reactions, 2) trauma and loss reminders, 3) traumatic loss and complicated bereavement, 4) secondary stresses and adversities, and 5) developmental impact. We quickly learned that the group members had their own therapeutic priorities that needed to be respected, with much of their concern focused on key adolescent developmental issues. For example, we learned that the adolescents immediately focused on the physical scars of their injuries and accompanying physical disabilities, not only as prominent daily trauma reminders but also as factors that often led to disturbances in their peer relationships. In addition, we came to appreciate the developmental importance of what we refer to as "the existential dilemma," when, during a life-threatening violent episode, these adolescents struggled between self-preservation and wishing to aid a friend who was in extreme danger or seriously injured. This revealed itself to be a critical shared experience, the disclosure of which galvanized group cohesion.

SETTING AND RECRUITMENT OF GROUP MEMBERS

Members of the group were selected from a larger screening for community violence exposure and associated distress in a sample of urban high school students referred for mental health services at a school-based clinic (Layne 1996). The clinic provides a range of free medical and psychosocial services at a multiracial public high school in the greater Los Angeles area. The school is located in an area characterized by high levels of gang activity, other forms of community violence, and marked socioeconomic disadvantage. What is most disconcerting is that this pilot group was formed from a much larger group of students who had been shot, stabbed, or beaten with baseball bats.

From the larger student body screening, we learned that those who had been shot and/or witnessed the shooting injury or death of a friend had the highest mean PTSD scores, which fell within the severe or very severe range. We also discovered that few of the adolescents who had been shot had been either identified as possibly needing mental health services or, if identified, provided the services, despite the availability of counseling and medical services at the clinic. For example, one group participant worked as a volunteer assistant in the nurse's office. He was referred for assessment only after he overheard the nurse discussing the screening study and pulled up his trouser leg to reveal a bullet scar. When interviewed, this student recounted an extensive history of traumatic experiences (Table 8–1) and reported some of the most elevated symptom scores of any student in the larger screening study.

Six students (hereafter designated as Students A through F) were recruited from the screening on the basis of three selection criteria. First, each student reported that he or she recently had sustained and/or witnessed violent injury or had witnessed the violent death of a close friend or family member. Second, each student reported current moderate to severe levels of PTSD, with five of the six meeting the full DSM-IV diagnostic criteria for that disorder as determined by a systematic clinical interview. Third, each student appeared to be at high risk of developmental disturbance, as indicated by marked posttrauma disruptions in important peer and family relationships, decreased academic performance, and abandoned future aspirations. Students were recruited into the group after a pregroup individual clinical interview. Group sessions were co-conducted by the first author and the third author, who served as the clinic mental health director, with weekly consultation provided by the second author.

Screening and Assessment Instruments

Screening and assessment instruments included

1. Survey of Children's Exposure to Community Violence (J. E. Richters and W. Saltzman, "Survey of Children's Exposure to Community Violence: Child Report," Child and Adolescent Disorders Research, National Institute of Mental Health, Rockville, MD, unpublished measure, 1990)
2. Impact of Events Scale (Horowitz et al. 1979)
3. UCLA Grief Inventory (K. Nader, R. S. Pynoos, and C. Frederick, "UCLA Grief Screening Survey," University of California, Los Angeles, unpublished measure, 1990)
4. Center for Epidemiologic Studies Depression Scale for Children (Falstich et al. 1986; Weissman et al. 1980)

TABLE 8–1. Chronology of chronic trauma exposure: history of a 17-year-old participant in a school-based pilot group psychotherapy program

Age	Traumatic experience
Childhood	Learns that his grandmother, as a child, watched helplessly as her father was forcibly taken by Pancho Villa's men, hanged from a tree in front of the family home, and shot.
Childhood	Aunt dies in a drowning accident.
Childhood	Uncle accidentally drives off a cliff and is killed.
Childhood	Uncle is killed in an earthquake in Mexico.
12 years	Sees a woman's leg severed when she is hit by a car near his home.
13 years	Witnesses police confront, shoot, and kill an armed suspect, who dies on a neighbor's lawn.
14 years	Witnesses an attempted murder–suicide outside his school in which a man tries to run over his estranged wife with a truck and then gets out, picks up a large rock, and repeatedly bashes her and then himself in the face.[a]
15 years	Brother is imprisoned for 1 year for aggravated assault.
15 years	Witnesses an intoxicated girl being raped at a party.
16 years	Witnesses his friend being shot by gang members, who then shoot him in the leg; he is forced to abandon his injured friend to save his own life.[b]

[a]Experience identified by adolescent as the "most traumatic."
[b]Referent trauma.

5. Hopelessness Scale (Beck et al. 1974)
6. A pilot version of the UCLA Traumatic Expectations Scale (C. M. Layne and R. S. Pynoos, "Traumatic Expectations Scale," University of California, Los Angeles, unpublished measure, 1999)

Pregroup Clinical Interview

The pregroup clinical interview is a critical step between the screening of a general student population and appropriate assignment to the school-based group intervention. It provides a more in-depth clinical evaluation and facilitates transition into group treatment. The goals of the clinical interview are summarized as follows:

A. Prepare the group therapist by gathering information about the adolescent's trauma history, psychosocial functioning, and environment.
   1. Review conditions of voluntary participation and confidentiality.
   2. Jointly create a subjective narrative of the referent traumatic event that includes both objective (e.g., physical injury, duration, frequency, relationship to the perpetrator) and subjective features (e.g., perceived life threat, helplessness, horror).
   3. Systematically screen for other lifetime trauma. If more than one traumatic event is identified, rank the events according to the degree of subjective distress and adverse developmental impact.
   4. Assess attributions of meaning and associated emotions pertaining to the most traumatic experience (e.g., persistent feelings of guilt, rage, shame, and revenge; formation of traumatic expectations; loss of confidence in the social contract).
   5. Assess severity of trauma-related distress, including PTSD, grief, and depression; regulation of psychological and physiological reactivity to trauma and loss reminders; and degree of trauma-specific patterns of avoidance.
   6. Assess level of psychosocial functioning, giving special emphasis to signs of developmental disruption (e.g., disturbances in family and peer relationships, decreased academic functioning, lack or loss of future orientation).
   7. Assess psychosocial circumstances and resources. Focus especially on adversities and resources that may promote or exacerbate recovery efforts (e.g., family functioning, physical disabilities, peer stigmatization, current trauma and loss reminders).
   8. Assess risk for suicide, self-harm, or other high-risk behaviors.

B. Initiate a therapeutic alliance.
   1. Establish a compassionate, nonjudgmental therapeutic atmosphere in which youths can disclose their subjective experiences and distress
   2. Begin to construct a shared vocabulary that facilitates open communication and understanding concerning the most traumatic experience.
   3. Prepare the adolescent to explore the traumatic experience within the group.
   4. Call attention to the ongoing developmental impact of traumatic experiences.
   5. Provide a conceptual framework that helps the adolescent to organize his or her trauma-related experiences in a therapeutically meaningful manner.

C. Evaluate the appropriateness of the adolescent for group work.
   1. Evaluate personal issues and material that would make participation in the group more difficult for the adolescent and assist in selecting appropriate personal material to reveal.
   2. Assess the degree of similarity between the student's experiences and those of other candidate group members in order to enhance group cohesion and group processes (Cutrona and Russell 1990).

D. Prepare the adolescent to join the group.
   1. Convey basic psychoeducational information concerning the adverse effects—both symptomatic and developmental—of traumatic experiences.
   2. Validate and normalize the adolescent's distress reactions, adversities, and developmental disruption by portraying them as understandable, expectable, and commonly shared by other youths exposed to trauma.
   3. Provide direct feedback about the results of the assessment, including diagnostic status.
   4. If the adolescent does not appear to need therapeutic intervention, emphasize how well he or she is doing, praise adaptive coping, review the supportive resources he or she has available, and leave an open invitation to see you as needed.
   5. If the adolescent appears to need other forms of therapeutic intervention, make an appropriate referral and follow-up.
   6. If the youth is an appropriate candidate for group work, provide an incentive to participate in treatment by expressing therapeutic concern over a) significant distress symptoms, b) developmental

disruption, and c) potential future risks given the current developmental trajectory.

E. Secure the adolescent's commitment to join the group.

1. Increase motivation to participate in treatment by explaining how being with other trauma-exposed youths can help young people cope with the aftermath of trauma, including interpersonal difficulties, distress symptoms, and life adversities. Personalize the description by emphasizing the adolescent's particular problems.

2. Describe the group format, composition, schedule, setting, and rules of confidentiality.

3. Extend the invitation to participate in the group.

4. As needed, address resistance issues, including avoidance, denial, distrust, fear of stigmatization, familial opposition, and negative attitudes toward help seeking.

Several important clinical observations emerged from conducting the pregroup clinical interviews. First, most students' descriptions of their traumatic experiences were remarkably candid and detailed. For example, Student E, a 17-year-old female, disclosed the following highly traumatic event:

> I saw my boyfriend get shot two months ago. We were at my girlfriend's birthday party—I had talked him into going. We were dancing and I left for a minute. When I came back, my boyfriend was arguing with another boy who was from another gang. My girlfriend and me tried to get them to stop. They did, and shook hands, but I decided that we should leave anyway. I left to say goodbye to the hostess, and when I came back they were arguing again. His brother and me pushed him to the car. I was standing in front of him, saying "bye" to my friend and apologizing for the argument, when they started shooting. I felt him slump back and I knew he was shot. I pushed him into the car—he was lying sideways on the front seat and his feet were sticking out the door. I kneeled down on the passenger's side in front of him and tried to hold the door closed but I couldn't close it, so I tried to hold him there. There was blood everywhere. He got shot under the chin and it came out of the top of his head. His eyes were open but they were staring—he didn't react when I talked to him. I thought he was dead. We drove very fast to the hospital, but when his brother turned the corner I couldn't hold the door closed, and he fell out into the street and hit his head and scraped up his leg. I was crying and screaming. Some people at a parking lot helped us put him back in the car. At the hospital, they took him, but then the nurse tried to get me to go in too, because she saw that I had been shot in the shoulder—I didn't know it until then—but I wouldn't because I wanted to make sure they helped him first. I went in later and got treated, but I kept asking about him. They told me he was just hanging on and that they didn't

think he would make it. I was crying a lot. I was released from the hospital three hours later and went over to see my boyfriend—the priest was performing the sacrament for him. Then the police took me to the station, where I stayed awake until 7 o'clock in the morning, and they interviewed me. My boyfriend lived, but now he can't move his left side and he talks like a baby.

Second, students recounted multiple lifetime exposures to violence. As a result, we asked them to rank these experiences in terms of which were most upsetting. A number of the students identified an experience other than the referent trauma as their "most traumatic." Several students ranked an earlier incident of witnessing violence higher than the subsequent experience of being shot; these rankings appeared to be strongly weighted by the developmental impact of the event. For example, Student A described her experience of witnessing a gang rape at age 13 and its impact on her psychosexual development:

Some nights, I think about "doing it" with a guy. But sometimes what happens is it turns into the rape that I saw. The guy's face turns into the face of the guy who was on top of that girl. I remember how the guy was smiling in a mean way, and how the girl was helpless and crying and screaming and how disgusted she looked. Then I start feeling sick, like I don't want to have nothing to do with a guy.

She then described renouncing her previously cherished goals of romantic relationships and marriage and expressed a newly formed resolve to adopt several children and raise them on her own.

Third, students consistently focused not only on their actual traumatic experiences but also on painful subsequent disruptions to close personal relationships. Significantly, each of the six group participants was victimized in the presence of at least one friend or family member, and even when there was no death, the victimized adolescent described the loss of that relationship through estrangement.

Fourth, we learned the importance of identifying special circumstances that may lead a student to decline participation in the group. For example, one student faced the predicament of being held accountable by his deceased friend's parent because he was the driver of the car in which their son had been shot by another driver in an incident of "road rage." He described how the father of the deceased had flinched and shrunk backward when they met at the funeral. The youth was subsequently warned to stay away from the family. He stated, "I want to drop out of school and start working so I can be distracted, so I won't think about what happened. We're just here to work and suffer, like from death and diseases." In such a case, when there are recriminating charges of culpability, special additional individual assistance may be required before the youth participates in a group. In a second case, an adolescent girl declined participation because she feared that a rekindling of her distress over an earlier tragic event—the accidental death of a sibling—would, in turn, worsen her mother's unresolved grief. In this situation, it may be necessary to conduct a sensitive family intervention before the adolescent consents to group participation.

GROUP CONTENT AND PROCESS

The present intervention used a semistructured approach, with specific goals for each session. In what follows, we describe each of the six group sessions in terms of its goals and processes, placing special emphasis on significant themes that emerged during the session. It is important to note that these session-by-session processes reflect the group themes as they emerged and fluctuated across sessions.

Session 1

Goals

1. Introduce the purpose, format, and rules of the group.
2. Make introductions and welcome the students to the group.
3. Provide an opportunity to briefly recount one's referent traumatic experience within a supportive group context.
4. Model sympathetic listening, understanding, validation, and caring.
5. Build trust and group cohesion, and reduce perceptions of deviancy and estrangement, by emphasizing the similarities among group members' traumatic experiences and subsequent difficulties.
6. Establish group members as a new reference group with whom to make normative comparisons regarding trauma-related experiences and reactions.

Process

The therapists began the group by greeting the students, introducing themselves, and explaining the purpose of the group. Group rules were then discussed in detail. Particular emphasis was given to explaining the necessity of keeping confidentiality in order to allow group members to develop trust in each other and to have confidence that the group is a safe place to talk about experiences that have had a very powerful effect on their lives. Group members were then invited to introduce themselves and to describe, in as much detail as they felt comfortable, the experience they had come to work on in the group. The therapist who had conducted the pregroup interviews gently facilitated these narratives. Notably, several members began their narratives by showing their scars to the group, and then commented on how challenging it was to explain these scars to their friends and classmates. These narratives were received with respectful attention by the other group members, who made subdued, empathic exclamations of support and, occasionally, surprise. This emotional identification with the intensity and import of one another's experiences initiated empathic responses among group members.

As the narratives progressed, it became apparent that each group member had been victimized in the presence of at least one significant friend. Led by the therapists' identification of this common theme, the group spontaneously expanded its discussion to an animated exploration of trauma-related disruptions in the members' important relationships. For example, Student A described the loss of her best friend:

> My friend who got shot was really upset. Whenever I tried to talk to her, she got really mad. She would say, "You don't understand what I went through. You didn't get shot." I told her it wasn't my fault that she got shot, and that I was really sorry. I told her that she was too selfish, and that she didn't understand what I went through being there and seeing her get shot. But she kept getting angry at me, so I stopped caring. Now, we don't even talk to each other any more.

An additional insight into trauma-related developmental conflicts in romantic relationships was illustrated by Student E's disclosure about the social obligation to care for her physically disabled boyfriend: "I need to move on—I wanted to break up even before he got shot, but now I feel like I can't because he's hurt. His family thinks that I should be with him all the time."

Insight into the impact of trauma on family relationships was illustrated by Student B's disclosure, in which he described his feelings of guilt for hurting his family: "I was stupid to be in a gang, because that's why they shot me. When I was lying in the hospital and saw how scared and hurt my mom was, I realized what my being in the gang was doing to my family." Becoming teary-eyed, Student B then described how belittled and misunderstood he felt as his fellow gang members trivialized the most terrifying moment of his life:

> They came and visited me in the hospital, but they weren't serious, and they joked about what happened. My friend who was with me when I got shot, he liked to talk about it like it was an adventure. It made me mad, and I told him that I almost died and that he didn't understand. I told them I didn't want to be "in" anymore. I didn't see them after that.

This description contained the first display of intense emotion within the group and assisted in defining the therapeutic contract, which was interpreted to mean, "I'm in this group because I want what happened to me to be taken seriously."

These disclosures then prompted Student C to relate a previously undisclosed and highly personal experience:

> The day after I got shot, I was thinking about killing myself, because I couldn't take the pain. That's what happens when you've got no insurance to buy medicine. I was pounding the walls, it hurt so bad. I even crawled to the kitchen looking for a knife when my family wasn't home, but I couldn't find one that was sharp enough.

Student C's remarks served to introduce the question of whether the group could tolerate and address these "worst" kinds of feelings and actions. This disclosure, coupled with the group's empathic response, served to strengthen the therapeutic contract among group members.

Student C then described his estrangement from his friend, who at the time they both got shot was a "wanna be" gang member. After the shooting, his friend, who now limped, became more invested in gang affiliation. Student C commented, "They brainwashed him. I told him, 'You're dumb to be in a gang—there's no future in it.'" A brief, spontaneous discussion then ensued about gangs and the deception that occurs when new members are recruited without informing them of the accompanying danger.

To conclude the session, the therapists recapitulated its primary theme: the distressing loss of a close relationship. This theme was used to underscore the role of the group as a unique source of understanding and support, and to emphasize how the ordeal of their traumatic experiences had prepared them to understand and help each other.

Session 2

Goals

1. Use members' experiences of physical injury, pain, and residual scars as a metaphor for introducing the concepts of psychological injury, distress, and persistent symptoms.

2. Introduce a therapeutic framework for conceptualizing psychological distress symptoms, reactivity to trauma and loss reminders, and secondary adversities.
3. As appropriate, invite group members to briefly describe their personal experience and its impact on their lives.
4. Continue to construct, explore, and further elaborate the students' trauma narratives, while recognizing that this material may serve as trauma reminders to other group members.
5. Introduce needed social skills to contend with trauma-related interpersonal interactions and to enhance social support in the face of reminders.
6. Continue identifying common themes across the narratives to challenge perceptions of deviancy and isolation.

Process

The second session was characterized by greater disclosure and expressions of support. It began with the introduction of a new member, Student F, who had a prominent surgical scar from a near-fatal stab wound. In his introductory trauma narrative, Student F related how frightened he felt when the paramedics began administering intravenous fluids, because it signaled that he had lost much blood and might die. He then highlighted the role played by his ever-present scar as a trauma reminder: "The scar reminds me of what happened. When I look at myself in the mirror and see the scar, sometimes I can see the hand with the knife, and me putting up my hand to stop it but I can't, and then I see it go in, and then I feel really scared."

Following this theme, Student B then raised his shirt to reveal a prominent scar across his torso, resulting from the surgery in which his bullet-shattered kidney had been removed. He then related the subsequent adverse developmental impact of his physical disability: "I used to wear muscle shirts, but now I don't because of my scar. I used to play soccer, too. I wanted to play on our school team, but my doctor said I couldn't play any more because I have only one kidney and it might get damaged." Encouraged by the group leaders, Student C then described the considerable secondary medical and physical adversities he experienced after being shot. Following, Student A discussed the social stress and recurrence of symptoms generated by inquiries from others after she returned to school.

> As much as you try to take it off your mind, people keep on asking you about it. For a week afterwards, everyone asked me about it every day, all day long. It gets on your nerves. It brought back flashbacks. Flashbacks

would come with no warning—a picture would pop into my mind. I would see her face screaming, "Why me? Why me? I'm gonna die!" Once I ran out of class and went and talked to a counselor. I started to gain weight, too.

These descriptions highlighted the issue of trauma reminders and secondary adversities and their role in perpetuating distress. The group leaders first focused on the theme of developing social skills for communicating with peers in response to inquiries and for explaining their behavior in response to trauma reminders.

- "If people ask you about your scars, what do you tell them?"
- "If you don't want to talk to people about what happened, what do you say?"
- "When something reminds you about something bad that has happened, do you want other people to help you feel better? How do you tell them?"

A portion of the session was then dedicated to modeling social skills that allowed the group members to have a genuine, yet self-protective voice in personal communication about their traumatic experiences. The group leaders role-played responses that conveyed the essence of the group members' feelings about the experience and of its impact on their lives but that prevented the disclosure of distressing and graphic material that would distress both themselves and their listeners.

The concept of secondary adversities was then extended to a psychoeducational presentation on posttraumatic symptoms. The group leaders used physical injury, pain, and residual scars as metaphors to introduce the concepts of psychological injury, distress, and persistent PTSD symptoms. To increase the relevance and persuasiveness of the presentation, the group leaders presented each symptom in terms of the group members' personal experiences, and group members experiencing that symptom were invited to briefly describe its phenomenology and impact on their lives. Several members offered that the presence of gang members at school served as a constant and unavoidable trauma reminder. They also realized that one reason for their estrangement from friends who had been with them during the trauma was that each of them was serving as a trauma reminder to the other.

The session concluded with the therapist's recapitulation of the common theme of disruption in important relationships, praise for members' courageous disclosures, and reassurance that such sharing would help them regain the trust they had lost. In addition, the group members were invited to provide support to one another when experiencing reminders in order to reduce reactivity and to increase tolerance and regulation, especially in preparation for more in-depth exploration of their traumatic experiences.

Session 3

Goals

1. Co-construct and conduct a detailed exploration of the trauma narratives.
2. Focus on the worst moments of these experiences, with special attention given to conflicts over one's own actions and the actions of others.
3. When appropriate, point out links between traumatic experiences and posttrauma behavior, especially in regard to disrupted relationships and changes in goal orientation.
4. Continue identifying common themes across the narratives.

Process

Overall, the third session was marked by an increasing level of involvement. Members not only listened intently to each other's descriptions but began to more actively disclose their symptoms and to ask for clarifications. The therapists began the third session by inviting the members to tell their narratives with as much detail as they felt comfortable sharing, including what was happening both outside and inside of them. What followed was remarkable, both in its emotional intensity and in the courage displayed as members explored the most terrifying moments of their lives.

The first theme to emerge in the narratives involved an intense moment of decision between life and death. Students B and C, both of whom had been shot and believed that death was imminent, recounted a moment in which they contemplated whether to passively resign themselves to death or to summon a will to live that motivated an active response. Student B, who had been shot in the kidney by a rival gang, related two such moments with great intensity and attention to detail:

> I tried to get up but I couldn't. I yelled to my friend, "Come back!" I was on my hands and knees, crawling. Then I heard a dog barking, and I had heard that dogs bark when they sense death. I looked around to see if Death was coming—I thought he was like a person. I thought, "No! I don't want to die!" I thought that if he was coming for me, I should fool him about where I was at, so I crawled to a different place.

> Then the ambulance came. I heard the attendants guessing about if I was going to die or not, and I got really scared. In the ambulance, I could see a small light in my head, like a dot, and it was getting smaller, and I was afraid it would shrink to nothing and I would never see light again. So I fought to stay alive again.

Student C recounted a similar moment of decision while he was fleeing for his life: "After they shot me in the leg, I was just thinking of getting to my friend's house. I was limping and I thought I was gonna fall because I had no power in my leg. But I guess I thought about my life—I didn't want to die right there."

A second theme emerged from the narratives of students who had been exposed to a traumatic event in the company of another person. Each of these students reported being thrust into a deeply distressing existential dilemma: In the midst of their terror, confusion, vigilance to further harm, and helplessness, these members had been forced to make a split-second, irrevocable, and agonizing choice between self-preservation and seeking to protect and care for their companion. This dilemma was experienced both by students who were violently injured and by those who witnessed the injury of others but refrained from directly intervening because they feared for their own safety, because they perceived that they would be unable to effectively intercede, or because they were prevented from doing so by others.

Repercussions stemming from this existential dilemma appeared to have exerted a significant developmental impact on the lives of the group members. This impact was partly manifested in the form of alterations in their self-perceptions in terms of being courageous or cowardly, loyal or traitorous, and efficacious or helpless. Several students angrily disclosed that their companions had failed them; others expressed remorse that they had failed their companions. For example, Student C's account clearly portrayed the dilemma and its adverse impact on both his self-image and his friendship with a fellow victim. Wounded and instinctively running for his life, he recounted:

> As I was running, I heard them shoot my friend again, and I turned around to go pick him up. I thought he was dead, and I was just waiting for them to shoot me. I was thinking, "I ain't gonna go out like this and leave him." Then I see the guy point the gun at me again and shoot, but he missed. I could see the sparks hit the ground. After that I ran. I couldn't do nothing—I thought he was dead. I was thinking that I could be "down" for [loyal to] my friend, but then I thought, "There's a difference between 'down' and stupid, and stupid I ain't." When I saw my friend afterwards, he said, "Why'd you leave me there like that?" I told him,

"There was nothing I could do, except get killed myself—I thought you were dead." He was really pissed off at me and told me I was no friend of his.

Student F's narrative depicted a profound sense of betrayal and distrust stemming from his friend's decision to run away without warning him of an imminent attack:

> It hurts to trust people, like my friend who ran away and let me get stabbed. After that, he tried to talk to me, but I thought he was a liar, and we went our separate ways. I feel like he betrayed me. I haven't trusted anyone since.

A remarkable feature of the narrative construction process was the pivotal role of a therapeutic focus on the existential dilemma in breaching traumatic estrangement. More specifically, the mutual disclosure and exploration by group members of their common anguish over the dilemma, the meaning ascribed to their behavior and that of others, and its subsequent disruption to their close relationships drew out a new level of trust, intimacy, and self-acceptance among the members. These interactions set the stage for the use of cognitive restructuring methods to challenge attributions of culpability by portraying the dilemma as an agonizing predicament for which there was no satisfactory solution. Humor was used, as appropriate, to emphasize the irrational nature of attributions (e.g., assuming a grandiose personal responsibility for what occurred) and the grim absurdity of the alternatives available at the time. For example, in response to Student C's disclosure, the therapist stated: "How many people were shooting at you? Gang #1 shoots you and your friend, then Gang #2 hears the shooting and sees you limping away, so they figure it's you, and *they* start chasing you and shooting at you as well! Can we add anything else to this scene to make it even *more* dangerous and crazy? [the group laughs together]." The group then discussed what it is like to be in a life-threatening situation where there is "no good solution."

For other students who had voluntarily exposed themselves to great danger or endured great distress in order to assist another victim, the therapeutic goal was to clarify the temporary suppression of fear for oneself and to validate the risks taken. The therapists' remarks were directed at assisting students to rediscover the appropriate use of fear for themselves and to validate their own needs for comfort and assistance.

The existential dilemma served as a concluding metaphor for encouraging commitment to the group, where getting involved has required courage and a willingness to risk caring for each other.

Session 4

Goals

1. Continue co-constructing the traumatic narratives; extend the narrative construction process to traumatic experiences other than the referent trauma.
2. Continue to elucidate common themes; focus especially on the existential dilemma and the meaning attributed to human agency in violent injury and loss.
3. Explore the links between traumatic experiences and posttrauma behavior, including reactivity and avoidance, irritability and estrangement in family/peer relationships, and loss of academic motivation.
4. Encourage efforts to reduce traumatic avoidance and to improve skills to manage trauma and loss reminders.
5. Provide emotional relief for negative self-attributions and associated emotions, especially guilt and shame, through reframing members' traumatic predicaments.
6. Call attention to the resulting developmental disruption emerging within the life and evolving personality of the adolescent.

Process

A notable feature of Session 4 was the spontaneous expansion of group members' narratives to include previously undisclosed traumatic experiences—ones that primarily occurred earlier in adolescence. In addition, the members carried out these exercises with less therapeutic assistance than was previously needed. As is depicted in Student C's narrative of witnessing an attempted murder–suicide, the students demonstrated the ability to identify salient traumatogenic elements and to describe the existential dilemmas inherent in those experiences:

> I was coming home from school with my friend. We saw all this screaming and running across the street, and we ran to see. Someone told us that a man had hit a woman with his truck, and that she fell and he got out and grabbed a giant rock and threw it in her face. When I got there, I couldn't see her face because of all the blood that was running down. She was standing there and crying, and she was trying to find her son and she did, and she was running away with him, but at the same time she was trying to stop the man from killing himself. He was standing in the middle of the street, hitting himself in his face with the giant rock, trying to kill himself. After a while you couldn't see his face because it was covered with blood. And what upset me the most was that you could hear the crunching sounds from the bones in his face getting busted. My friend was crying,

just looking at him do that. And when I seen my friend cry, that's what got me scared, and I was shaking and felt like I wanted to throw up. And, because we were the only boys there, I felt I should have run and kicked him—tried to stop him from hitting himself—but I was too scared, because I thought he was on drugs and he would try to kill me. Then the teachers from the school came out and saw him and started crying, and then the police came and started hitting him in the legs with batons to make him stop so they could handcuff him. My aunt said later that the lady was divorcing the man and that's why he did that.

Therapist comments during the narratives were directed toward eliciting clarifying information, elucidating the dilemmas inherent in the traumatic situations, exploring the subjective meanings attributed to important aspects of the events, and identifying ongoing and future reminders. After the narratives were completed, the therapists identified common elements and themes across all the narratives to increase group cohesion and to elucidate the links between trauma-related experiences and reminders, avoidant behavior, and current relationship and motivational problems. Group members were then invited to share their reactions to these reflections and interpretations. One theme was a sense of heightened personal vulnerability. A second was a loss of faith in the social contract, and a third was the experienced historical discontinuity in the emerging personalities of the adolescents. After the identification and processing of these themes, illogical assumptions were identified and challenged. For example, Student A's narratives contained a recurrent pattern of traumatic death, with an implicit assumption that she was a "jinx" who brought death to those close to her:

It sounds like you decided that it was better to be lonely than to try again to be close to people. That way, you told yourself, they won't die, and you won't have to risk getting hurt again by losing someone else. Considering how bad being lonely makes you feel, that decision to be alone is a big sacrifice on your part. But it doesn't make a lot of sense to think that your uncle and your friend died simply because you cared for them. Your love isn't deadly or dangerous. You have known and cared about lots of people, including us in the group, and we haven't died! So you are clearly not the Angel of Death. Besides, think of the people whom you could be close to right now who are missing out on having a really good friend.

Other group members were invited, as appropriate, to provide corrective feedback and encouragement. Challenging these catastrophic assumptions initiated the important task of addressing trauma-related avoidance and introduced the aim of resuming interrupted developmental progression.

Session 5

Goals

1. Explore the developmental impact of traumatic experiences.
2. Facilitate restoration to a normative developmental trajectory in critical life domains.
3. Encourage and monitor the generalization of skills developed within the group to outside settings.
4. Introduce and explore termination issues.

Process

Session 5 began with descriptions of efforts to address interpersonal estrangements and to initiate or resume age-appropriate activities. The therapists focused on the developmental impact of the students' traumatic experiences by identifying and exploring the links between traumatic experiences and posttrauma behavior and life goals. Special attention was given to family relationships, peer relationships, and academic motivation. For example, Student B, who had made evident progress during the group, described how his increased appreciation for being alive had changed his relationship with a family member: "The other day I felt really happy to be alive, so I hugged my brother. He started telling me I was crazy. I told him that I was just happy to be alive." Later, in the fifth session, Student A reported that she had accepted a date from a boy she liked and expressed confidence that she would be able to accept dating invitations from other boys.

The group discussion then spontaneously progressed to an exploration of issues of ambition, motivation, and impediments to pursuing life goals. Several members described feeling derailed from actively taking charge of their lives and plans for the future. Student E disclosed that she had lost her motivation for doing well in school and for attending college, and expressed the fear it might not return. The therapeutic response was to highlight the courage and commitment that Student E had shown within the group and to garner the group's expressions of confidence that Student E could do the same with respect to the challenge of higher education. Thereafter, the session was devoted to problem-solving obstacles to pursuing life goals. The concluding portion of the session was devoted to exploring termination issues. Topics included concerns about having come to rely on the group's support, and concerns about being able to find other sources of support after the group ended.

Session 6

Goals

1. Continue to explore the developmental impact of traumatic experiences, placing increased emphasis on motivation, ambition, future expectations, and planning.
2. Continue to monitor and encourage the generalization of skills outside the group.
3. Review the group experience, emphasizing members' progress to foster reflection on treatment gains and to increase perceptions of efficacy in realizing personal goals.
4. Process termination issues, emphasizing the contrast between voluntary and traumatic separations.
5. Formally evaluate the group by essay and questionnaire.

Process

Session 6 was marked by the shift of therapeutic focus away from the disruption of peer relationships to issues concerning future ambitions, plans, and motivation. After reminding the group that this was their last session, the leaders then reviewed the various ways in which members' development had been derailed. They then contrasted these with a review of each member's progress since joining the group. These commentaries focused to some extent on symptom reduction, but also, to a greater extent, on gains in the ability to trust, initiation of age-appropriate activities, and investment in interpersonal relationships. With moderate therapist direction, each group member then commented on his or her experience as a group member and reflected on the progress he or she had made since joining the group. Most students expressed surprise, in retrospect, at realizing how deeply their adolescence had been wounded by these experiences. They also remarked on how important it had been to recover from their most distressing traumatic reactions in order to regain a sense of self-efficacy and better emotional regulation. They also noted that the therapeutic experience of the group served to enhance their future orientation. For example, Student C commented,

> In the group, the violence has happened to everybody. You hear what happened to other people and how they are dealing with it and recovering from it, and I felt like I can do it, too. I hear how they have plans for the future and what they want to become, and I want to do the same things. The group helped a lot—I'm not going to let getting shot stop me—it's not going to hold me back.

The group then problem-solved by projecting into the future their management of traumatic reminders, especially moments of perceived vulnerability, and coping with future life stresses.

Last, the group participated in a termination exercise that involved sharing what the group experience meant to them. The members were assisted in differentiating this termination from the acute interpersonal estrangement and experience of loss that occurred after their trauma. They were also supported in their interests to become involved in peer mentorships at their high school and to help refer other students who they thought might benefit from a similar intervention. Several members expressed interest in organizing peer groups to address the wanton violence in their community and school environment. Sufficient time was left at the end of the session to ensure a proper leave-taking, with each member relating his or her plans for the summer and following year, and offering expressions of good will toward each other.

CONCLUSION

From postgroup evaluative essays, self-report measures, and a 13-month follow-up interview, we found that significant progress was made by group members in achieving the therapeutic goals. For five group members, there was a moderate to dramatic reduction in PTSD, hopelessness, and depression. One student who experienced an intervening violent trauma during the year postgroup reported significant new-onset PTSD symptoms. The essays were poignant in their descriptions of the importance of the group to recovering their adolescence and overcoming traumatic avoidance, which had so perniciously undermined their expected developmental achievements. The essays also revealed the importance of the group modality in addressing trauma recovery among adolescents, especially in terms of recovering from interpersonal estrangement and feelings of being isolated, abnormal, and frozen in time. The 13-month follow-up served to provide some perspective on the recovery of aspirations and future planning. The students reiterated how powerful the role of the group had been in helping them to restore their developmental progression. Three of the members had recovered their prior academic aspirations and regained their previous levels of academic functioning, with resumed plans after graduation to attend community college. Two students had participated in student events aimed at violence prevention, in which they spoke about the impact of violence on adolescents' lives.

This pilot work demonstrates the feasibility of school-based screening and intervention, even for the most extremely and acutely traumatized adolescents. As we have previously argued, the school is an especially appropriate and effective site to deliver mental health services related to these types of trauma and loss (Pynoos et al. 1998). Expanding on this pilot work, we have developed a more extended, structured, manualized group intervention for adolescents that focuses on trauma and grief. The intervention includes specific instruments designed to assess and monitor recovery along the five dimensions of the treatment foci. We previously reported that intervention aimed at these foci can produce treatment gains that are sustained over a considerable time period (Goenjian et al. 1997). The UCLA Trauma Psychiatry Program is currently field testing this extended treatment protocol among urban youth in high schools in the Los Angeles region and among war-traumatized youth in Bosnia–Herzegovina. A rigorous evaluation of the efficacy of these programs is planned for the 2000–2001 school year. As society seeks to stem the epidemic of violence among our youth, we hope this chapter will increase attention to the urgent need of providing for the mental health needs of the many thousands of young people whose adolescence has been wounded by violence.

REFERENCES

American Psychiatric Association: Diagnostic and Statistical Manual of Mental Disorders, 4th Edition. Washington, DC, American Psychiatric Association, 1994

Beck AT, Weissman A, Lester D, et al: The measurement of pessimism: the hopelessness scale. J Consult Clin Psychol 42:861–865, 1974

Bell CC, Hildreth CJ, Jenkins EJ, et al: The need for victimization screening in a poor outpatient medical population. J Natl Med Assoc 80:853–860, 1988

Boney-McCoy S, Finkelhor D: Psychosocial sequelae of violent victimization in a national youth sample. J Consult Clin Psychol 63:726–736, 1995

Cutrona CE, Russell DW. Type of social support and specific stress: toward a theory of optimal matching, in Social Support: An Interactional Perspective. Edited by Sarason BR, Sarason IG, Pierce R. New York, Wiley, 1990, pp 319–366

Falstich ME, Carey MP, Ruggiero L, et al: Assessment of depression in childhood and adolescence: an evaluation of the Center for Epidemiologic Studies Depression Scale for Children (CES-DC). Am J Psychiatry 143:1024–1027, 1986

Fitzpatrick KM, Boldizar JP: The prevalence and consequences of exposure to violence among African-American youth. J Am Acad Child Adolesc Psychiatry 32:424–430, 1993

Goenjian AK, Pynoos RS, Karayan I, et al: Outcome of psychotherapy among pre-adolescents after the 1988 earthquake in Armenia. Am J Psychiatry 154:536–542, 1997

Horowitz MJ, Wilner N, Alvarez W: Impact of Event Scale: a measure of subjective stress. Psychosom Med 41:209–218, 1979

Kilpatrick DG, Saunders BE, Best CL, et al: Violence, PTSD, and substance abuse: national survey of adolescents results. Poster presented at Traumatic Stress Studies, Boston, MA, October 1995

Kilpatrick DG, Acierno R, Saunders B, et al: Risk factors for adolescence substance abuse and dependence: data from a national sample. J Consult Clin Psychol 68:19–30, 2000

Layne CM: Effects of community violence on minority high school students. Unpublished doctoral dissertation, University of California, Los Angeles, 1996

Murphy L, Pynoos RS, James CB: The trauma/grief focused group psychotherapy module of an elementary school–based violence prevention/intervention program, in Children, Youth and Violence: Searching for Solutions. Edited by Osofsky J. New York, Guilford, 1998, pp 223–255

Pynoos RS, Steinberg AM, Wraith R: A developmental model of childhood traumatic stress, in Manual of Developmental Psychopathology. Edited by Cichetti D, Cohen DJ. New York, Wiley, 1995, pp 72–93

Pynoos RS, Goenjian AK, Steinberg AM: A public mental health approach to the post disaster treatment of children and adolescents. Psychiatr Clin North Am 7:195–210, 1998

Weissman MM, Orvaschel H, Padian N: Children's symptom and social functioning self-report scales: comparison of mothers' and children's reports. J Nerv Ment Dis 168:736–740, 1980

III

LEGAL ASPECTS

9

Duty to Foresee, Forewarn, and Protect Against Violent Behavior

A Plaintiff Attorney's Perspective

MICHAEL BREEN, J.D.

America is unsurpassed as the most litigious culture in the history of humankind. Although Americans abhor what they perceive to be a climate of runaway lawsuits, when personally aggrieved they are insistent on availing themselves of the civil justice system with unparalleled aplomb. Regardless of what anyone's personal convictions or opinions about the matter may be, every clinician, in conducting his or her professional affairs, must be cognizant of how deeply legal accountability and its consequent financial implications are embedded in American society.

The last 5 years alone have given rise to monumental liability claims heretofore considered legally untenable. Payments to claimants, including governmental authorities, have run into the billions. The tobacco industry, long thought to be invincible in the courtroom, is but the latest defendant to succumb to the siege of tort jurisprudence. It should come as no surprise, therefore, that principles of tort liability are being vigorously applied in lawsuits that have been filed in the wake of the epidemic of secondary school shootings.

Such lawsuits are the natural evolution of liability theories that are well established in the law but of relatively recent moment in terms of practical application in the courtroom. These types of cases, called *third-party liability actions*, are brought by the victims of violence against persons said to have actual or constructive knowledge of a perpetrator's violence. The person with foreknowledge is considered the first party, the perpetrator the second party, and the victim the third party. Financial liability attaches as between the first and third parties if the first party fails to reasonably act on threats made by the second party.

The implications for mental health care professionals are considerable, because they will be among the primary courtroom targets when the perpetrator has a history of mental health treatment. Because of these professionals' expertise in the pathology of mental disorders, parties who bring lawsuits (hereinafter plaintiffs) will quickly claim that the care provider should have recognized and acted on pre-incident conduct predictive of violence. Because school violence is so emotionally volatile to the public, even an unmeritorious claim against a clinician can be ruinous.

That we have an epidemic of school murders and aggravated assaults should come as no surprise. Studies of recent origin describe a staggering number of assaults, rapes, murders, and drug-related crimes, not to mention a pervasive culture of gang organization and membership (The Annie E. Casey Foundation 1994; National Center for Educational Statistics 1998). School massacres should be seen as the inevitable fruit of rampant juvenile crime and not as some spontaneous and unexplained phenomena.

The commonplace nature of school crime has significant implications in the legal arena. The more widespread the problem, the more readily courts will impute knowledge or notice to all who have contact with perpetrators, including behavioral science professionals, because heightened awareness of the pervasiveness of violent conduct equates with the increased foreseeability of criminal conduct. The failure to protect against criminal conduct will likely result in a viable liability claim against the professional.

In this chapter, I offer a plaintiff's attorney's perspective of the legal consequences of the failure to foresee and forewarn of violent behavior. The chapter begins with a discussion of general legal duties, including the concept of foreseeability. I then describe a hypothetical yet realistic case against a clinician. The chapter concludes with suggestions about minimizing exposure to the legal claims that will inevitably follow in the aftermath of violence. The emphasis, therefore, will be on the practical and not the academic.

A LIABILITY PRIMER

A *tort* is a wrong committed by someone who owes a legal duty of care to another and breaches that duty. The word itself is an Old French derivative from the Latin *tortus*, meaning twisted or wrung. If a recognized duty of care is breached, then the at-fault party is liable for money damages. As applied to the field of medicine, if a doctor fails to observe the standard of care for a patient and harm follows, then the doctor is liable.

Historically, lawsuits have been allowed only for breaches of specifically recognized duties such as the negligent operation of a motor vehicle or a deviation from a medical standard of care. However, the last 20 years have seen the development of a broad legal doctrine called the *universal duty of care*. It simply states that "every person owes a duty to every other person to exercise ordinary care in his activities to prevent foreseeable injury" (*Grayson Fraternal Order of Eagles, Aerie No. 3738, Inc. v. Claywell* 1987).

This concept is an acknowledgment of the extraordinary dynamic of human interactions. Relationships between people have become especially complex, and the opportunity for harm has increased correspondingly. Rather than fashioning a Byzantine set of liability rules that are case-specific, courts are electing to rely on a single rule echoed in the medical profession: do no harm unto others. In the context of juvenile and other violent events, the universal duty of care opens new vistas for professional negligence claims.

The law has traditionally been reluctant to impose liability on first parties for second-party conduct. Generally speaking, no one owes any legal duty to prevent someone from harming himself or another. A citizen is perfectly free to sit on a pier, smoke a cigar, and watch another drown in the middle of the lake so long as the viewer did not put the drowning person in peril in the first place (Restatement [Second] of Torts 1965). Similarly, the law historically has been reluctant to hold a person accountable for the criminal conduct of another.

Moreover, third-party liability cases involve difficult issues of foreseeability. Before liability may attach, the actor must be able to reasonably anticipate that harm will follow the conduct in question. For example, how can a clinician be legally liable for failing to warn the victim of a crime when clinical studies demonstrate a notorious unpredictability as between the threat and actuality (Roth and Meisel 1977)? By definition, it would seem to be unreasonable to require a clinician to foresee what is clinically unpredictable.

However, third-party liability has been gaining momentum coincidental to the advent of the universal duty of care. In *Tarasoff v. Regents of the University of California* (1976), a case well known to the mental health community, the California Supreme Court found a duty of care owed by the criminal's therapist to the subject of the criminal's death threats (see Chapter 5, this volume). Specifically, the *Tarasoff* court held:

> When a therapist determines or pursuant to the standards of his profession should determine that his patient presents a serious danger of violence to another[,] he incurs an obligation to use reasonable care to protect the intended victim against such danger. The discharge of this duty may require the therapist to take one or more of various steps depending upon the nature of the case. Thus it may call for him to warn the intended victim or others likely to apprise the victim of the danger to notify the police or to take whatever other steps are reasonably necessary under the circumstances.

Because this is very strong stuff, it is worthwhile to reflect on the practical aspects of *Tarasoff*. *Tarasoff* is a true third-party liability case: it recognizes a specific duty to prevent harm owed to a person other than the patient. *Tarasoff* has been widely reported in the literature as a case that creates a duty to warn the target of the threats (Melonas and Hinton 1998; Roth and Meisel 1977). Although true, this characterization is a gross understatement of *Tarasoff*'s holding. *Tarasoff* states that the clinician must take *whatever* steps are reasonable under the circumstances to *protect*, not just *warn*, the victim. Therefore, a warning may not be enough to discharge the legal duties owed the victim. Indeed, the therapist in *Tarasoff* sought commitment and warned law enforcement of the threat but did not warn the victim.

Reasonableness of conduct, therefore, is fact- and case-specific and will not be evaluated by the courts in a mechanical fashion; liability will follow if it is proven that a warning or other action was insufficient. Moreover, actual knowledge of a threat is not required. If the law deems that the reasonable therapist *should have known* about a threat, notice and knowledge will be imputed and liability will follow.

The *Tarasoff* court also considered many of the objections to disclosure raised by the mental health community. Among those were the low incidence of actual commission of the threatened crime, the unpredictability of violent behavior, and the importance of patient confidentiality. The court found that the societal interest in the prevention of harm outweighed these considerations and that disclosure was a small price to pay for public safety.

Tarasoff has also been interpreted as meaning that a clinician has a duty to act only when a specifically identifiable threat has been made against a specifically identifiable victim. This interpretation is consistent with the concept of foreseeability; vague or generalized threats are insufficient to impose an obligation to prevent harm. However, this should be of little comfort to the clinician. Tort liability is dynamic and evolutionary; it is not difficult to anticipate the judicial expansion of clinical duties to third parties. The spadework for this has already been done. A leading legal treatise recognizes a broad duty to refrain from conduct that creates "an unreasonable risk of harm to another through the conduct of the other or a third person . . ." (Restatement [Second] of Torts §302B). This generalized expression of the duty of universal care is an invitation to the plaintiff's attorney to broaden the *Tarasoff* rule.

A NOT-SO-HYPOTHETICAL CASE AGAINST THE MENTAL HEALTH CLINICIAN

By now it should be apparent that the legal system places the mental health clinician in the liability headlights. The clinician is in an exquisite medico-legal dilemma. On the one hand, the clinician has an ethical responsibility to put the interests of the patient at the forefront. A bedrock principle of any successful treatment is confidentiality, and any breach of that confidentiality may undermine the therapy (American Psychiatric Association 1998). Even the mere disclosure of the physician-patient relationship is considered extremely sensitive. On the other hand, the clinician has a legal duty to protect third persons from aggressive patients. The universal duty of care is the golden rule of liability law, and the law trumps psychotherapeutic principle. The clinician, therefore, has coexisting obligations to the patient and the putative victim; the conflicts between these two duties can lead the clinician to make bad choices about to whom allegiance is owed.

Herein lie the seeds of exploitation in the litigation setting. Clinicians have been extensively trained in recognizing the value of the therapeutic relationship but have little concern with their duty to the public. The courtroom argument will be made that clinicians have a "patient obsession disorder" and rarely look beyond their immediate relationship with the patient to the larger interests of the common good.

The psychiatric literature reflects this preoccupation with the patient. Authors have decried how "[t]he psychiatrist's social control functions are expanded at the expense of therapy" (Roth and Meisel 1977, p. 509). Some astounding practice recommendations also have been made for the sake of preserving the therapist-patient relationship. For example, it has been suggested that because actual violence is rare, "the psychiatrist may prefer to rely on the odds and to hope for the best, rather than warning a potential victim or attempting to hospitalize the patient involuntarily" (Roth and Meisel 1977, p. 511).

Moreover, a major study on threat management that analyzed post-*Tarasoff* notifications found that therapists rarely did anything to protect others (McNeil et al. 1998). The authors of this study also concluded that therapists were probably ignoring the law, even though the massive post-*Tarasoff* intrusion on the confidentiality of private practice feared by many had not materialized.

Even the American Psychiatric Association's own annotations to *The Principles of Medical Ethics* can be characterized as wanting (American Psychiatric Association 1981, 1998). The annotations seem obsessed with the propriety of sexual relationships with patients as opposed to anything else. Paragraph 8 of Section 4 contains a modest authorization to reveal confidences when the risk of danger is deemed to be significant. However, the import of Paragraph 8 is watered down in Paragraph 9, in which it is stated that even within the framework of the law, all doubt is resolved in favor of the patient. Interestingly, the authorization for the disclosure of confidences appears under the principle that deals with patient confidentiality and not in Section 3, which addresses respect for the law.

The principles are not proactive and contain no affirmative statements about the societal obligation to disclose and prevent patient violence. Indeed, the body of psychiatric literature itself is largely silent about therapists' duties when a patient is putatively violent. No guidelines, committees, or substantial research has addressed the burgeoning threat of third-party violence committed by patients, even though the *Tarasoff* ruling occurred more than 20 years ago. What can be inferred, therefore, about the psychiatric community's attitude toward public safety? Where do its loyalties lie?

Given this setting, let us construct a realistic hypothetical that results in a lawsuit against a psychotherapist:

> A 14-year-old white male from an upper-middle-class family has been in therapy for 6 months. The patient has an IQ of 120, performs sporadically in school, and describes feelings of rejection by his peers. The diagnoses of dysthymic disorder and schizotypal personality disorder have been made.
>
> During therapy, the patient reveals that he avidly views pornographic and occult materials and reads and writes stories that deal with graphic death and violence, including stories in which the patient murders others. He denies any delusional thinking. The patient ultimately tells his thera-

pist that he is considering shooting his classmates at school. The therapist discourages the patient from doing so, and the patient agrees. The therapist tells no one.

Within weeks the patient commits a multiple homicide at school. The parents of the dead children sue the psychotherapist in a highly publicized lawsuit, claiming that the therapist neglected his *Tarasoff* duties.

The first thing any seasoned plaintiff's attorney would do is hire a forensic psychiatrist as an expert witness. They are easy to find, and legal periodicals are full of advertisements for their services. Whether we like it or not, the forensic psychiatrist is a legally acceptable hired gun who will be used to prove negligence—namely, that the therapist knew or *should have known* of the serious potential for violence and did not discharge his or her *Tarasoff* duties. Remember, *Tarasoff* does not require actual knowledge of the threat; if the therapist unreasonably fails to perceive a serious threat, then knowledge will be imputed.

Naturally, the therapist will claim that none of the behavior shown by the juvenile patient was reasonably predictive of murder. After all, violent behavior is notoriously unpredictable, and juvenile homicide is extremely rare. The recent school shootings are an unprecedented psychiatric phenomenon and atypical as to juvenile homicides heretofore described in the literature (Benedek and Cornell 1989). Therefore, the therapist could not have anticipated the shootings in question, and patient treatment was best served with confidentiality. Further, an agreement with a patient not to commit violence is an accepted practice, and, after all, the shooter was just a child and not to be taken seriously.

The plaintiff will argue that the threat to commit murder was plain enough and that the therapist's *Tarasoff* duties were obvious. However, the plaintiff's attorney and the forensic psychiatrist will also comb the patient's history and the relevant professional literature for evidence that can be used to aggravate the liability picture.

The therapist's own background will also be probed for qualifications, other litigation, and disciplinary action. Is the therapist a patient? Was the therapist ever a patient as part of his training? If so, what medications, if any, were prescribed? Are medications being taken now? What does the *Physicians' Desk Reference* say about the effects of those medications? Was the therapist's judgment clouded by them? What guidelines did the therapist consider in making the decision not to tell anyone about the juvenile's threat? And so on.

Authoritative psychiatric and psychological literature also can be effectively used by the plaintiff's attorney. For example, DSM-IV (American Psychiatric Association 1994) states that patients with schizotypal personality disorder may experience transient psychotic episodes that can last for hours. It also states that "[i]n some cases, clinically significant psychotic symptoms may develop that meet criteria for Brief Psychotic Disorder, Schizophreniform Disorder, Delusional Disorder, or Schizophrenia" (p. 642). Persons diagnosed with dysthymic disorder feel inadequate and have subjective feelings of irritability and anger. Major depressive episodes are likely to follow.

Moreover, in this hypothetical case, the patient actually communicated a threat against a readily identifiable target (i.e., his classmates). He is preoccupied with violent and pornographic imagery and is vicariously living out his violent tendencies by writing gruesome stories. Given this history and the recognized potential for serious psychopathologies to develop, what right-minded therapist would not communicate the threat to the authorities and school officials? Why not play it safe and warn law enforcement and the victim? Why not commit the patient?

That is what the forensic psychiatrist and the plaintiff's attorney will say to a jury in a community that has lived in the emotionally charged aftermath of the murders. Violence in school hallways, striking at the very last bastion of perceived safety in a society plagued by violence, is intrinsically revolting to our culture. How is a jury going to feel about the therapist who could have prevented it all with a few phone calls but opted in favor of patient confidentiality?

But it does not end here. The clever plaintiff's attorney will turn the case into an indictment of the entire profession. The facts are compelling. It has been more than 20 years since the *Tarasoff* ruling, but the mental health community has done nothing to address a genuine threat to public safety. The plaintiff's attorney will argue to the jury that the therapist has access to something few people ever do: the ability to detect and prevent violence. But, ladies and gentlemen of the jury, that is not important to psychiatrists, psychologists, and other mental health clinicians. They are more worried about their patient. Their own peer-reviewed literature says that it is all right to roll the dice and take chances. In an article in a prestigious journal (Roth and Meisel 1977), the authors noted with approval an actual instance in which an agitated drug-addicted individual showed up at a clinic with a gun threatening to kill. The staff got the gun away from him. And what did they do? They took the bullets out of the gun and gave it back to him! What were they thinking? That they are smarter than the rest of us? To make matters worse, psychiatric studies have shown that disclosing patient threats does nothing to undermine therapy, but therapists are still ignoring their *Tarasoff* duties (McNeil et al. 1998). Who do they really care about? What do they really care about?

What has the profession done to address the problem? Where are the assessment criteria? Where are the disclosure guidelines? Where are the committees to address this terrible problem? Why hasn't the profession bothered to change its ethical principles to address the epidemic of violence in our country?

Mental health professionals, the plaintiff's attorney continues, have a pathological problem with gambling. They want to plays craps with people's lives. They are obsessed with patient confidentiality and have forgotten about the rest of us. Well guess what? They came up snake eyes this time. People have died and will die because of this attitude unless you do something. Ladies and gentlemen of the jury, you are here to cure them of this affliction and tell the psychiatrists, psychologists, and other mental health clinicians to heal themselves, and you do that by awarding punitive damages.

This is the stuff of which ruinous headline verdicts are made. And it is a realistic version of how a *Tarasoff* case would be made to a jury, since it is a common and effective tactic for attorneys to make the case larger than the immediate parties.

SUGGESTIONS ON HOW TO DISCHARGE TARASOFF DUTIES

So wherein lies the middle ground? Can mental health clinicians effectively treat patients and meet their duties to the public? The answer must be yes.

By demanding that the clinician protect third persons, all *Tarasoff* really asks for is meaningful action by the clinician that draws on all the resources and skills of his or her profession, as well as good judgment. Absolute prevention of the crime itself by the clinician is not required, and the law recognizes this. Many states have enacted statutes that immunize a clinician from liability if law enforcement is notified or the patient is committed (see, e.g., Kentucky Revised Statutes §202A.400 [1986]). Consequently, the duty to protect may often be fulfilled by the therapist's notifying those who have the wherewithal to meet the threat and warning those who may be in danger. But exigent circumstances may require more, such as commitment, as an adequate measure of protection.

However, the most serious problem facing mental health professionals is the absence of any clear standards for dealing with a *Tarasoff* threat—a somewhat disquieting fact considering the abundance of diagnostic criteria for psychopathologies. This lack of clear standards makes little sense from a legal perspective. To prove liability in a *Tarasoff* situation, the plaintiff must prove a deviation from the applicable standard of care. The law prescribes no such standard; it only articulates the duty of care. Instead, the formulation of the standard of care is reserved to those best skilled to establish it: the mental health professionals themselves. If the profession establishes a standard of care that is met by a clinician, there can be no liability. Establishing such a standard is infinitely preferable to having the plaintiff's forensic expert tell the jury his or her version of the standard, which, of course, is tailor-made for the plaintiff's theory of liability. This opportunity should not go unheeded, since it allows the profession to establish realistic ground rules and avoid much of the fluidity of a creative plaintiff's attorney.

What follows are some suggestions for mental health clinicians faced with a *Tarasoff* problem:

- **Make disclosure a part of the contract with the patient.** Doing so eliminates many medicolegal considerations that may inhibit action on a threat. A responsible patient genuinely interested in improvement may not like such an arrangement, but he or she will respect disclosure (see Chapter 5, this volume). If the patient does not respect the therapist's duty to disclose, how can the therapist have a meaningful treatment relationship in the first place? Have a written contract to memorialize this, and give the patient a copy.
- **Consult with another mental health clinician.** A course of action confirmed by another qualified clinician shows reasonableness and concern. Consider a referral for a second opinion.
- **Establish a committee in your hospital, clinic, or local medical association available on an emergency basis to evaluate patient threats.** As with consultation with another clinician, if a course of action is approved by a committee, the clinician has an excellent basis for claiming that he or she acted reasonably. It may make sense to make the committee interdisciplinary; such an approach can inject other perspectives into the matter and obviate charges of bias or partiality.
- **Forget about playing the odds; the law won't let you get away with it.**
- **Forget about insisting that the patient rid himself or herself of weapons.** While it may sometimes make sense clinically, a juror will not understand how a clinician believes that he or she might be able to talk an aggressor out of a possessing a weapon or of committing a violent act.
- **Maintain documented contacts with the patient.** The advent of managed care has sometimes resulted in an attenuated relationship with the

patient. Some psychiatrists may not be the primary therapist, engaging instead in "medication management" in conjunction with another therapist who sees the patient the most. Such an arrangement may result in the unwitting exposure of the psychiatrist to *Tarasoff* liability. If the primary therapist neglects his or her *Tarasoff* obligations, the managing psychiatrist may be an inviting target for a charge that, had more time been spent with the patient, the danger signs would have been detected and appropriate actions would have been taken. Regular contacts with the patient may help prevent this situation.

- **Be an aggressive risk manager, especially with juvenile threats of violence.** Juvenile threats often are serious and should not be taken lightly (Melonas and Hinton 1998). In a country that has been traumatized by the epidemic of school shootings, a jury will have no trouble punishing the clinician who dismisses adolescent threats as incredible. Also, be alert for a history indicative of violence. Patients with a history of noncompliance, substance abuse, antisocial behavior, or volatile domestic circumstances are all candidates for proactive measures (McNeil et al. 1998).
- **Keep precise documentation.** There can never be a substitute for adequate documentation. This documentation includes a verbatim recitation of the threats themselves, persons the clinician consulted with, options considered and reasons for their rejection, and patient compliance or noncompliance (Melonas and Hinton 1998).
- **Do not be reluctant about involuntary commitment.** The law will be reluctant to penalize a clinician for a judgment that errs on the side of avoiding violence. What the law will not forgive is the clinician who forsakes safety for the sake of the therapist-patient relationship.
- **Do not be reluctant to contact victims.**
- **Do not be reluctant to contact law enforcement.**
- **Establish a liaison with law enforcement.** Liaisons with law enforcement can be established through your local association, hospital, or clinic to help ensure that a skilled and rapid response can be made by the authorities.
- **Be aggressive with threat and victim identification.** Although most post-*Tarasoff* laws require that the clinician receive a specific threat against an identifiable victim, it is not difficult to foresee that courts may relax this standard. Threats that appear to be vague may become clear on further investigation, or ill-defined threats may be the beginnings of a notion that evolves into an actual menace. No clinician wants to become a test case for this theory of liability.
- **Consider aggressive therapies in conjunction with the above steps.**

REFERENCES

American Psychiatric Association: The Principles of Medical Ethics, With Annotations Especially Applicable to Psychiatry, 1981 Edition. Washington, DC, American Psychiatric Association, 1981

American Psychiatric Association: The Principles of Medical Ethics, With Annotations Especially Applicable to Psychiatry, 1998 Edition. Washington, DC, American Psychiatric Association, 1998

American Psychiatric Association: Diagnostic and Statistical Manual of Mental Disorders, 4th Edition. Washington, DC, American Psychiatric Association, 1994

The Annie E. Casey Foundation: Kids Count Data Book. Baltimore, MD, The Annie E. Casey Foundation, 1994

Benedek EP, Cornell DG (eds): Juvenile Homicide. Washington, DC, American Psychiatric Press, 1989

Grayson Fraternal Order of Eagles, Aerie No. 3738, Inc. v Claywell, 736 SW2d 328 (Ky 1987)

Kentucky Revised Statutes, §202A.400, 1986

McNeil DE, Binder RL, Fulton FM: Management of threats of violence under California's duty-to-protect statute. Am J Psychiatry 155:1097–1101, 1998

Melonas JM , Hinton M: Experts share advice on reducing risk when treating potentially violent patients. Psychiatric News, October 2, 1998. Available at www.psych.org/pnews. Accessed May 2000

National Center for Education Statistics: Violence and Discipline Problems in U.S. Public Schools: 1996–97. Washington, DC, U.S. Department of Education, 1998

Restatement (Second) of Torts. Washington, DC, American Law Institute Publishers, 1965, Section 314, Comment c, and Section 302B

Roth LH, Meisel A: Dangerousness, confidentiality and the duty to warn. Am J Psychiatry 134:508–511, 1977

Tarasoff v Regents of the University of California, 17 Cal 3d 425, 551 P2d 334, 131, (1976)

10

Duty to Foresee, Forewarn, and Protect Against Violent Behavior

A Psychiatric Perspective

ROBERT I. SIMON, M.D., P.A.

THE TARASOFF DUTY

As a matter of law, one person has no duty to control the conduct of a second person in order to prevent that person from physically harming a third person (Restatement [Second] of Torts 1965). Applying this rule to psychiatric care, psychiatrists traditionally have had only a limited duty to control hospitalized patients and to exercise due care upon discharge. Within the last two decades, this rule has changed (see Chapter 9, this volume). After *Tarasoff v. Regents of the University of California* (1976) (referred to hereafter as *Tarasoff*), the therapist's legal duty and potential liability substantially expanded. In *Tarasoff*, the California Supreme Court recognized that a duty to protect third parties was imposed only when a "special relationship" existed between the victim, the individual whose conduct created the danger, and the defendant.

The court in *Tarasoff* held that

> once a therapist does in fact determine, or where applicable professional standards should have determined, that a patient poses a serious danger of violence to others, he bears a duty to exercise reasonable care to protect

the foreseeable victim of that danger. While the discharge of this duty of care will necessarily vary with the facts of each case, in each case the adequacy of the therapist's conduct must be measured against the traditional negligences standard of the rendition of reasonable care under the circumstances. (17 Cal 3d at 439; 551 P2d at 345)

The court did not state explicitly what actions the psychiatrist or therapist was required to take in order to protect the victim. The court stated generally:

The discharge of this duty may require the therapist to take one or more of various steps, depending upon the nature of the case. Thus, it might call for him to warn the intended victim of the danger, to notify the police or to take whatever other steps are reasonably necessary under the circumstances. (17 Cal 3d at 431; 551 P2d at 340)

The court further stated:

We recognize that in some cases it would be unreasonable to require the therapist to interrogate his patient to discover the victim's identity or to conduct an independent investigation. But there may also be cases in which a moment's reflection will reveal the victim's identity. The matter thus is one which depends upon the circumstances of each case, and should not be governed by any hard and fast rule. (17 Cal 3d at 439, n.11; 551 P2d at 345, n. 11)

Following *Tarasoff*, courts in other jurisdictions have interpreted the case variously. Some states have adopted the *Tarasoff* holding, whereas others have limited or extended its scope and reach. In a majority of states, psychotherapists have a duty, established by case law or statute, to act affirmatively to protect an endangered third party from a patient's violent or dangerous acts. A few courts have declined to find a *Tarasoff* duty in a specific case, while some courts have simply rejected the *Tarasoff* duty (*Evans v. United States* 1995; *Green v. Ross* 1997). In *Thapar v. Zezulka* (1999), the Texas Supreme Court ruled that the state statute *permits* but does not *require* disclosures by therapists of threats of harm to endangered third parties by their patients.

SITUATIONS IN WHICH THE TARASOFF DUTY ARISES

A duty to exercise reasonable care to protect others arises when a psychotherapist determines, or should have determined, on the basis of standards of the profession, that a patient poses an *imminent threat* of *serious harm* to an *identifiable third party.* The duty to protect has been criticized by legal commentators as vague and open to interpretation. Determining what the "standards of the profession" are in evaluating an imminent threat (i.e., predicting dangerousness) is controversial at best. Practitioners find that the revised duty to protect gives more latitude for treatment interventions than the duty to warn. Except in states with immunity statutes limiting the responsibility of therapists for their patients' violent acts, no hard-and-fast rules exist about how the duty to protect should be exercised. In jurisdictions where no duty to warn or protect currently exists by case law or statute, case law from other states may be applied in deciding suits that allege such a duty.

If professionals fail to exercise their clinical judgment and think they are excused from doing so by an immunity statute, serious legal consequences may be incurred (Beck 1990, p. 19). If a patient seriously injures another person and the therapist failed to exercise due care, a court likely will find a way to hold the therapist liable, even in the presence of an immunity statute.

Mental health professionals at all levels of training and experience frequently perform evaluations of children and adolescents. Even if the clinician does not undertake the treatment of a potentially violent person, if violence occurs toward others, the evaluation process may be deemed sufficient to have created a "special relationship" that gave rise to a *Tarasoff* duty.

DISCHARGING THE DUTY

Courts and state statutes that have addressed the duty-to-protect doctrine usually require that an identifiable victim be warned and/or the police be notified (Appelbaum et al. 1989). The law favors the duty to warn in defining the clinician's duty to protect endangered third parties from violent patients. Courts typically focus on whether the violence was foreseeable and if a sufficient element of control was present. Three key steps should be followed by the clinician in a potential duty-to-protect situation:

1. Assess the imminence and seriousness of the threat of violence to another.
2. Identify the potential object of that threat.
3. Implement some affirmative, preventive act.

In discussing the duty to protect, courts have been divided on the issue of therapists' ability to control outpatients. The law assumes that violence is preventable if it is foreseeable. *Foreseeability* is a legal term of art. It is a commonsense, probabilistic concept rather than a scientific construct. Legally, foreseeability is defined as the reasonable anticipation that harm or injury is a likely result from certain acts or omissions (Black 1990). For example, if the practitioner determines that a patient is at significant risk of harming others, it is reasonable to expect that harm will occur to third parties unless preventive measures are undertaken. Such a determination does not imply an ability of clinicians to predict violent behavior. Also, foreseeability should not be confused with *preventability*. By hindsight, some violent acts seem preventable that were clearly not foreseeable.

Assessing Threat

The law requires that therapists exercise reasonable care in making threat assessments, even though psychiatrists cannot accurately predict the occurrence of violence. The evaluation requires compliance only with ordinary assessment procedures used in the profession. A thorough pretreatment history, inquiry about and exploration of past or present violence, and attention to factors reasonably thought to contribute to violent behavior are likely to satisfy a reasonable standard of care (Simon 1998).

Identifying the Intended Victim

When the practitioner determines that a threat of violence to others exists, it is clinically and legally necessary to determine which person or persons might be the object of the threat. A majority of court decisions have held that the duty to protect applies only when there is a "specific or identifiable threat to a specific or identifiable victim" (*Brady v. Hopper* 1984; *Thompson v. County of Alameda* 1980; *White v. United States* 1986). A small minority of courts have broadened this finding by requiring the duty to protect whenever there is a "foreseeable risk of harm" to the general public (*Lipari v. Sears, Roebuck & Co.* 1980; *Schuster v. Altenberg* 1988). Thus, if a specific victim is not identified, it is essential for the clinician to act in some affirmative way to safeguard against a potential risk of harm to unidentified third parties.

Taking an Affirmative Action

The broad language contained in the current case decisions regarding the duty to warn and protect affords a therapist certain latitude in determining "what[ever] steps are reasonably necessary" to discharge that duty. The legal reasoning applied in cases involving the duty to warn and protect suggests a number of factors, discussed later in this chapter, that should be considered in order to reduce the risk of potential liability from patients who threaten harm to others.

SPECIAL ISSUES

Time Limitations

Courts have not specifically addressed the time limits to a therapist's duty to protect. Instead, the reasonableness of a therapist's evaluation of a patient's potential for violence plays a more important role in a court's finding of liability. The amount of time elapsing between the last therapy contact and the injury of a third party does not seem to be a determining factor. For example, in *Naidu v. Laird* (1988), the Delaware Supreme Court found that an inpatient psychiatrist was negligent in failing to foresee a former patient's potential to commit a violent act 5½ months after discharge. The court stated that the lapse of time, by itself, was not a bar to recovery, but one factor to be weighed by the jury.

Confidentiality and Liability

Even in jurisdictions affirmatively endorsing the duty to warn, the therapist could still be sued for breach of confidentiality. The disclosure about the patient must be made with discretion and in a manner that preserves the patient's privacy as much as possible while preventing potential harm. The disclosure also must be based on a reasonable risk of harm. Courts not recognizing the duty to warn, and thus adhering to the common-law recognition of doctor-patient confidentiality, will likely favor a reasonable clinical alternative to breaching patient confidentiality such as hospitalization.

Unforeseeable Violence

Liability for injury to third parties will not be imposed if the assessment that a patient was at low risk for violence is based on reasonable clinical data and judgment. When liability is found, despite a clinical judgment of a low risk of violence, the evidence usually shows that the therapist's evaluation and treatment procedures were substandard or that the therapist substantially departed from acceptable clinical practice.

Risk of Patient Self-Harm

A psychotherapist does not have a duty to inform another party if a patient is going to harm himself or herself (*Bellah v. Greenson* 1978; *Lee v. Corregedore* 1996). The danger of physical harm by patients must be to others, not to themselves. Nevertheless, sound clinical practice may require that the family be brought into the treatment of the suicidal patient, especially with children and adolescents.

Unreachable Identified Victims

If the patient is judged to be a threat to a third party but the third party cannot be reached in order to be warned, the therapist should consider notifying the police or contacting someone in close relationship with the potential victim. Appropriate clinical interventions also should be used. Documenting that the therapist was unable to reach the identified victim and that alternative methods and clinical interventions were implemented may prevent liability.

Liability

Although potential liability for violence has expanded significantly, only a few psychiatrists have been found guilty of negligence. Nonetheless, the *Tarasoff* decision should be considered a national standard for clinical practice affecting psychiatrists and other mental health clinicians in every jurisdiction (Beck 1987). Monahan (1993) provides guidelines for limiting therapist exposure to lawsuits in *Tarasoff* cases.

Since *Tarasoff*, a number of psychiatrists, psychotherapists, hospitals, and other health care facilities have been sued for allegedly breaching the duty to protect. Beck (1990) estimated that approximately 50 psychiatrists are sued each year for breach of the duty to protect. Of these cases, roughly two-thirds are settled before trial. Of the 17 trials, approximately two-thirds resulted in defendant verdicts, leaving 6 psychiatrists a year that are found liable. For a psychiatrist who is a member of the American Psychiatric Association, Beck estimated that the odds of being sued for breach of the duty to protect, going to trial, and being found liable are 5,800 to 1 in any one year.

TARASOFF AND CLINICAL PRACTICE

The duty to warn and protect was originally applied to outpatient cases. The same legal duty to protect individuals and society from harm also arises in the release of potentially violent patients. The majority of courts have held that the therapist's control of the outpatient is insufficient to establish a duty to protect without a foreseeable victim. In the outpatient setting, the *Tarasoff* duty generally is applicable when there is evidence, through either expressed or implied threats or acts, that the patient has the potential to commit a violent act against a specific, foreseeable victim. The potential violence must be imminent and substantial and involve serious bodily harm or death. If no threats or potentially violent acts are uncovered after careful clinical evaluation, a basis for liability is unlikely to exist, even if violence occurs.

In inpatient release cases, the courts have held that there is a duty to control the patient with or without a foreseeable victim if there is reasonable evidence that the patient may be potentially violent. The duty to evaluate the patient for potential violence would obviate a *Tarasoff* duty, because continued dangerousness based on mental illness would require continued hospitalization. If the court releases a patient who is assessed to be at high risk for violence, the clinician should go on record and document the concern about the patient's high risk for potential violence. Psychiatrists are successfully sued much more frequently for the negligent release of violent patients than for the failure to warn and protect endangered third persons in outpatient cases.

The therapist should attempt to integrate the *Tarasoff* duty into the clinical interaction with the patient. In some states, statutory provisions that limit the *Tarasoff* duty to warning an endangered, identifiable victim may distract the practitioner from providing a full spectrum of clinical interventions (Appelbaum 1985). Warning, by itself, often is insufficient. Additional clinical interventions usually are required.

Beck (1985) observed that once the clinical assessment is made that a patient is potentially violent, three basic options are open to the clinician:

- Address the violence in the therapy.
- Warn the victim and/or call the police.
- Hospitalize the patient, either voluntarily or involuntarily.

If after conducting a careful assessment the clinician is satisfied that the patient will not commit violence before the next scheduled appointment, the clinician can continue to treat the potential violence as a purely therapeutic matter. If the therapist determines that the patient will likely become violent within 24–48 hours, hospitalization is the treatment of choice. If an intermediate situation exists in which the therapist believes that violence is a distinct possibility but is not imminent, the best course is to warn the victim. Warning may also be the intervention of choice if it appears that a patient may become violent before the next session but refuses hospitalization and is not committable. However, in addition to warning, other clinical interventions likely will be needed.

Violence Risk Assessment

The standard of care requires that the clinician competently assess the *risk* of violence. No professional standard exists for the *prediction* of violence. Short-term risk assessments of violence are more accurate because the parameters that influence future occurrences can be specified with greater precision. For long-term assessments, the clinician loses the ability to specify both psychological and environmental determinants of behavior and, thus, to assess with reasonable accuracy the likelihood of particular outcomes. Accordingly, potentially violent patients should be seen frequently, and their risk factors for violence should be reassessed at each of these visits. Violence risk assessment is a process, not an event. Information must be gathered continuously and evaluated, and the probability assessment must be updated accordingly.

Documentation that a violence risk assessment was carefully conducted demonstrates that the clinician adhered to the standard of care. In treating the potentially violent patient, the clinician can ensure only the process of assessment, not the outcome of the assessment. Violence risk assessment is not merely an academic exercise. Its main purpose is to guide patient management for the purpose of identifying treatable violence risk factors and for providing safety for the patient and others. As Appelbaum (1985) correctly observed, "Clinicians have learned to live with *Tarasoff*, recognizing that good common sense, sound clinical practice, careful documentation, and a genuine concern for their patients are almost always sufficient to fulfill their legal obligations" (p. 106).

Long before *Tarasoff*, psychiatrists warned and protected endangered third parties as part of their professional and ethical duty. The duty arose when the therapist possessed "insider information" developed from the patient's treatment about the potential risk of violence posed by the patient to others. Therapists should not become mesmerized by the duty to warn at the expense of implementing other clinical interventions that are likely to be more effective. Most potentially violent patients can be managed through sound clinical interventions.

Warning Endangered Third Parties—Is It Enough?

A number of states have defined the *Tarasoff* duty in statutes (mostly in duty-to-warn language) and have narrowed exposure for liability. Nonetheless, the therapist who does not exercise reasonable professional judgment in managing the violent patient may still be vulnerable to a lawsuit. In states offering no such guidance, health care providers are required to use the clinical judgment that will accomplish the objective of protecting the object of the patient's threat. As stated earlier, simply issuing a warning to discharge a legal duty usually is not enough in managing the violent patient. Clinical efforts to manage and control the patient's risk of violence should be attempted before a warning to the intended victim is issued. The patient's treatment often ends when a warning is made to an endangered third party. At that point, the therapist's clinical intervention options are severely limited or nonexistent. Involuntary hospitalization may be an appropriate clinical intervention for potentially violent, treatment-refusing patients who meet the substantive criteria—namely, mentally ill and dangerous—for civil commitment.

Therapists have a professional, ethical, and legal duty to protect patients and their potential victims. From a clinical perspective, the legal duty is obviously important but incidental to the therapist's professional duty. Accordingly, when the duty to warn is implemented, every effort should be made to include it as a treatment issue by engaging the patient in the warning process.

Warning endangered third parties can be perilous. Even assuming that a victim is able to escape or to evade the violent patient, the predictability of violence is inaccurate, causing individuals to be falsely warned. Receiving a letter or a phone call from a therapist warning of serious violence is extremely disturbing. Warned individuals may become severely distressed and psychologically harmed by the duty to warn. Warning can also become an empty gesture when police are reluctant to act before a crime is committed. Preventive detention is not constitutionally permitted. What happens if the endangered person is out of town? Should a letter be sent? Should it be sent by e-mail, certified mail, express mail, or special delivery? How long will delivery take? Trying to locate potential victims can be an impossible task.

If the therapist decides to warn, a phone call should be made. A phone call permits the potential victim to ask questions. Nuances and difficulties in communication can also be recognized and corrected by both parties. Making the phone call in the patient's presence helps to temper exaggerated remarks by the therapist, who may be overreacting to the threat of violence. The patient's presence also tends to preempt distrust that the psychiatrist is acting duplicitously. The warning should be given clearly. The clarity of the warning has been the subject of second-guessing by some courts. The rationale for and the content of a warning should be carefully documented in detail.

The psychology of victimization is relevant to the decision to warn (Levin and Hill 1992). For example, the psychodynamics of victim–victimizer in which one party is being abused may require moving the victim toward a sheltered environment instead of warning the abuser that the abused person is considering retaliatory violence. Issuing a warning to the abuser may seriously endanger the patient or precipitate mutual violence.

How the warning is given, not whether one is given, is the more crucial factor. When the clinician discusses warning endangered third parties with the patient before giving the warning, the clinical result is often positive. Failing to discuss the warning with the patient likely will harm the therapeutic alliance and the therapy. Potential victims should be warned by the therapist in a clinically supportive manner. If potential victims feel that evasive action can be taken and that the therapist is acting in a responsible, genuinely concerned manner, the warnings are likely to be received constructively.

Generally, courts have refused to impose a duty on psychiatrists to warn the foreseeable victim when the latter knew of the potential violence from a patient (Simon 1992, p. 302). In *In re Estate of Heltsley v. Votteler* (1982), the plaintiff had knowledge of the patient's previous aggressive behavior but contended that a warning from the psychiatrist would have made her appreciate the significance of the threat. The Iowa Supreme Court rejected this argument. On the other hand, in *Jablonski v. United States* (1983; overruled, *In re complaint of McLinn* 1984), the defendant's wife, who was killed by the patient, had received warnings about the patient from her priest, her mother, her attorney, and a hot-line service. She had even voiced her fears to the psychiatrist, but, nonetheless, the court imposed liability.

The therapist should not assume that an endangered person who previously has been threatened or harmed by the patient fully appreciates the current danger of his or her situation. Denial may cause the person to minimize or ignore the threat. Depending on the nature of the case and of the relationship between the patient and the potential victim, the therapist may nevertheless decide to warn the endangered person of the specific threats made by the patient, despite that person's prior knowledge.

An important, evolving trend is the application of the *Tarasoff* duty to sexual abuse cases by an alleged pedophile. A psychiatrist was successfully sued for not reporting to the medical school that his patient was a pedophile (*Garamella for Estate of Almonte v. New York Medical College* 1998). The patient, a psychiatric resident, eventually molested a child at a hospital crisis center. However, the defendant psychiatrist's control over the psychiatric resident was far greater than in the typical psychiatrist-patient relationship. A *Tarasoff* duty was also found when a spouse had knowledge of her husband's sexually abusive behavior against children in the neighborhood (*J.S. v. R.T.H.* 1998; *Touchette v. Ganal* 1996). In another case, one involving the parents of a babysitter who sexually assaulted a child in his care, the court found that a *Tarasoff* duty could exist but declined to find the parents liable for their son's dangerous sexual behavior (*People v. Rose* 1998). The court determined that no evidence existed that the parents knew of their son's proclivity to commit a sexual assault.

CONFIDENTIALITY VERSUS THE DUTY TO PROTECT

Trust is the cornerstone of psychotherapy. Without trust, the therapeutic alliance cannot develop. In the real world, confidentiality, like trust, is never absolute. Exceptions to the maintenance of confidentiality exist that protect both the patient and society. In *Tarasoff*, the court was mindful of the importance of preserving as much confidentiality as possible in the therapist-patient relationship when warning a victim of threatened violence. Generally, confidentiality should not be breached by warning a third party unless the threat of harm is serious and imminent and an identifiable victim is endangered. Nonetheless, a plaintiff may allege breach of confidentiality when a therapist issues a warning. Resolving the tension between the need to maintain confidentiality and the duty to protect others from patient violence often is a difficult judgment call that must be applied to the clinical fact pattern of individual cases. When treating potentially violent children or adolescents, the duty to warn and protect usually requires involving parents or other caretakers.

The Principles of Medical Ethics, With Annotations Especially Applicable to Psychiatry states, "Psychiatrists at times may find it necessary, in order to protect the patient or the community from imminent danger, to reveal confidential information disclosed by the patient" (American Psychiatric Association 1998, §4, p. 6). The exception to confidentiality represented by the duty to warn and protect is part of the same public policy exception requiring the reporting of, for example, contagious diseases, suspected child abuse, and gunshot wounds for the welfare of the patient and society. The tension between confidentiality and the duty to protect may also arise concerning some patients' ability to drive an automobile. A *Tarasoff* duty has been found in cases where patients have injured third parties with their vehicles (Pettis 1992). Generally, courts do not impose liability unless the physician had significant control over the patient (e.g., inpatient vs. outpatient) (Foreman 1999).

Mental health professionals should be familiar with the legal regulation of confidentiality in their jurisdiction. Although the *Tarasoff* duty arises only occasionally, the maintenance of confidentiality is a continuing duty in clinical practice whose breach occurs much more frequently in other clinical contexts. In 1996, the United States Supreme Court ruled, in *Jaffe v. Redmond* (1996), that communications between psychotherapist and patient are confidential in federal cases under the Federal Rules of Evidence. Perlin (1999) pointed out that a footnote in *Jaffe* states an exception to the privilege when a serious threat of harm exists to the patient or others that "can be averted only by means of a disclosure by the therapist" (pp. 20–21). Perlin commented that "[t]he relationship of this footnote to the *Tarasoff* doctrine has not yet been fully explored" (pp. 20–21).

Some therapists give defensive Miranda-type warnings to new patients about the therapist's duty to warn or protect third parties against violent threats (Simon 2000). Starting a treatment with a proscriptive warning casts a pall over the fledgling therapeutic process. Patients who already are frightened by their aggression may find that such a warning confirms their own worst fears. Secretive, resistive patients may seize on such a warning in order to withhold verbal expression of violent feelings. When the protection of others from patient violence is necessary, clinical interventions usually allow for the preservation of confidentiality, making Miranda-type warnings to patients a gratuitous gesture.

In a further erosion of confidentiality, recent court cases have required the therapist to testify, in the case of a patient who later becomes a criminal defendant, about a *Tarasoff* warning issued during the patient's therapy. The confidential treatment information that formed the basis for the warning was deemed to lose its privileged status once a third party was warned. Thus, the warning of endangered third parties has resulted in therapists being compelled to testify in criminal trials of their own patients on behalf of the prosecution (Leong et al. 1992). Once confidentiality is lost in the therapeutic situation, it cannot be regained in litigation.

PROTECTING ENDANGERED THIRD PARTIES— THE GOLD STANDARD

Whenever possible, the therapist should apply clinical principles in the management of the potentially violent patient. There is no inherent conflict between the professional duty to treat the patient and the legal duty to protect third parties. Above all, therapists must not feel so threatened by legal issues that they become distracted from providing good clinical care. Although therapists should have a working knowledge of the law as it applies to clinical practice, they need not become lawyers.

Whereas *Tarasoff I* emphasized the duty to *warn* exclusively, *Tarasoff II* stated that the psychiatrist must exercise his or her own best judgment (consistent with that reasonable degree of skill, knowledge, and care ordinarily exercised by psychiatrists under similar circumstances) to *protect* the victim from the foreseeable violence of dangerous patients. The law does not require perfect skill, but only the reasonable skill exercised by therapists in similar circumstances. The duty to protect permits a broad and meaningful clinical approach to the management of violent patients. Although warning can be part of a therapist's intervention strategy, it rarely should be relied on initially or exclusively.

CONCLUSION

The clinician should consider the legal duty to warn and protect endangered third parties from threatened harm by his or her patient to be a national standard. The risk of harm must be serious, imminent, and directed toward an identifiable person. The management of duty-to-warn-and-protect cases is primarily clinical. The duty to protect allows greater treatment latitude than the duty to warn alone, while also preserving confidentiality. Courts closely examine the specific facts of a case to determine whether a duty to warn and protect exists.

REFERENCES

American Psychiatric Association: The Principles of Medical Ethics, With Annotations Especially Applicable to Psychiatry, 1998 Edition. Washington, DC, American Psychiatric Association, 1998

Appelbaum PS: Implications of Tarasoff for clinical practice, in The Potentially Violent Patient and the Tarasoff Decision in Psychiatric Practice. Edited by Beck JC. Washington, DC, American Psychiatric Press, 1985, pp 98–108

Appelbaum PS, Zonana H, Bonnie R, et al: Statutory approaches to limiting psychiatrists' liability for their patients' violent acts. Am J Psychiatry 146:821–828, 1989

Beck JC: The psychotherapist and the violent patient: recent case law, in The Potentially Violent Patient and the Tarasoff Decision in Psychiatric Practice. Edited by Beck JC. Washington, DC, American Psychiatric Press, 1985, pp 10–34

Beck JC: The psychotherapist's duty to protect third parties from harm. Mental and Physical Disability Law Reporter 11:141–148, 1987

Beck JC: Current status of the duty to protect, in Confidentiality Versus the Duty to Protect: Foreseeable Harm in the Practice of Psychiatry. Edited by Beck JC. Washington, DC, American Psychiatric Press, 1990, pp 9–10

Bellah v Greenson, 81 Cal App 3d 614, 146 Cal Rptr 535 (Cal Ct App 1978)

Black HC: Black's Law Dictionary, 6th Edition. St Paul, MN, West, 1990, p 649

Brady v Hopper, 751 F2d 329 (10th Cir 1984)

Evans v United States, 883 F Supp 124 (5D Miss 1995)

Foreman T: Physicians do not have duty to third-party drivers. J Am Acad Psychiatry Law 27:637–639, 1999

Garamella for Estate of Almonte v New York Medical College, 23 F Supp 2d 167 (D Conn 1998)

Green v Ross, 691 So2d 542 (Fla App 1997)

In re Estate of Heltsley v Votteler, 327 NW2d 759 (Iowa 1982)

Jablonski v United States, 712 F2d 391 (9th Cir 1983), overruled, In re complaint of McLinn 739 F2d 1395 (9th Cir 1984)

Jaffe v Redmond, 1165 Ct 1923 (1996)

J.S. v R.T.H., 714 A2d 924 (NJ 1998)

Lee v Corregedore, 925 P2d 324 (Haw 1996)

Leong GB, Eth S, Silva JA: The psychotherapist as witness for the prosecution: the criminalization of Tarasoff. Am J Psychiatry 149:1011–1015, 1992

Levin RB, Hill EH: Recent trends in psychiatric liability, in American Psychiatric Press Review of Clinical Psychiatry and the Law, Vol 3. Edited by Simon RI. Washington, DC, American Psychiatric Press, 1992, pp 129–150

Lipari v Sears, Roebuck & Co. 497 F Supp 185 (D Neb 1980)

Monahan J: Limiting therapist exposure to Tarasoff liability. Am Psychol 48:242–250, 1993

Naidu v Laird, 539 A2d 1064 (Del Super Ct 1988)

People v Rose, 573 NW 2d 765 (Neb 1998)

Perlin ML: Tarasoff at the millennium: new directions, new defendants, new dangers, new dilemmas. Psychiatric Times, November 1999, pp 20-21

Pettis RW: Tarasoff and the dangerous driver: a look at driving cases. Bull Am Acad Psychiatry Law 20:427–437, 1992

Restatement (Second) of Torts. Washington DC, American Law Institute Publishers, 1965, §315(a)

Schuster v Altenberg, 144 Wis 2d 223, 424 NW2d 159, 1988

Simon RI: Clinical Psychiatry and the Law, 2nd Edition. Washington, DC, American Psychiatric Press, 1992

Simon RI: Concise Guide to Psychiatry and Law for Clinicians, 2nd Edition. Washington, DC, American Psychiatric Press, 1998, pp 165–198

Simon RI: Defensive psychiatry and the disruption of treatment boundaries. Israel Journal of Psychiatry 37:124–131, 2000

Tarasoff v Regents of the University of California, 17 Cal 3d 425, 551 P2d 334 (1976)

Thapar v Zezulka 944 SW2d 635 (Tx 1999)

Thompson v County of Alameda, 27 Cal 3d 741, 614 P2d 728, 167 Cal Rptr 70 (1980)

Touchette v Ganal, 922 P2d 347 (Haw 1996)

White v United States, 780 F2d 97 (DC Cir 1986)

PREVENTION

11

Prevention of Firearm Fatalities and Injuries

Public Health Approach

GEORGE J. COHEN, M.D.

Firearm injuries are a major cause of death and disability of American youngsters. In 1996, almost 14% of the 34,000 gun fatalities in the United States were of people younger than 20 years. In 1995, firearm deaths were four times more frequent in the United States than in any other industrialized nation (National Center for Health Statistics 1997). From 1985 to 1992, firearm deaths doubled among those younger than 20 years, and in 1996 there was a death from firearms every 1.9 hours in this age group (National Center for Health Statistics 1998). A nationwide survey found 105 school-associated violent deaths from 1992 to 1994; 80% of those deaths were due to homicide, and more than 75% were due to firearms (Kachur et al. 1996). From 1990 to 1994, in Milwaukee, Wisconsin, 89% of firearm homicides and 71% of firearm suicides were committed with handguns, the most com-

This chapter is an updated version of a paper presented at the International Seminar on Violence and Adolescence, Jerusalem, Israel, November 16–18, 1999, that appeared with the other seminar presentations in a special issue of the *International Journal of Adolescent Medicine and Health* (Vol. 11, No. 3–4, 1999).

mon being a .25 caliber handgun (Hargarten et al. 1996). Firearms were reported to cause more deaths than motor vehicles in six states in 1996 (Jeter
1999).

NONFATAL FIREARM INJURIES

From June 1992 through May 1994, more than 34,000 unintentional nonfatal firearm injuries were treated in hospital emergency departments: 61%
were in 15- to 34-year-olds, and 87% were in males; 70% were self-inflicted,
and 57% were due to handguns (Sinauer et al. 1996).

A study in Washington State of self-inflicted and unintentional firearm injuries and deaths of children and adolescents younger than 19 years
found that a gun at home accounted for two-thirds of suicides and one-
fourth of unintentional firearm injuries (Grossman et al. 1999). In a 1995
survey of middle school children in North Carolina, 14% reported carrying
a club or knife to school and 3% reported carrying a gun. Early onset and
frequency of substance use were strongly associated with weapon carrying (DuRant et al. 1999).

ECONOMIC COSTS

The economic costs of firearm injury are staggering. From data from hospital discharges, the National Electronic Injury Surveillance System, and
the National Spinal Cord Injury Statistical Center, it was estimated that
gunshot injuries produced $2.3 billion in lifetime medical costs, of which
almost half was paid by taxpayers. The mean medical cost per injury was
estimated to be $17,000, and gunshots during assaults accounted for al-
most three-fourths of total costs (Cook et al. 1999). The average total cost
of a gun-related crime was estimated to be almost $270,000, with most of
the cost borne by taxpayers (Lengel 1997). Additional indirect costs (e.g.,
lost potential earnings) have been estimated at $19 billion (American Col-
lege of Physicians 1998).

EMOTIONAL COSTS

Emotional costs are difficult to estimate in dollars but are significant in
terms of functioning in both children and adults. Even infants and toddlers

demonstrate traumatic stress disorder symptoms, namely, reexperiencing of the traumatic event, numbing of responsiveness, and hyperarousal. In addition, they also may develop new fears and aggressive behavior (Zeanah and Scheeringa 1996). Common stress symptoms are likely to vary according to the age of the child. Preschoolers may become more clingy and have decreased appetite, sleep disturbance, and regression in bowel and bladder control, as well as fear of the dark and increased thumb sucking. Elementary school children often show irritability, aggressiveness, clinging, nightmares, poor concentration, school avoidance, and withdrawal from normal activities and social contacts. Young adolescents are likely to avoid contact with friends, complain of somatic symptoms, perform less well in school, and have disturbance of sleep and appetite (see Chapter 8, this volume). Older adolescents show many of the responses of younger adolescents but are more likely to appear agitated or lethargic and to engage in irresponsible or delinquent behavior (Waddell and Thomas 1999).

PUBLIC HEALTH PROBLEM

Given the toll in lives, chronic disability, psychological dysfunction, and monetary costs, youth firearm injury should be viewed as a national epidemic and approached as a public health problem (see Chapter 11, this volume). First, the problem must be defined in terms of its impact on the population. Second, risk factors and resilience or modifying factors must be identified so that appropriate corrective interventions can be formulated and tested. Third, successful pilot interventions should be implemented on a broader scale so that societal outcomes can be evaluated and the best interventions can be continued and expanded. With a public health approach, risk and protective factors can be classified as host factors, environmental factors, and agent factors, although it should be recognized that a degree of overlap is inevitable.

Host Factors

Host factors relate to both perpetrators and victims of youth firearm violence and include previous aggressive and/or violent behavior; being a victim of abuse (physical, sexual, psychological); viewing violence at home, in the media, and in the community; brain damage and mental illness; impulsiveness; anger; and fear (American Academy of Child and Adolescent Psychiatry 1996). In American Indian and Alaska Native youths, suicide attempts were associated with friends or family members attempting or completing suicide, somatic symptoms and health concerns, being in a special education class, gang involvement, and gun availability, as well as abuse, substance use, and treatment for emotional problems (Borowsky et al. 1999).

Environmental Factors

Environmental factors include poor parenting and violence in the media. A magazine poll found that more than half of those polled agreed about these two factors ("Gun War Comes Home" *Newsweek* 1999). It has long been known that gangs and peer pressure encourage a variety of antisocial behaviors in teenagers. Poverty, with its frequent association with poor housing, poor schools, poor recreation facilities, and stressed parents, frequently has been identified with behavioral, emotional, and antisocial activities of young people. A study of firearm storage practices in 1994 found that in one in five homes with guns, the firearms were kept loaded. In fewer than half of the homes with both guns and children were stored firearms unloaded and locked (Stennies et al. 1999).

Agent Factors

The agent in this public health approach is, of course, the firearm and its ammunition. Both availability of firearms and increasing lethality of weapons and bullets are definite risk factors. With more than 200 million guns available and more than one-third of American families having at least one gun, it is easy to see why firearms are so often used in dangerous ways and by those who should not have access to them ("Guns in America" *Newsweek* 1999). A study of incarcerated offenders ages 13 to 18 years found that 84% acquired their first gun before they were 15 years old. Almost all these individuals said that it was easy to get a gun on the street. If they purposely obtained their handgun, they were more likely to be frequent or constant carriers. Forty percent said they felt safer and/or more powerful when carrying a gun (Ash et al. 1996). A gun in the home increased the risk of suicide fivefold (Kellerman et al. 1992) and the risk of domestic homicide threefold (Kellerman et al. 1993). The plethora of high-powered weapons, such as TEC-DC9 handguns, 9mm Uzis, Glock 9mm pistols, .30 caliber hunting rifles, and now .50 caliber sniper rifles, as well as armor-piercing and hollow-point expanding bullets, are increasingly cause for concern ("America's Weapons of Choice" *Newsweek* 1999c; Vobejda and Ottaway 1999).

PREVENTING FIREARM INJURY

Approaches to preventing firearm injury of children and youth fall into several categories: educating and counseling parents, identifying adolescents at risk, mentoring at-risk adolescents and children, providing educational programs for children and adolescents in school, enacting legislation, strictly enforcing gun control laws, publicizing public opinion (polls), and pursuing litigation.

Educating and Counseling Parents

Although 98% of pediatricians surveyed in one study believed in counseling parents who had guns at home about gun safety, only 55% believed in counseling all parents (Becher and Christakis 1999). Moreover, the pediatricians' estimate of parent gun ownership was only 65% sensitive. Becher and Christakis (1999) stated that pediatricians should ask all parents about firearm ownership. A survey of pediatricians in Washington, D.C., and six mid-Atlantic states revealed that two-thirds of the respondents counsel sometimes and were most likely to do so if they had treated a patient for a firearm injury, practiced in a rural or poor urban area, or were themselves gun owners (Rosenquist et al. 1998).

In 1992, the American Academy of Pediatrics published a policy statement on firearms and adolescents in which they recommended legislative and regulatory measures to reduce the availability of guns to adolescents. All adolescent health care providers were urged to counsel about gun-safe homes, identify high-risk teens so that age-appropriate services could be provided, and develop community-based coalitions to address methods of reducing firearm injury and death, school curricula aimed at violence prevention and coping skills, and active research on prevention strategies (Beach et al. 1992). In addition, the Academy of Pediatrics, with the Center to Prevent Handgun Violence, developed the STOP program, which includes an educational brochure for parents and counseling tips, both written and on audiotape, for pediatricians (*STOP: Steps to Prevent Firearm Injury* 1996).

Identifying Adolescents at Risk

In efforts to identify adolescents at risk, a number of organizations have published useful material. The American Psychological Association has a brochure for adolescents that notes factors that contribute to violent behavior such as peer pressure, need for attention or respect, feelings of low self-worth, early childhood abuse or neglect, witnessing violence, and easy access to weapons. The brochure also offers teenagers advice on dealing with anger and violence in self and others (American Psychological Association "Warning Signs," undated).

The American Academy of Child and Adolescent Psychiatry (1998) offers families advice about children's threats and points out that threats about hurting or killing self or others, threats of running away from home, and threats of damage or destruction of property must be taken seriously and professional help must be sought.

In response to recent school shootings, DeBernardo and McGee (1999) described characteristics of the classroom avenger and interventions for dealing with him. The authors characterized him as a sullen, angry, seclusive youngster with average school grades and expressed fantasies and plans of revenge. They recommended direct, active cognitive-behavioral techniques focusing on anger management and social skills training and point out the need for family therapy and close monitoring of the patient.

Mentoring At-Risk Adolescents and Children and Providing Educational Programs for Schoolchildren

Mentoring programs have demonstrated success in changing negative behaviors of teenagers. For example, Big Brothers/Big Sisters has reduced antisocial activities by 27%–45%, improved school performance slightly, decreased skipping 36%–52%, decreased lying to parents by 36%, and improved peer and family relationships slightly (Grossman and Garry 1997). Adapting a gang model of mentoring in a violent inner-city community resulted in less support for violence among the mentored children than among control children, whose behavior scores worsened (Sheehan et al. 1999). The U.S. Office of Juvenile Justice and Delinquency Prevention reviewed research reports, initiatives, and more than 50 programs aimed at reducing youth gun violence, many of which were demonstrated to have positive outcomes (Bilchik 1996). An example is Straight Talk About Risks (STAR), a comprehensive curriculum in both English and Spanish for children and adolescents in prekindergarten through twelfth grade designed to help prevent gun violence. Twenty-one New Jersey school districts implemented the curriculum in the 1992–1993 school year, and surveys revealed generally positive and effective evaluations (Bass et al. 1993).

Enacting Legislation

Legislative efforts go back at least to 1934 with passage of the National Firearms Act, which regulated automatic weapons and sawed-off shotguns because of their use in gang violence during the Prohibition era. Other federal legislation includes banning mail-order sales of firearms and import of handguns; prohibiting felons and mentally ill persons from owning firearms; prohibiting possession of a firearm within 1,000 feet of a school; requiring a waiting period and background check of prospective gun buyers (the Brady bill); banning (in 1994) the sale, manufacture, and import of certain assault weapons; performing background checks at gun shows; and requiring child safety locks on guns (Pianin 1999). Although some of these laws were struck down by federal courts, states and local jurisdictions have passed their own gun control laws. Carrying concealed weapons was outlawed in some states and authorized in others. In Virginia, a law limiting purchases of guns by an individual to one per month has reduced by over 50% the illegal interstate transfer of firearms (Weil and Knox 1996). More recently, a bill has been introduced in the Senate to expand research on mental illness links to teen suicide and violence (Domenici 1999). A successful approach to enforcement of existing laws is Project Exile in Richmond, Virginia, where it is illegal to carry a gun while in possession of drugs; more than 500 guns have been confiscated and more than 200 violators have been jailed, and the homicide and robbery rates have dropped about 30% ("Guns in America" *Newsweek* 1999).

Strictly Enforcing Gun Control Laws

Public opinion is showing increasing support for stricter gun control measures; polls show that almost three-fourths of Americans support further restrictions on the sale and handling of guns (Pianin 1999). A *Newsweek* poll indicated that 74% supported registration for all handgun owners and 93% favored a mandatory waiting period for those wanting to purchase handguns ("Gun War Comes Home" *Newsweek* 1999a).

The main obstacles to gun control legislation have been the profits earned by manufacturers as they produce and sell ever more weapons and lobby legislators who do not pass stronger gun control measures. The National Rifle Association does much of this lobbying, using as a rationale the Second Amendment to the U.S. Constitution. They consistently quote only the latter part of the amendment ("the right of the people to keep and bear Arms, shall not be infringed") but always ignore the first part ("A well regulated Militia, being necessary to the security of a free state . . ."). The courts have repeatedly denied that the meaning of the Second Amendment authorizes unlimited personal ownership of firearms. Until recently, public apathy or lack of concern has been seen by opponents of gun control activities as tacit approval of their opposition.

Publicizing Public Opinion

Public opinion appears to be moving in the direction of more gun control and antiviolence action, as noted earlier. Statistics on firearm-related injuries are encouraging, although cause and effect cannot yet be defined accurately. From 1993 to 1995, among injuries treated in emergency departments, nonfatal firearm-related injuries declined more than 11% (with a decline of 5% among 15- to 24-year-old males), injuries from assaults were down more than 6%, and unintentional injuries decreased almost 29% (Mitka 1998). From 1995 to 1996, total firearm deaths dropped 5%, and firearm deaths among youth younger than 19 years declined 12% (National Center for Health Statistics 1998). Firearm homicides from 1993 to 1995 in the 15- to 24-year-old population declined between 4% and 15%, depending on the size of the city (Fingerhut et al. 1998). Among high school students, between 1993 and 1997, the percentage of students who carried a gun decreased 25%, the percentage who got in a fight on school property dropped 9%, and the percentage who carried a weapon on school property declined 28% (Brener et al. 1999). During the 1997–1998 school year, approximately 30% fewer students were expelled for bringing weapons to school than in the previous year (Kalb 1999).

There is now evidence that the entertainment industry is responding to public opinion and reducing the volume of depictions of violence in the media. According to one poll, more than 75% of respondents stated that media violence was at least partly responsible for recent mass shootings (Leland and Brown 1999).

As encouraging as these statistics seem, the continued large number of firearm injuries and deaths among our young people and the population at large indicates that we cannot become complacent. For example, although firearm homicide decreased almost 15% from 1997 to 1998, murder rates actually rose in cities with populations of 10,000 to 24,999 during that time (Adams and Vise 1999). Attorney General Janet Reno recently said, "There is no one reason for the continued drop in crime." She indicated that more police on the streets, collaboration among law enforcement agencies, efforts to keep guns out of criminal hands, and a balanced approach, including prevention, intervention, punishment, and supervision, have all been factors (Adams and Vise 1999).

Pursuing Litigation

A variety of litigation against firearm manufacturers is being pursued. The premises behind this litigation are that 1) the lack of locks and other safety features on guns causes injury and death and 2) manufacturers know that the only purpose of many of their products is to kill people and the products are so advertised. It is too early to predict the outcome of these efforts.

It is hoped that the prevention approaches discussed in this section will result in further decline in the epidemic of violence and firearm injury of children, adolescents, and adults. When all of us can live in less fearful environments, we can expect our young people to be healthier, happier, and more productive.

REFERENCES

Adams L, Vise DA: Crime rates down for 7th straight year. Washington Post, October 18, 1999, A2

American Academy of Child and Adolescent Psychiatry: Understanding Violent Behavior in Children and Adolescents (Facts for Families #55). Washington, DC, American Academy of Child and Adolescent Psychiatry, 1996

American Academy of Child and Adolescent Psychiatry: Children's Threats: When Are They Serious? (Facts for Families #65). Washington, DC, American Academy of Child and Adolescent Psychiatry, 1998

American College of Physicians: Firearm Injury Prevention. Ann Intern Med 128: 236–241, 1998

American Psychological Association: Warning Signs (brochure). Washington, DC, American Psychological Association, undated

America's weapons of choice. Newsweek, August 23, 1999, pp 36–37

Ash P, Kellerman A, Fuqua-Whitley D, et al: Gun acquisition and use by juvenile offenders. JAMA 275:1754–1758, 1996

Bass D, Gannon N, Ferguson L, et al: Straight Talk About Risks: Final Report and Evaluation. Washington, DC, Center to Prevent Handgun Violence, 1993

Beach R, Boulter S, Felice M, et al: Firearms and adolescents. Pediatrics 89:784–787, 1992

Becher E, Christakis N: Firearm injury prevention counseling: are we missing the mark? Pediatrics 104:530–535, 1999

Bilchik S: Reducing Youth Gun Violence: An Overview of Programs and Initiatives (NCJ 154303). Washington, DC, Office of Juvenile Justice and Delinquency Prevention, U.S. Department of Justice, 1996

Borowsky I, Resnick M, Ireland M, et al: Suicide attempts among American Indian and Alaska Native youth. Arch Pediatr Adolesc Med 153:573–580, 1999

Brener N, Simon T, Krug E, et al: Recent trends in violence-related behaviors among high school students in the United States. JAMA 282:440–446, 1999

Cook P, Lawrence B, Ludwig J, et al: The medical costs of gunshot injuries in the United States. JAMA 282:447–454, 1999

DeBernardo C, McGee J: Preventing the classroom avenger's next attack. On The Move 4(2):1–5, 1999

Domenici P: Public health response to Youth Suicide and Violence Act of 1999. Congressional Record, August 5, 1999

DuRant R, Krowchuk D, Kreiter S, et al: Weapon carrying on school property among middle school students. Arch Pediatr Adolesc Med 153:21–26, 1999

Fingerhut L, Ingram D, Feldman J: Homicide rates among US teenagers and young adults. JAMA 280:423–427, 1998

Grossman J, Garry E: Mentoring C a proven delinquency prevention strategy. Juvenile Justice Bulletin, April 1997, 1–7

Grossman D, Reay D, Baker S: Self-inflicted and unintentional firearm injuries among children and adolescents. Arch Pediatr Adolesc Med 153:875–878, 1999

Gun war comes home. Newsweek, August 23, 1999, p 26

Guns in America. Newsweek, August 23, 1999, pp 23–25

Hargarten S, Karlson T, O'Brien M, et al: Characteristics of firearms involved in fatalities. JAMA 275:42–45, 1996

Jeter A: Firearms take over as leading cause of injury-related deaths in Md. Montgomery Journal, March 16, 1999, A3

Kachur S, Stennies G, Powell K, et al: School associated violent deaths in the United States, 1992 to 1994. JAMA 275:1729–1733, 1996

Kalb C: Schools on the alert. Newsweek, August 23, 1999, pp 42–44

Kellerman A, Rivara F, Somes G, et al: Suicide in the home in relation to gun ownership. N Engl J Med 327:467–472, 1992

Kellerman A, Rivara F, Rushforth N: Gun ownership as a risk factor for homicide in the home. N Engl J Med 329:1084–1091, 1993

Leland J, Brown C: A lower body count. Newsweek, August 23, 1999, pp 46–48

Lengel A: The price of urban violence. Washington Post, December 28, 1997, B1

Mitka M: Good news on guns—but not for everyone. JAMA 280:403–404, 1998

National Center for Health Statistics: 1995 Firearm Deaths. Hyattsville, MD, National Center for Health Statistics, July 1997

National Center for Health Statistics: 1996 Firearm Deaths. Hyattsville, MD, National Center for Health Statistics, 1998

Pianin E: In push-pull of gun debate, suburban areas are pivotal. Washington Post, June 13, 1999, A3

Rosenquist G, O'Donnell R, Cheng T, et al: Firearm counseling by practicing general pediatricians. Ambulatory Child Health 4:13–19, 1998

Sheehan K, DiCara J, LeBailly S, et al: Adapting the gang model: peer mentoring for violence prevention. Pediatrics 104:50–54, 1999

Sinauer N, Annest J, Mercy J: Unintentional, nonfatal firearm-related injuries. JAMA 275:1740–1743, 1996

Stennies G, Ikeda R, Leadbetter S, et al: Firearm storage practices and children in the home, United States, 1994. Arch Pediatr Adolesc Med 153:586–590, 1999

STOP: Steps to Prevent Firearm Injury, 2nd Edition. Washington, DC, American Academy of Pediatrics and Center to Prevent Handgun Violence, 1996

Vobejda B, Ottaway D: On streets, firepower for an army. Washington Post, August 17, 1999, A1

Waddell D, Thomas A: Disaster: Helping Children Cope. Communique, Special Edition. Bethesda, MD, National Association of School Psychologists, 1999

Weil D, Knox R: Effects of limiting handgun purchases on interstate transfer of firearms. JAMA 275:1759–1761, 1996

Zeanah C, Scheeringa M: Evaluation of posttraumatic symptomatology in infants and young children exposed to violence. Zero to Three 16(5):9–14, 1996

12

Problems With and Solutions for School Violence

The Philadelphia Experience

PAUL J. FINK, M.D.

Violent behavior among children and adolescents in schools is not unique to Philadelphia or any other single community, large or small, as illustrated by the Littleton, Colorado, tragedy and those that preceded it, such as in Pearl, Mississippi; Paducah, Kentucky; and Springfield, Oregon (see Chapters 6 and 7, this volume). School violence also is certainly not limited to the inner city or a single ethnic group.

School violence is a problem that is much bigger than the school environment (see Chapter 4, this volume). This problem may seem to be solely related to school because attention is focused only on students' misbehavior, inattentiveness, and disruptiveness in the classroom. The reality is that mental and emotional disturbances in some families and youth, as well as social and environmental determinants, have overwhelmed the schools and led to the neglect of the multiple causes of violent behavior. School personnel generally have believed that the only way to deal with these problems is through punishment, transfer to another school, suspension, or expulsion of the student.

School violence is not a problem that can be solved by the schools alone. Rather, it is a multidimensional problem that must be addressed by multiple agencies working together. This premise is gaining acceptance throughout the country with the understanding that the solution takes communication, cooperation, and collaboration (the three C's).

Using the three C's, I look here at some examples of dealing with high school violence not only in Philadelphia but also in New Haven, Connecticut; Boston, Massachusetts; and Chicago, Illinois (see Chapters 2 and 13, this volume). I discuss ongoing projects in these cities to illustrate that communication, cooperation, and collaboration, with a foundation of trust and good will and the involvement of a group of high-minded, seriously motivated people, can make schools safe for children and adolescents; schools can then be places where children can learn without disruptions from problems created by the violence in our society, in our homes, and among our youths.

The Problems

If we try to examine the matrix that leads children and adolescents to act in a violent way and attempt to determine how we can prevent these behaviors, we must look at the home, street, and school environments. We also must look at the attitudes conveyed in the greater society—through, for example, parenting and parental behavior and television and other media—and, above all, at many Americans' reliance on violence to solve problems. Other underlying causes of school violence that need to be examined are domestic violence, the increased drug use among ever younger children over the last two decades, the availability of guns, the litigious and argumentative nature of our society, and the failure of children to get adequate care and love in their lives, leading to great reservoirs of anger and hate.

The media are filled with negative stories—stories of murders, rapes, serial killers, white-collar crime, and assaults—of "man's inhumanity to man." America is a violent society. Recent statistics show that a murder occurs every 24 minutes, a woman is battered every 12 seconds, 1.3 women are raped every minute, and an aggravated assault occurs every 29 seconds. In addition, the American family is violent. Hitting children is almost universal in this country. Around 25% of infants between the ages of 1 and 6 months are hit, and the proportion of infants who are hit increases to about 50% between the ages of 6 and 12 months (Straus 1994). In 1993, there were estimated to be 2.8 million abused and neglected kids in America. Abuse of females and domestic violence are rampant. It should be clear that children learn violent behavior at home and that they transfer the feelings they develop as a result of being either victims of violence or witnesses to it. Their responses to violence vary enormously and are manifested in their behaviors at home and at school.

During the last decade, America has embraced the concept that trauma is an important etiological factor in the development of emotional disturbance and mental illness. We now know that changes in brain chemistry result not only from being a victim of violence but also from witnessing a traumatic or violent event, as well as from other, more subtle activities in the life of the child (see Chapter 3, this volume). Rene Spitz (1965) said, "Infants without love, they will end as adults full of hate" (p. 300). This aphorism is important because it directs us away from the school and to the family for some better understanding of how the child learns to behave in a disruptive and destructive way.

SCHOOL EFFORTS TO PREVENT VIOLENCE

In the 1980s and into the early 1990s, schools left to their own devices used precious dollars that should have been directed to educational activities to address the problem of school violence. In many cases, schools were misguided and did too little too late. They failed to look for the underlying reasons for violent behavior; they merely tried to prevent the behaviors in whatever way they could.

The rise in the number of school police in big cities has been extraordinary. Many high schools and some middle schools have installed metal detectors at their doors to prevent weapons from coming into the schools. Legislatures have passed harsh laws to deal with children who bring guns into the schools (i.e., they must be expelled) (see Chapter 2, this volume). Massive amounts of money have been spent on support teams, psychological testing, in-service training for teachers, special education projects, and segregation of children with behavioral problems. Overprescription of psychostimulants is common for youths whose behavior is difficult, some of whom may not even have attention-deficit/hyperactivity disorder (ADHD). Often, school teachers and administrators, particularly in the inner city, "give up" and "write off" these youths. Their antagonism in their battles with the these students intensifies, and they tend to develop methods of controlling the class that are clearly self-protective and not useful in creating a true learning environment.

There are a great many schools where well-intentioned faculty try to work together to try to address specific problems of children and adolescents. But, because there has not been cooperation among various agencies, these teachers feel unsupported when they cannot get help for a child who is in trouble. They often feel that their hands are tied, that they have no tools, and that they were not trained to work with children with such severe behavioral and emotional problems.

CHILDREN'S LIFE EXPERIENCES AND THE SCHOOL

One small anecdote may be helpful in demonstrating the nature and extent of the problem of school violence. Two days after the shootings in Littleton, Colorado, a father went into the bedroom of his 7-year-old son and found him crying. He asked what was wrong and the child answered, "I don't want to go to school." The father asked why, and the child answered, "Because I might get killed." This family lives in an affluent area of the city, a safe area, where there is very little crime or disturbance compared with what one finds in other parts of the city (see Chapters 1 and 7, this volume). This child's response clearly relates to the repeated imagery that all kids see on television of body bags; bloodied, wounded children; children running and screaming; parents crying; and everyone expressing pain in reaction to the violent event. Events like the Columbine shootings become part of a much broader socialization of children, so that children learn from the environment things that most adults would rather they did not learn and that many adults do not know they are learning. This fear, accidentally uncovered by this caring and loving father, might have passed by unnoticed and merely been absorbed into the private world of this child.

Children transport the violence they see at home to the schoolyard. The problem of bullies has been around for a long time. But the nature of the bully's behavior and the response of the children who are bullied are important to observe (see Chapter 15, this volume). Part of what must be done if we are going to reduce violence in schools is to drastically reduce domestic violence. There are suggestions in the literature that one form of abuse in a household is a good predictor of the presence of another form (Browne and Finkelhor 1986, pp. 143–179; Finkelhor et al. 1983, p. 22). At least half the men who abuse their wives also abuse their children. Mothers are eight times more likely to hurt their children when they are in battering relationships than when they are in nonbattering relationships.

Research indicates that the effects of children's witnessing domestic violence are varied. Among the many things we know, however, are that these children often take on the responsibility for the abuse of their parent, bear a tremendous anxiety that another beating will occur, have guilt for not being able to stop the abuse or for loving the abuser, blame themselves for not preventing the violence or possibly for causing it, and have an enormous fear of abandonment. The personal, internal disasters that the children experience are innumerable, including regression, eating disorders, excessive compliance, aggression, attachment disorders, somatic complaints, depression, anxiety disorders, weakened academic performance, truancy, and delinquency (see Chapter 5, this volume). Although we know, scientifically, through many studies, that domestic violence has these effects, we also should understand that the school staff may have no knowledge that such violence is happening at home and may be totally unaware of the stress and distress that the child brings to school with him or her every day.

In recent times, trauma theory has become a major part of our scientific effort to understand human behavior. Although the idea that trauma results in emotional problems was one of the cornerstones of Freud's early thinking, this conceptualization fell into disfavor; only in the last 10–15 years has the idea been revived through the development of a better understanding of how trauma affects children. Similar work by Finkelhor et al. (1983), Putnam (1996), Straus (1994), and many others have demonstrated how traumatic events, including physical, sexual, and emotional abuse of children, have a profound, long-term effect on the way children operate. Witnessing trauma is also known to have long-term effects: children who witness abuse of their parents, murders, and deaths often become disturbed, withdrawn, or delinquent in adolescence (see Chapters 2, 3, and 8, this volume).

In recent times, because of the extraordinary advances in technology, such as positron emission tomography (PET), the discovery that traumatic events, including witnessing trauma, change brain chemistry also has allowed us to think differently about how development changes behavior. In two seminal studies, Baxter et al. (1996) and Brody et al. (1998) discovered that two samples of patients with obsessive-compulsive disorder, one treated with psychotherapy and the other treated with drugs, had the same brain changes after successful treatment. This discovery changed the arguments based on the dichotomies of nature versus nurture and genetics versus development, to acknowledge that genetics and development simultaneously contribute to children's behavior and build on each other.

In minority communities, children often are traumatized daily and see things that most adults have never seen. In some classrooms, large percentages of the children indicate that they have seen shootings and murders. In one class that I visited, every child in the class talked about hearing gunshots every night, while fearing and ultimately sensing that they were not safe. African American males in particular have a sense that they are not going to survive through their youth to any life beyond. Feeling afraid and angry and expecting to die before they reach adulthood is a common clinical finding in my experience.

I once had the opportunity to chair a panel with eight children: two white boys, two white girls, two African American boys, and two African American girls. At one point, when each of them was talking about their future, one of the African American boys said, "I am going to be a businessman, if I make it." For 12-year-olds, thinking "if I make it" has a devastating effect on self-esteem, ambition, and the resulting expectation that life will be good and will take them into some powerful and positive space. This devastating remark from a 12-year-old—one that shows he is already feeling that his life may not last and that there is a tentative quality to his world—is in contrast to the experience of those of us who grew up never doubting for a moment that we would be able to fulfill every dream and anticipating reaching an optimistic end to great expectations for a full and happy life. "If I make it" is not an idea that most middle-aged and older people ever thought of when they were growing up. It was not "if I make it," it was "when I make it." It was not "maybe I'll live to see my 20th birthday," it was "I am going to live forever." The idea of dying was not part of the general ethos of children with this hopeful sense of a future. Many children are "throwaways"; they grow up in poverty and they never feel valued. The task of adults in our society is to make children feel safe at home, on the streets, and in school. That does not happen with regularity in inner-city areas or some rural areas, or in every corner of the nation.

SOCIAL FACTORS RELATED TO SCHOOLS

In today's world, many schools, particularly in lower- and lower-middle-class neighborhoods, have a large number of disturbed, disruptive, withdrawn, and traumatized children. The neighborhoods from which these schools draw have large numbers of single-parent homes and a significant amount of poverty. But children with these problems are found not just in economically disadvantaged areas. In almost every part of America, there are significant numbers of latchkey children. The high divorce rate speaks to antagonism between parents, resulting in a great deal of domestic violence as opposed to tranquility. Children and their parents—and children and adults in general—have difficulty communicating with each other. As a result, teachers are spending more and more time trying to calm children and to develop order so they can teach.

Changes in the value system in our nation have altered the way children view school. Respect for teachers, once automatic, has diminished, and this erosion of respect, in some cases, has aided and abetted truancy. These developments have led to a cadre of teachers who are less interested in the children and more often angry and frustrated. School districts often offer only punitive solutions.

In Philadelphia, as in many other cities, the usual and prevailing method of dealing with difficult and disruptive children during the past three decades was to move them to another school, suspend them, or expel them. These methods are still frequently used. No effort is made to understand why the child is behaving badly. There are no collaborative efforts with other agencies that could help the schools to deal more appropriately, therapeutically, and reparatively with children with damaged lives. We also have to take into consideration the great unknowns: How many children in each class were born with cocaine addiction or fetal alcohol syndrome? Was the child a victim of the parents' drug use? Does the child have biological impairment that might be a part of the behavioral problem?

SOLUTIONS TO SCHOOL VIOLENCE

Addressing the problem of school violence and finding a solution are based on the following two overriding premises. First, agencies must collaborate with members of the school faculty and the school administration, with a maximum of communication, to foster an understanding that education will not take place where there is anxiety, emotional disturbance, or fear of being unsafe and in danger. Second, there must be a communal agenda, similar to the agenda in therapy, with the underlying assumption that if all parties—schools, parents, children, public agencies, private groups, and volunteers—work together in the best interests of the children, the results will be dramatically different.

A good example of such a collaborative approach is the Alternative Learning Center that I developed at a middle school in Philadelphia. Previously, the room where the center was established had been used generally for in-house detention and was called "the time-out room." Upon first entering the room, I saw children lined up doing busywork, filling out problem papers, and the teacher was reading the newspaper in the corner. The students and teacher did not look at each other, nor did they speak to each other. As a psychiatrist, I believed that this was an extraordinary waste. Here were children who had gotten into trouble and no one was talking to them, either about what they were feeling, why they had caused disruption, or what their reaction was to the generally punitive environment. It was clear that in this dark and dreary room they were essentially neglected.

The principal of the school and I worked to turn the room into the Alternative Learning Center. She made the room brighter and more inviting and furnished it differently. We selected teachers with enormous amounts of empathy and the capacity to relate emotionally to the children. The busywork was set aside; instead, the children and the teacher engaged in a group discussion on values, affects, problems, and issues that were burning in these children's minds but that they had never openly discussed. The result was a series of important changes in the way these children behaved in the school. The children learned that the two teachers at the center were their friends. When the students did have problems, they could go to these teachers, with or without being assigned to the Alternative Learning Center.

Getting everybody on the same page may be the most important thing we can do in changing the nature of the schools. A collaborative approach will enable us to get away from the belief that the only purpose of schools is reading, writing, and arithmetic and to develop a rapport that is more akin to the twenty-first century than to the nineteenth century.

SPECIFIC EFFORTS TO PREVENT SCHOOL VIOLENCE

The Philadelphia Story

The central focus of the Philadelphia experience is the establishment of the Youth Homicide Committee, an interdisciplinary group interested in understanding the murders of children. As chairman of this committee, I have met monthly with other committee members for the past 5 years to examine the death of every child and adolescent under age 22 years in Philadelphia. Our purpose was to see if, first, the murder was preventable and, second, any public policy changes should be made as a result of what was learned.

Addressing Truancy

Among the first things we learned is that one of the earliest indicators of trouble in almost every child who was either a victim or a perpetrator of homicide was truancy. As a result of that finding, and working through the District Attorney's office and the courts, we were able to convince the Administrative Judge of Juvenile Court to expand the truancy hearings from 2 days a month to 4 days a week. The hearings were decentralized to the schools—a change that allowed teachers and parents to attend the hearings more easily.

This cooperative effort between the courts and the schools was the beginning of a new era in which both groups could take credit for greater attention to those kids who were not in school. Up to that time, the teachers and the schools heaved a sigh of relief when a disruptive and difficult child was not in school. Now, the sense was that it was their duty to educate these children and that a new approach was needed. The willingness of the court and the schools to put out a great deal of effort and money into addressing truancy changed the situation.

At the end of the first year of decentralization of truancy hearings, which certainly was not complete, the results were phenomenal. The city went from 2,000 hearings a year to 10,000 hearings. The threshold of absenteeism was reduced from 50 days to 25 days. After 1 year, 4,000 more children attended school *each day* than in the year before.

As the success of this venture became more evident, the police decided to join in and began to pick up kids on the streets or in the subways who were not in school. A central location for the police to take these children to was designated by the school district, or the police could take the children to the children's own school if it was close by. The result has been a quiet but cooperative link between the school district and the police that was not seen before.

The most important effect was that the entire faculty in the school district felt that truancy court had become effective instead of ineffective and accessible rather than inaccessible.

Dealing With Gun-Carrying Youths

It was clear to the Youth Homicide Committee that guns were the most frequent cause of deaths—more than 80% of children and adolescents killed were killed with guns (see Chapter 11, this volume). Efforts to deal with guns in Philadelphia were weak until the mayor and the police department made a real push to address the problems of straw purchases (i.e., sale of guns illegally to minors and others who cannot get a license to purchase) and illegal availability of guns. A number of high schools have installed metal detectors, and the number with such equipment will triple over the next 2 years.

It became clear that something had to be done with children and adolescents who were extremely violent and who scared the rest of the student body and the teachers. To address this problem, we developed a program called VUFA (Violation of the Uniform Firearms Act) for youths who were first-time offenders caught with a gun. VUFA is an intensive educational program with 30 hours of training in the consequences of gun carrying, which includes a trip to the morgue, 40 hours of community service, and assignment of a mentor. Assignment to this program was in lieu of the previous approach, namely, assignment to an overworked probation officer who already had many and more serious cases. In the past, the youth was essentially neglected and often went on to bigger and more serious crimes.

The VUFA has been extraordinarily successful. Of the first 50 youth in the program during the first year, 47 had no offenses after the training period. For those of us who know that these children and adolescents generally escalate their negative behavior, the results of this program seemed too good to be true.

Identifying Children and Adolescents at Risk

Statistics on the 1995 group of children who were victims or perpetrators of homicide reviewed by the Philadelphia Youth Homicide Committee have some interesting implications. Eighty percent of the perpetrators and 52% of the decedents (the percentages were this low because infants and small children were included) had been arrested at least once between ages 10 and 14. It was clear to the committee members that we needed to identify at-risk children earlier. We needed to deal with children who were disruptive in kindergarten, first, second, and third grades. If some were already being arrested in fifth grade, they clearly would have been identifiable prior to that time.

One program that resulted from these statistics is *middle-school summits*. The School District of Philadelphia is divided into 22 clusters: one for each high school, its feeder junior high schools, and the elementary schools feeding into those junior high schools. In the Audenreid Cluster, I was able to work with the cluster leader to involve all 11 schools in a project that ostensibly was intended to identify at-risk children but that has had many other benefits. The Audenreid Cluster contains two middle schools. At each of these middle schools, we organized a monthly meeting that is attended by the counselors and other school personnel, such as school nurses, assistant principals, and principals from the middle school and the feeder elementary schools; a representative from the high school also attends. Also attending these meetings, in addition to myself as the moderator, are representatives from the Department of Human Services, the local community mental health center, the Student Assistance Program, probation department, and other neighborhood agencies that are working in the schools to address the needs of children and adolescents.

A counselor from any of the schools can present a case to the group. The group then sets up a treatment plan. Not all children need mental health treatment. Many other aspects, such as an educational plan, are included in the treatment plan. For the most part, we end up further investigating the child, the family, the home, the circumstances of the misbehavior, and his or her aggressiveness and try to resolve these problems by assigning specific persons to work on interventions. The number of children actually discussed is small; the results are much larger. We discuss approximately 60 children a year at these two summits, 3 at each summit per month for 10 months.

The most important thing we have done is empowering the schools to resolve problems in a positive direction on their own. The summits have helped the schools learn to know the members of their local community mental health center or the Department of Human Services supervisor, make calls directly around and beyond the usual bureaucratic approaches, and, most important, assume that there is a positive solution for the children if efforts are put forward more meaningfully. For instance, a child was prescribed methylphenidate for ADHD, but the parents did not fill the prescription, failed to regularly medicate the child, and would not bring the medication to school for the nurse to dispense. We resolved this problem by establishing that the parents' actions were considered medical neglect and having the Department of Human Services worker tell the parents that if they did not comply, the child would be removed from the home. Believe it or not, that was never a way the school had addressed such problems. Often the nurse would complain to the principal, who would throw up his hands in disgust, and the child would continue to be hyperactive and disruptive.

Replication of the summit project in the other 21 clusters in Philadelphia is constantly being discussed. Visitors from other clusters come to the meetings to see how the summit works. Efforts to either replicate our method or develop a new method are being made at the school level, at the cluster level, and at the district level. Helping children rather than continuing to let them deteriorate is an important process in addressing not only the emotional but the sociocultural, family, and community problems that plague communities and our youths.

What is important for us to realize is that these programs that appear to less directly involve the schools are critical to making the schools safer places where education can take place. They should not be seen as irrelevant to the child psychiatry community. While the major goal of the Youth Homicide Committee is saving children's lives, the approaches are multiple and the effort is global. Reducing the number of kids out on bench warrants who obviously are not attending school was a task undertaken by the Youth Homicide Committee in cooperation with the courts and the District Attorney's Office. This effort resulted in clearing hundreds, if not thousands, of kids on bench warrants and not only locating them but also, in some cases, returning them to the community.

Interdisciplinary programs and interagency efforts such as I.C.E. Violence (I Can End Violence) are an important part of what we do. In 1998, the staff at I.C.E. Violence, an interdisciplinary volunteer organization consisting of representatives of a significant number of community-based agencies, addressed 42,000 children in the schools on issues of violence and safety.

Efforts of the Philadelphia City Council and the Department of Recreation to address one of the other factors discovered at the Youth Homicide Committee resulted in a significant change. The committee looked at the time of day when youth acted out or got killed; we found that homicides occurred most frequently between 3:00 P.M. and 8:00 P.M. (see Chapter 4, this volume). In response to these findings, the Department of Recreation developed 150 after-school programs in its recreation centers over a 1-year period—a significant intervention that will definitely save lives.

Finally, it became clear that disruptive families who essentially are unavailable to children who are very needy were helped by the involvement of mentors. The city already had a good mentoring program for kids who showed promise, but few mentoring services were available for children who were disruptive and difficult. In cooperation with the Philadelphia Bar Association and the School District's Volunteer Program, an attorney mentoring program was developed. Sixty attorneys, 10 for each of six middle schools, were matched with children who the schools felt needed some help. The result has been a massive educational program within the legal community that addresses the kinds of problems these children and adolescents face before they appear in court and before they get into serious legal difficulties.

The New Haven Program

A decade ago, Steve Marans and his colleagues at the Yale Child Study Center developed a program called the Police Mental Health Collaboration in New Haven (Marans et al. 1995) (see Chapter 2, this volume). This program was started to address the immediate needs of children who had been traumatized. In a cooperative effort between the police and the child mental health community, children who had witnessed serious trauma were seen immediately, in situ. They were evaluated and their needs were assessed. This program was incredibly successful. Not only did it deal with the serious problem of children's witnessing trauma (with changes in a child's brain starting within 72 hours of the event), but it led to a massive education of the entire police department with regard to mental health and sociocultural issues. It also led to an exchange that allowed the police to speak freely about the distress they feel, the difficulties of their job, and the inability to move from their major purpose, law enforcement and crime investigation, to what in their minds is a much less serious issue, the child who witnesses the act of violence. Marans et al.'s (1995) book *The Police–Mental Health Partnership*, in which they describe the New Haven program, has led to efforts to replicate their work in many places around the country, and Marans and his associates have helped communities in developing similar collaborative efforts.

New Haven started the program with a grant of $350,000 from the federal government and was able to gradually go about the process of educating the police before implementing the project. In Philadelphia, where we tried to do it without any funding and with volunteers, it was very difficult to get the project under way. The participating parties were unable to put in the necessary energy and effort with no funds available to pay for people's time and no central office to report the findings and make recommendations for treatment.

What first alerted the Youth Homicide Committee to the need for something like the New Haven program was a case discussed at one of our meetings. A 28-year-old man entered an apartment and shot and killed his lover and her 16-year-old sister. During our discussion, it was discovered that the 7-year-old brother had been in the room during the murders and had witnessed this horror. As we went around the room to see if any of the agencies had ever had contact with the brother or if the school had any record that this child had received help, we found no evidence that anyone had been involved in helping this child. This child's plight alerted us to the need for some community effort to deal with children who are harmed in this way.

In most cases, when children who witness a trauma return to school, no one in the school is aware of what has occurred. The children often have no way to communicate their distress. The teacher may notice that there is a slight change in behavior—a withdrawal and more negative activity or complaints of physical illness—but no real effort is made to determine whether the child has been hurt in some way, as either the victim of or a witness to violence. We must keep in mind that 70% of men who beat their wives also beat their children. Children injured in this way cannot learn and are distracted from their major purpose in being in school.

In Tucson, Arizona, for over 25 years, the community has used volunteers to go to the site of traumatic events and deal with issues faced by children and their families while the police are conducting the investigation. This project has become a sophisticated operation, having its own vehicles and a cadre of more than 1,000 volunteers on which to draw. Whether done by paid staff members or by trained volunteers, the effort is important because something has to be done about the festering pain experienced by traumatized children that effects serious personality changes.

Yale also produced Jim Comer and his extraordinary activity in designing and evaluating school-based mental health clinics (Comer 1980). This innovative and far-sighted idea has still not been universally adopted, although it is of great value for children in need and at risk. Some school districts have established school-based mental health clinics, and it is hoped that this concept will be understood as a vital and cost-saving use of resources (see Chapter 2, this volume).

The difficulty is that even when inner-city children have access to mental health services, frequently they are merely evaluated and actual therapy is scarce. Development of working relationships among a psychiatrist, clinic personnel, the school nurse, faculty, and administrators makes treatment more informed and, it is hoped, more successful. Among the new careers for both psychiatrists and clinical psychologists is working in schools as consultants or in school-based mental health clinics.

The Chicago Plan

Chicago has been blessed with Carl Bell, M.D., and other activist psychiatrists and psychologists who have worked diligently for more than a decade to make significant changes in the school system and in the way children's emotional and behavioral problems are handled at the school and community levels (see Chapter 13, this volume). They also have had the benefit of a direct collaboration with the superintendent of schools in a huge school district and have made enormous strides by developing an array of approaches to address serious problems (C. Bell, S. Gamm, P. Vallas, et al.: "Strategies for the Prevention of Youth Violence," unpublished Chicago Public Schools report, 1999). Dr. Bell, who manages a community mental health center, has been able to rally the mental health community to work with the school community so that children who need care can get it. In many communities, evaluations are in abundance, but minimal or no treatment is available. We know that the children have problems, but we do not find effective ways to deal with those problems.

Chicago's Violence Prevention Strategic Plan frames violence as a public health issue and contains a coordinated and a systematic citywide approach to combating the disease. Consistent with this approach, Chicago Public Schools (CPS) has developed multidisciplinary strategies to ensure that schools and communities are safe for children and youth. These strategies utilize community-based and governmental resources that transcend those traditionally used by schools to address today's realities. By implementing the following violence prevention strategies, CPS plays a central, stabilizing role in the community and enables schools to serve as a safe environment for serious learning.

Segregating troubled and violent youths into learning disabled and emotionally disturbed classes, though useful in terms of having them in smaller groups with highly educated teachers and separating them from other, nondisruptive kids so that the latter can have a more intensive learning experience, is not sufficient. What Chicago has done is bring the mental health community into the schools, and the schools have welcomed the development of a significant number of projects to help children who are in trouble, who create trouble, and who augment an antagonism that festers in both the children and the faculty.

The Boston Experience

Perhaps no other city has done more to develop a safe environment for children through the cooperation of public agencies than Boston (see Chapter 2, this volume). In what has been called the "Boston Miracle," the city was able to reduce the murders of children under the age of 18 to zero for 2½ years. This effort has led many representatives from other cities to go to Boston to see what the city did and how it was able to make the streets safe for children and make the police, courts, probation, and other public safety agencies credible in the community so that the community could trust them. The results are clearly evident, not only in the reduction in murders but in the way in which the community now looks and reacts when traumatic events occur.

Two people, a very dedicated police sergeant and his friend, a valued and long-term probation officer, decided they would ride together in the evening and pick up adolescents who were breaking their probation by being out on the street. The premise was simple: the police officer could arrest, but the probation officer could not; the probation officer knew who was on probation, but the police officer did not. Up until this seminal event, probation officers worked from 8:00 A.M. to 4:00 P.M., and the police were on duty 24 hours a day. Now, with this effort, called the Police/Probation Sweep, changes could take place that would ensure the safety of not only the probationers but also the community. The kids were delighted, although they could not admit it, to have the probation officer say, "Get off the street." They could then tell their friends they could not come out because the probation officer was around and would put them back in jail.

Although impossible to describe in its entirety, the Boston activity was a combination of FBI-like intelligence; street workers engaged diligently with the kids and the police; the faith community, which got rid of the "race card" (by viewing the issue in terms of law-abiding citizens vs. criminals) and fought the drug activity in the inner city; and an enormous cooperative effort among police, probation, and the courts.

Every big city in America would give anything to have the kind of record that Boston has established. Zero murders of children on the streets and from guns, reduction in the visibility of the drug trade, and availability of the open air and the streets to the children—all these effects do appear to be miraculous. But these results were possible only through massive cooperation and a belief that if people spoke to one another, worked with one another, and filled in the enormous bureaucratic gaps that can occur in these kinds of situations, changes would take place.

The Hawaii Experience

Although the following story about what happened in Hawaii may seem to have nothing to do with school-based efforts to help children, it is included in this chapter because addressing the needs of children only after they reach school age may be insufficient to resolve the problems appropriately.

The most important primary prevention for violence is good parenting. The availability of someone who loves the child and understands child development enough that he or she does not run counter to the normal and expected needs and behaviors of infants and children is an extremely valuable premise on which to address antiviolence efforts for children in the community long before they get to school. The success of Head Start programs shows that if we can get to children when they are preschool age instead of waiting until they enter school at age five, we will make tremendous advances in changing their lives.

The work of Dr. Henri Parens and colleagues (Parens et al. 1993), in his psychoanalytic approach to parenting education, demonstrates, albeit in a small sample, that miraculous changes can take place in at-risk children.

These children will avoid many of the damaging events of adolescence and will lead successful lives.

In the Hawaii Healthy Start program, systematic hospital-based screening was established to identify 90% of high-risk families of newborns from a specific geographic area. Using a list of risk indicators developed by the Hawaii Family Stress Center, the early-identification workers analyzed the records of eligible mothers. If a screened record was positive, the mother was interviewed by a worker who had been intensively trained.

Risk indicators used in the early identification process were

1. Marital status (single, separated, divorced)
2. Unemployed partner
3. Inadequate income (per patient) or no information regarding source of income
4. Unstable housing
5. No phone
6. Education under 12 years
7. Inadequate emergency contacts (e.g., no immediate family contacts)
8. History of substance abuse
9. Late (after 12 weeks) or no prenatal care
10. History of abortions
11. History of psychiatric care
12. Abortion unsuccessfully sought or attempted
13. Relinquishment through adoption sought or attempted
14. Marital or family problems
15. History of or current depression

Mothers who looked as if they were potential child abusers because they fit some or all aspects of this pattern were visited at home in the first week postnatally. The visits continued if there appeared to be some danger of disruption, frustration, or abuse by the mother.

Since implementation of the Hawaii Healthy Start program, child abuse has been reduced by 80% in the state of Hawaii. Although seemingly incredible, this figure has been validated, and the Hawaii experience is clearly an important lesson in terms of primary prevention. Children who are not violated are children who function reasonably well in school.

Most parents raise their children the way they themselves were raised. If they were raised with shame, then they will shame their children; if they were raised with brutality, they will be brutal to their children. Ninety-five percent of Americans hit their children, and 52% continue to hit those children into adolescence. Yet people in general seem surprised that children are treated so badly. Using techniques of shame, humiliation, guilt, demeaning remarks, lack of encouragement, and failure to respond to good things, parents dominate and overcontrol their children. The greater the fear parents have that their children will either repeat their own mistakes or become wild and uncontrollable in adolescence, the more assiduous they become in trying to overcontrol and dominate their 2-, 3-, or 4-year-old. Although discipline in general is not abuse, some discipline can be very abusive; in these cases, the parent may harm the child, sometimes to the point of killing him or her.

When rage in a child is unrequited, unresolved, and not followed by loving, caring, hugging, and caressing from parents, I believe it accumulates and is dissipated in a number of pathological ways. In many, it becomes stored up to be displaced in adolescence on any unsuspecting "weaker" victim. For some, this pattern of behavior lasts for a lifetime. For others, it is transformed into psychosomatic illness, masochism, depression, and a variety of other psychopathological conditions essentially ruinous to human beings. Even those born with the best temperaments can be filled with rage if they grow up in a loveless home.

In Philadelphia, we are attempting to find a way to increase our capacity to provide excellent parenting education. Such education must take into account not only the psychodynamic understanding of child development but also the problems faced by parents with few parenting skills and little knowledge about kids. Through this education process, it is hoped that these parents will learn to be more loving toward their children. Keep in mind Spitz's admonition that children raised without love will become adults filled with hate. It is necessary to reduce the need for parents to overcontrol children at the wrong ages and to reduce cognitive dissonance between children and parents, as well as find a way to train people to be more physically loving and emotionally supportive.

The Hawaii Healthy Start program gives hope that we can find ways to get into the lives of people with minimal knowledge of childrearing. Several years ago, the Pew Foundation issued a report on parenting education that was almost entirely related to family support (Carter and Kahn 1996). It had very little to do with parenting education. It was clear that even an agency of this importance in the country was unable to understand the difference between food, clothing, and shelter and the socioemotional needs of children. It is important that we as child psychiatrists, psychologists, and other professionals trained with extensive knowledge of children and child development enter the fray and find a way to work with parents at every level to enhance their knowledge of children and their capacity to parent well.

While the often-used euphemism "increase parent involvement" covers everything from holding parent-teacher association meetings to paying parents to be hall monitors in the schools, it does not really address the needs of the child or the parent-child relationship. Efforts that do not address these needs are not forms of primary prevention and, of course, do not result in lasting change.

CONCLUSION

The basic premises on which school and preschool interventions for school violence need to be developed are as follows:

1. Parenting education is the most important element in primary prevention for future violence, disturbance, and antisocial behavior. Child mental health professionals can play a major role in this area.
2. The major task of adults in the community is to make sure that the child is safe at home, on the streets, and in schools.
3. The earlier at-risk children can be identified and their needs addressed, the more likely it is that we will have a safer community and a population of adolescents who will be less likely to commit murder, be antisocial, and undermine the community.
4. The most important principle in addressing the needs of schoolchildren is that schools cannot do it alone. Maximizing cooperation between the schools and public and private agencies in the community, including the mental health community, is essential to finding appropriate and effective solutions to the extraordinary problems confronting thousands of schools across America.
5. Empathy, remorse, and a good conscience cannot be developed in adolescence. Children who kill apparently have no conscience and no remorse and do not understand the enormity of taking another person's life. Parenting education, which includes the capacity for parents to give love and care, is essential for the growth and development of infants and children.
6. Communication, cooperation, and collaboration are the major ingredients of any program's efforts—whether by the schools alone or by the schools in cooperation with social service agencies, public safety agencies, and nongovernmental agencies. Those involved must desire to work together to help children grow up with an interest in education and a willingness to work hard to achieve.

The bottom line for dealing with disruptive and difficult children in schools is that the community must work together with a sense of optimism and a determination to succeed. The mental health community, including child psychiatrists, must move out of their offices into schools and into community agencies related to the schools to guide children in a lust for life, an expectation and hope that life will be fulfilling, and a willingness to work hard in order to achieve.

REFERENCES

Baxter LR Jr, Saxena S, Brody AL, et al: Brain mediation of obsessive-compulsive disorder symptoms: evidence from functional brain imaging studies in the human and nonhuman primate. Seminars in Clinical Neuropsychiatry 1:32–47, 1996

Brody AL, Saxena S, Schwartz JM, et al: FDG-PET predictors of response to behavioral therapy and pharmacotherapy in obsessive-compulsive disorder. Psychiatry Res 84:1–6, 1998

Browne A, Finkelhor D: Initial and long-term effects of sexual abuse, in A Sourcebook on Child Sexual Abuse. Edited by Finkelhor D. Beverly Hills, CA, Sage, pp 143–179

Carter N, Kahn L: See How We Grow: A Report on Parenting Education in the United States. Report Prepared for the Pew Charitable Trust, 1996

Comer JP: School Power: Implications of School Based Clinics. New York, Free Press, 1980

Finkelhor D, Gelles RJ, Hotaling GT, et al (eds): The Dark Side of Families: Current Family Violence Research. Newbury Park, CA, Sage, 1983

Marans S, Adnopoz J, Berkman M, et al: The Police–Mental Health Partnership: A Community-Based Response to Urban Violence. New Haven, CT, Yale University Press, 1995

Parens H, Bockoven D, Goldberg-Moore L: Prevention/Early Intervention Parent-Child Groups Follow-Up Study: Preliminary Report. Philadelphia, Department of Psychiatry, Medical College of Pennsylvania, 1993

Putnam FW: Child and adolescent posttraumatic stress disorder, in American Psychiatric Press Annual Review of Psychiatry, Vol 15. Edited by Dickstein LJ, Riba MB, Oldham JM. Washington, DC, American Psychiatric Press, 1996, pp 447–468

Spitz R: The First Year of Life. New York, International Universities, 1965

Straus MA: Beating the Devil Out of Them: Corporal Punishment in American Families. New York, Lexington Books, 1994

Strategies for the Prevention of Youth Violence in Chicago Public Schools

CARL C. BELL, M.D., F.A.C.PSYCH.
SUE GAMM, J.D.
PAUL VALLAS, M.A.
PHILLIP JACKSON, B.A.

Recently, the incidence of youngsters killing and wounding others in school has appalled the nation. Although a tragedy of this nature has not taken place in the city of Chicago, there is no question that Chicago youths experience violence in the community (Jenkins and Bell 1994). In mid-1995, the School Reform Board of Trustees took over the leadership of the Chicago Public Schools (CPS) and began to develop infrastructure and policies to help improve CPS education and to provide an environment that would allow students to learn. As a part of this effort, in 1998, the CPS began to implement its multidisciplinary violence prevention strategies to ensure that schools and communities are safe for youth. These strategies use community-based and governmental resources to transcend the traditional role of schools to address today's realities. By setting up the following violence prevention strategies, CPS plays a central, stabilizing role in the community and enables schools to be a safe environment for serious learning.

The purpose of this chapter is to underscore the principles necessary for any successful health behavior intervention. The principles highlighted here are rebuilding the village; providing access to health care; improving bonding, attachment, and connectedness dynamics within the community and between stakeholders; improving self-esteem; increasing social skills of target recipients; reestablishing the adult protective shield; and reducing the residual effects of trauma.

REBUILDING THE VILLAGE

In delivering public health interventions in communities that lack a well-developed social infrastructure, there has to be a facilitator that helps to develop community infrastructures by "rebuilding the village," that is, developing community partnerships and coalitions. Figure 13–1 illustrates how any player can bring other players to the table to build a vision of a healthier community (U.S. Department of Health and Human Services 1998). In this instance, the player who brought the other players to the table was the CPS and its leadership.

The CPS strategy involves partnering with community-based secular and nonsecular organizations to foster programmatic activities designed to reduce violent and disruptive behavior by and against youth in the schools and surrounding communities. Increasing parental involvement in school and increasing parental collaboration with school personnel have great potential in reducing risk of in-school violence (Elliott and Tolan 1999). Thus, CPS designed these partnerships to share the vision of a violence-free environment.

Partnership With Religious Community

By partnering with the religious community, CPS has increased attendance, improved school environments, provided positive role models, and created activities for youth. CPS provides support to religious school-community partnership networks in each of the CPS regions. Through these partnerships, CPS helps coordinate antiviolence marches with religious communities throughout the city. In addition, the network of secular and nonsecular organizations provides assistance in mentoring programs, off-site detention and community service programs, and after-school homework centers. One example of these partnerships is the CPS Near North Ministerial Alliance. The CPS Near North Ministerial Alliance Prevention Program is a community-based plan to reduce crime and violence in Cabrini Green schools. This program's intervention and prevention activities include efforts designed to ensure that youths comply with curfew laws

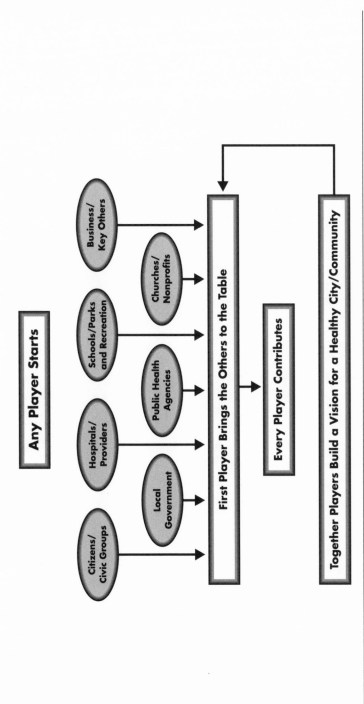

FIGURE 13–1.   Building a vision for a healthy community.
Source.   Reprinted from U.S. Department of Health and Human Services: *Healthy People in Healthy Communities: A Guide for Community Leaders.* Washington, DC, Office of Public Health and Sciences, Office of Disease and Health Promotion, U.S. Department of Health and Human Services, June 1998.

and procedures to reduce gang activity. The program also offers tutoring, family strengthening services, and social services. Further, a "Walking School Bus" recruits individuals to escort children to and from school.

Safe Schools, Safe Neighborhoods Summer

As part of the Safe Schools, Safe Neighborhoods Summer 1998 initiatives, CPS partnered with the community in developing the CPS Youth Outreach Workers program. This effort trained 100 violence intervention program specialists, comprising off-duty police, community members, parents, teachers, and social workers, to provide positive, alternative activities for youths in high-crime areas. Also, a newly created referral service network directed follow-up services for more than 2,000 referrals for recreational activities, job preparation, job orientation, job placement, gang detachment, and housing relocation over the summer. Follow-up services were also provided for referrals for suicide ideation. In addition, CPS youth outreach workers participated in collaborative partnerships with more than 50 governmental and city agencies and community-based organizations.

School-Community Activities

CPS has developed many school-community programs and activities, especially for schools in communities that experience high rates of violence. One example of such efforts is the CPS Logan Square Neighborhood Association, one of whose goals is to create up to five community learning centers to serve families in adult education, children and youth education, and recreational programming. The association also provides homework assistance, child care, and other family-focused activities. The Logan Square Neighborhood Association has trained more than 400 parents for placement in classrooms, where they tutor children and help the teacher. Several other community councils and alliances, consisting of local churches, organizations, residents, schools, and law enforcement, have been formed. These collaborations are helping parents to coordinate violence prevention activities, facilitating hiring and training of parent patrols and parent attendance officers, and guiding development of evening sports programs. The purposes of these efforts are to increase safety of students, parents, and school staff; increase attendance; and create a learning environment. Another CPS effort in developing community partnerships is the CPS Region Anti-Violence Workshops. These regional workshops, held in the summer, address violence issues affecting schools and their surrounding communities.

Mission-Driven Philosophy

By emphasizing the shared vision, a facilitator can encourage a "mission-driven" philosophy. Within this framework, diverse elements within society are encouraged to adopt the mission and place it above less important personal driving forces. Our experience is that by emphasizing the ecological relations among diverse elements in a community, a good facilitator can encourage attachment/affiliative/approach behaviors between the various elements. Emphasizing ecological relations also encourages the development of systems thinking.

Theoretical support for the development of community partnerships comes from the observation that communities with social fabric have less violence (Sampson et al. 1997). Shaw and McKay (1942), in their social disorganization theory, proposed that limited job opportunities, poverty, single-headed households, isolation from neighbors, and weakened community friendship networks and community institutions lead to reduced informal and formal social control. Elliott and Tolan (1999) note that community organization efforts are producing promising results, although applying traditional scientific criteria to community organization experiments is difficult.

HEALTH CARE

Evidence suggests that children with high exposure to lead may be predisposed to violence (Earls 1991). Further, there is evidence that children with attention-deficit/hyperactivity disorder (ADHD) may be predisposed to violence and conduct disorder (Klein et al. 1997). ADHD also may predispose children to engaging in other high-risk behaviors such as drug abuse and early onset of sexual behavior (American Psychiatric Association 1994). There is additional evidence that neuropsychiatric disorders may predispose individuals to violence (Lewis et al. 1985; Moffitt 1997). Clearly, treatment for individuals with psychiatric or behavioral disorders that predispose them to engage in high-risk behaviors is essential in promoting violence prevention.

When neuropsychiatry becomes more sophisticated, psychiatric diagnosis of some causes of impulsive and violent behavior will become more specific. In addition, as neuropsychiatry becomes more sophisticated, psychiatric treatment of some causes of risky behaviors will become more specific. For example, we constantly are discovering more specific treatments for drug addiction (see, e.g., American Psychiatric Association 1996).

If the infrastructure necessary to provide more sophisticated services is not developed, communities with the greatest need will be the last to receive appropriate health care that can prevent some causes of risky health behaviors. Unfortunately, experience teaches us that epidemics move across society in waves by first affecting the disadvantaged and then moving into more advantaged populations. Therefore, no one is safe from behavioral epidemics. The only way we can all be safe is to address the inappropriate health behaviors in disadvantaged populations before these behaviors spread to other segments of society (see Chapter 1, this volume).

While CPS is mandated to educate children who have psychiatric or behavioral disorders, CPS has also stepped up efforts to ensure that children have access to primary health care and social services to promote healthy social and physical development. Accordingly, CPS developed Healthy Kids/Healthy Minds, a service that provides free hearing aids, eye examinations, and eye glasses for under- and uninsured students. It also provides dental screening and cleaning for all elementary students. In addition, linkages between 300 schools and social service and health agencies have been established.

In a pilot school-based outreach program of the U.S. Department of Education, called "Kid Care," CPS is collaborating with community health agencies and the Illinois Department of Public Aid to facilitate enrollment of children eligible for Medicaid and public children's health insurance. Expanded coverage and enrollment enables children greater access to school-community health and social services.

BONDING, ATTACHMENT, AND CONNECTEDNESS DYNAMICS

Bowlby (1973) and Ainsworth (1973) theorized that failure to form a secure attachment with caregivers during infancy has a strong influence on an individual's ability to form trusting relationships later in life. Meloy (1992) provided ample evidence that individuals lacking in secure attachments during infancy form violent attachments resulting in chronically violent relationships. Similarly, Renken et al. (1989) found that youths who engaged in aggressive behaviors were the most insecurely attached to their families. Pinderhughes (1972) outlined the importance of attachment behaviors in violence prevention and intervention efforts. Empirical studies reveal that children who are connected to their family and school engage in less risk taking (Resnick et al. 1997). Borduin et al. (1985) noted that improving intrafamily relations—closeness, positive statements, communication clarity, and emotional cohesion—can reduce risk of serious antisocial behavior and violence.

Low levels of cohesion and parental warmth, acceptance, and affection and high levels of conflict and hostilities are associated with delinquent and violent behavior (Farrington 1989; Henggeler et al. 1992; Tolan and Lorion 1988). Aggressive children show more "insecure" attachment styles (Booth et al. 1992). Further, there is an association between delinquency and weak attachment bonds to parents. Eron et al. (1991) found that parental rejection was strongly related to youths' later criminal outcomes. Conversely, McCord (1983) found that parental warmth and affection buffered boys from criminal behavior despite increased risk of criminal involvement due to environmental disadvantages.

This evidence supports the age-old paradigm of medicine that encourages the establishment of rapport with the patient and upholds the wisdom of the need for good relationships to effect violence prevention. CPS seeks to increase bonding, attachment, and connectedness dynamics in different ways (see Chapters 5 and 8, this volume). CPS provides an opportunity for parents and youth to become attached to each other. In addition, it provides successful educational opportunities for children and their parents, creating the basis for an "Ah ha" experience or a sense of personal mastery. This allows for the development of a strong bond with or attachment to the educational service provider, whether that function is carried out by a parent or the school.

Parents as Teachers First

The CPS has developed several programs to increase bonding, attachment, and connectedness dynamics between parents and CPS and between parents and their children. One program, Parents as Teachers First, called for CPS to hire 300 parents from 75 schools to act as parent-tutor mentors. These parents' function is to mentor other parents in the latter's homes to prepare preschoolers for kindergarten by providing developmentally appropriate activities. Thus, preschoolers obtain academically enriched opportunities, including attention to socially appropriate behavior, and many parents receive an employment opportunity. This program served more than 1,000 preschoolers in the 1999–2000 school year. Parents as Teachers First thus serves a dual function: connecting parents to CPS and helping parents connect to their children by helping parents provide academically enriched opportunities for their preschoolers.

Cradle to Classroom

Another CPS program, Cradle to Classroom, provides opportunities for parents to bond with their infants. This long-range prevention strategy allows infants to grow up with basic trust and security. Trust provides the groundwork for later relationships in life that may be necessary to prevent or to intervene in violence. In addition, many teenage women with children lose connection with school, and the strategy used in this program helps teenage mothers remain in school. In collaboration with the Chicago Department of Public Health, six hospitals, and other agencies for pregnant and parenting teens, Cradle to Classroom trains teens in the development of parenting skills and in accessing community resources. It provides counseling to new mothers around issues of domestic violence and provides access to prenatal, nutritional, medical, social, and child care services.

Since pregnancy is the primary reason for high school dropout among urban teenage women (Dryfoos 1990; Furstenberg et al. 1987), Cradle to Classroom has significantly reduced dropout rates of teenage moms in CPS; none of the females in the program have dropped out to date. In the 1998–1999 school year, 1,100 young women with babies were in CPS, and 228 of them graduated, with 100 going on to college. These young women only had one child, despite having the child at a very young age.

CPS has also expanded early childhood services by increasing the number of classrooms for preschool children. As a result, approximately 31,000 preschool children, including children with disabilities, are receiving educational services. Thus, more preschool children will receive educational services through contractual arrangements with 45 private and public community-based agencies. By providing quality preschool activities for all children, children have an easier time getting attached and connected to school. In addition, these early childhood services allow for the identification of children with attachment disorders by providing Early Intervention and Head Start programs.

School-Based Summer and Afterschool Programs

Another strategy the CPS is using to increase attachment and connectedness dynamics is expanding the school year. For example, during the summer of 1998, CPS began holding their largest school-based summer program for Chicago students. Academic programs provide intensive structured instruction for children who did not meet academic promotion standards, for children with significant disabilities, and for children with limited English proficiency. In addition, regional competition and camping experiences provide athletic and recreational opportunities.

Other efforts, such as the Lighthouse Program (funded in part by Ronald McDonald Children's Charities), include expanding the school day by providing structured academic activities and recreational activities, including a nutritional dinner, for children after regular hours. These efforts also have served to increase community partnerships with parental involvement. Additionally, all high schools and many elementary schools have competitive and noncompetitive athletic and sports programs after school.

In addition, CPS promotes the use of school uniforms. Each local school council is required to vote on whether to enact a uniform or dress code policy for the school. Seventy-five percent of Chicago public schools have started a uniform or dress code policy, a strategy that prevents students from wearing clothing that indicates gang affiliation, such as trench coats. Further, such efforts help to identify unfamiliar, out-of-uniform kids in the schools.

Truancy and Dropout Prevention

Efforts are also directed at increasing student attendance and reducing the youth dropout rate, since poor attendance and dropping out are indications a student is not connected to his or her school. Accordingly, to help in truancy prevention, CPS developed a 24-hour hotline that takes calls from individuals to identify youths who are truant from school or have other issues that impact education. CPS truancy prevention services consist of at least two truancy outreach workers at every high school who follow up on students who have unexcused absences. The outreach workers provide counseling services, visit and call youths and parents at home, and monitor attendance daily. Further, regional staff work with all schools to provide assistance in developing programs designed to improve student attendance. In addition, a CPS Hispanic dropout prevention program addresses the high dropout rate among Hispanic teens. The program offers alternative educational and extracurricular activities to all at-risk students at schools where at least 48% of the student population is Hispanic.

CPS has developed relationships with alternative schools for youths returning to school. Thirty schools organized in cooperation with community and social services agencies provide educational services for students who return to school after having dropped out. These schools provide small class sizes and support services through individual learning plans for each student. Most recently, evening programs at 23 of CPS's 79 high schools offer coursework for students who are over 16 years of age and are out of school.

TABLE 13–1. Chicago Public Schools end-of-year membership and attendance: 1993–1994 through 1997–1998

School year	End-of-year membership	End-of-year attendance, %
1993–1994	407,241	88.7
1994–1995	412,921	89.2
1995–1996[a]	421,334	89.6
1996–1997	428,184	91.1
1997–1998	431,085	91.5
1998–1999	431,750	90.9

[a]School reform began in the summer of 1995.
Source. Office of Accountability of the Chicago Public Schools.

Bonding and Attendance

Practitioners seeking to develop an ability to change health behaviors would do well to read "Differential Bonding," an article by Pinderhughes (1979). In that article, Pinderhughes clearly explains the psychophysiology of bonding and attachment behaviors and why these behaviors are so important in developing influence over people (see Chapter 5, this volume). Common sense tells us that trying to teach someone when there is no relationship or when there is a negative relationship is a very difficult undertaking. It is much easier to teach someone when a good relationship has been established.

Table 13–1, which presents the CPS end-of-year membership and attendance figures for the 1993–1994 through 1998–1999 school years, shows the improvement in attendance in CPS since the efforts of the School Reform Board of Trustees began in mid-1995.

SELF-ESTEEM

Self-esteem is a feeling that comes from a sense of power (i.e., a feeling of being competent to do what must be done); a sense of uniqueness (i.e., acknowledging and respecting the qualities and characteristics about oneself that are special and different); a sense of models (i.e., having models that can be used to make sense of the world); and a sense of being connected (i.e., a feeling of satisfaction from being connected to people, places, and things (Bean 1992). We propose that improving the target recipients' self-esteem is a critical component in any successful prevention/intervention strategy to change health behavior. Bell (1997) suggested that constructive activities help youths develop social skills and self-esteem that reduce engagement in risky behaviors. This principle firmly grounds the CPS's prevention and intervention initiative in the idea that efforts at violence prevention are necessary in order to improve the self-esteem of their participants.

Sense of Power

One of the Chicago Board of Education's strategies to give youths a sense of power was to incorporate service learning requirements in the high school curriculum. Another strategy was to improve the academic performance of all students by requiring students, teachers, administrators, and schools to be accountable. Thus, providing learning outcome standards and relevant staff development supported the academic performance of all students. Accordingly, the board developed lesson plans consistent with the standards and made them available to teachers. With establishment of a rigorous high school core curriculum, junior and senior academies in high school also improved the academic performance of all students.

Students attending the six regional high schools with academic entrance criteria or the expanded International Baccalaureate programs can also obtain a sense of power. Motivated and able students can take college courses by attending local area city junior colleges, colleges, and universities with which CPS is collaborating.

For children having academic difficulty, providing individualized strategies increases their sense of power. Retained students can improve their deficiencies through tutoring services, smaller class sizes, and specialized curricula, all of which are provided by CPS. We suggest the academic performance of all students has improved because they need to be better prepared for the enhanced high school curriculum and because the academies have helped further to shift the schools' culture toward learning by their emphasis on academics.

Sense of Uniqueness

CPS's strategy for increasing a student's sense of uniqueness is to provide youths the opportunity to find their unique talent so they can acknowledge and respect their qualities and characteristics that are special and different. Accordingly, CPS provides a wide range of activities for students in the hope that each student can find an area in which his or her unique talent will shine forth. ROTC, organized athletic activities, academic clubs, and service clubs are being made available in Chicago public schools to enable youths to express their unique talents.

Sense of Models: Character Development

Character education gives youths a sense of models in prekindergarten through twelfth grade by providing educational strategies for strengthening and supporting positive character development. Models for conflict resolution are also provided. Further, the school curriculum contains information and practice—including instruction to reduce racial, ethnic, and religious intolerance—on how youths may avoid or prevent violence. Finally, by providing youths with constructive activities that encourage developing skills, such as communicating, solving problems, providing leadership, managing resources, removing barriers to success, and planning, we hope that youths will learn models that will help them avoid high-risk health behaviors of violence. Finally, in the 1999–2000 school year, CPS initiated its Mentor Connection Program and recruited more than 100 volunteer adults to provide support for individual students.

Sense of Being Connected

Finally, CPS hopes to increase students' sense of being connected by adopting some of the strategies discussed earlier in the section on bonding, attachment, and connectedness dynamics. We also are attempting to increase the feeling of satisfaction derived from being connected to people, places, and things by providing opportunities that encourage attachment to valued people and places and to activities such as mentoring, sports, ROTC, and academic clubs. Such activities also encourage delinquent youths to form relationships with prosocial peers rather than with antisocial peers—a strategy that works to reduce aberrant behavior.

The changes in academic achievements since the School Reform Board of Trustees took over, as measured by Iowa Tests of Basic Skills and Tests of Achievement Proficiency, are shown in Figures 13–2 and 13–3.

Social Skills

Weissberg, Elias, and Greenberg (Weissberg and Elias 1993; Weissberg and Greenberg 1997) have long been proponents of teaching social skills as tools to help youths avoid engaging in risky behaviors. Accordingly, CPS seeks to increase the social skills of the target recipients that would help in reducing their health risk–taking behaviors.

CPS' efforts to increase the social skills of its target recipients include providing educational opportunities for infants, toddlers, and preschool-

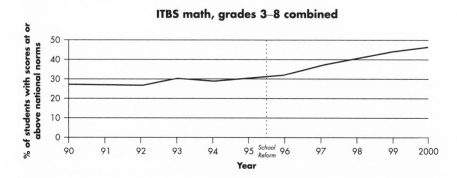

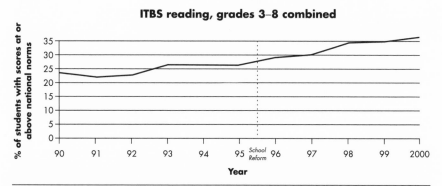

FIGURE 13–2. Performance on Iowa Tests of Basic Skills (ITBS) for mathematics and reading, grades 3 through 8 combined: Chicago Public Schools, 1990–2000.

Source. Office of Accountability of the Chicago Public Schools.

ers and their parents. Individuals are given the opportunity to develop life skills and social skills necessary to prevent and to intervene in violence. Giving youths opportunities to serve their community, resolve disputes peacefully, and develop leadership skills enables them to model and promote healthy alternatives to violence. By helping youths develop social skills, CPS hopes to help youth avoid the high-risk health behavior of violence. Thus, schools are providing opportunities to be involved with a Teen Court Program. In addition, the CPS Peer Leaders Program in elementary and high schools teaches students peer mediation, conflict resolution, and anger management skills. Further, the CPS Young Negotiators Program teaches student negotiation skills. In the CPS Peer Mediation Program, students learn from peers to manage conflict and disagreements through a diversity of techniques, thereby allowing them to avoid violence and

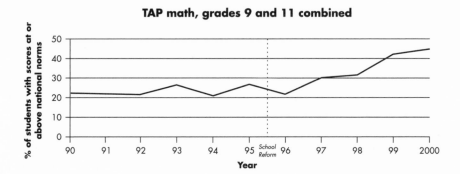

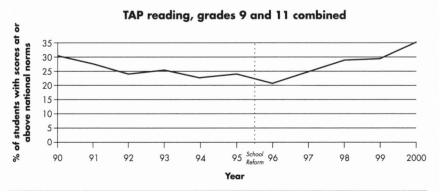

Figure 13–3. Performance on Tests of Achievement Proficiency for mathematics and reading, grades 9 and 11 combined: Chicago Public Schools, 1990–2000.

Source. Office of Accountability of the Chicago Public Schools.

other forms of aggressive and antisocial behavior. Finally, by being involved in mentoring programs and service clubs, youths learn additional social skills.

CPS also is providing support to school staff and parents to improve their ability to teach children appropriate social skills and to use positive interventions to decrease disruptive student behavior. Thus, CPS School Climate Teams help in the development of safety plans that schools include in their School Improvement Plans. School Climate Teams also cooperate with Crisis Intervention Teams, Religious Institutions Partnership, and School and Community Relations staff to help in school crisis situations. The CPS Boys Town Educational Model has been used to provide a social/ life skills curriculum training model that teaches intervention strategies to school personnel. The CPS Behavior Management Training Program provides training on request. Schools, teachers, and educational support staff are taught techniques to modify students' disruptive and aggressive behavior and to help students develop self-control and socially proactive behavior. School personnel in 20 schools receive training on how to help diffuse volatile behavior and to teach students proactive behavior. Finally, CPS Behavior Intervention Teachers are specialists who provide proactive assistance to teachers who need to enhance their behavior management skills to deal with violent and hostile behavior and to help school personnel in developing individual behavior management plans for students.

Reestablishing the Adult Protective Shield

Pynoos and Nader (1988) discussed reestablishing the adult protective shield as a psychological first-aid measure to deal with the symptoms of generalized anxiety when an individual is confronted with a traumatic stressor. The authors believe that this idea also is extremely useful in helping individuals make health behavior changes (see Chapter 8, this volume). As pointed out earlier, communities with an intact social fabric clearly have less "deviant behavior" because of the adult protective shield (Sampson et al. 1997). The social disorganization theory of deviance, which attributes reduced informal and formal social control to the deterioration of the community social fabric, can be interpreted as involving a deterioration of the adult protective shield (Shaw and McKay 1942). Reestablishment of the adult protective shield has been considered a key component in the violence prevention efforts in CPS.

Alternative Programs

By strictly enforcing disciplinary rules while providing a safety net of school-based educational opportunities for youths who have been expelled, who have violated probation, or who have committed serious but nonviolent first-time offenses, CPS reestablishes the adult protective shield. CPS Zero Tolerance/Alternative Programs contain a Uniform Discipline Code that establishes consequences for student misconduct. Students found to possess illegal drugs or firearms or other dangerous weapons face immediate consequences, including expulsion and referral to an alternative school. Fortunately, six alternative school sites are available for 300 students who are expelled from school or referred for chronically disruptive behavior, allowing for continual monitoring of youths with problematic behavior. These schools have small class sizes and provide support services through individual learning plans for each student. In addition,

CPS has a Saturday Morning Alternative Reach Out and Teach Program, or SMART. In this program, first-time drug or alcohol offenders, who would otherwise be expelled, are taught a curriculum that focuses on character education, leadership development, conflict resolution training, gang prevention and detachment, and substance abuse counseling. Students meet on eight consecutive Saturdays, with their parents participating in two of the meetings. Further, CPS expects each student to provide 20 hours of community service and to have a mentor. Students who do not successfully complete the program attend one of the alternative schools. In collaboration with the Cook County Probation Department, Operation Jump Start gives intensive support to youth who are under the jurisdiction of the probation department. Operation Jump Start also provides extensive instruction in social skills and back-to-school transitional support for youths who have had significant educational problems. After the 8-week program, youths attend either an alternative or a regular school.

Safety and Security Programs

CPS is reestablishing the adult protective shield by setting up safety and security programs designed to maximize school safety. More than 3,200 parents have patrols at 375 schools. In this initiative, parents patrol the streets before and after school to ensure safe travel. CPS trains parents in safety and security measures, and parents participate in workshops on safety, violence, and conflict resolution. CPS also has enhanced training and expansion of security personnel by assigning more than 1,990 professional security personnel to its schools.

Further, CPS, in collaboration with the Chicago Police Department, provides two-person teams of uniformed police officers who work eight-hour shifts at each high school. The Chicago Police Department and the Office of Specialized Services provide training to enable the officers to work proactively with students and the school community. Targeted training includes cultural awareness, diversity, sensitivity, internal and external school linkages, positive intervention techniques, de-escalating aggressive behavior, referral procedures and resources, and communication skills. Schools also are assisted in the development of individualized school security programs.

CPS also has initiated Operation S.A.F.E. (Schools Are for Education), a system of rapid response teams consisting of officers in a mobile tactical unit who patrol the vicinity immediately surrounding high schools and can respond quickly to any emergency calls. A rapid response team, composed of part-time police officers, supplements the high school mobile tactical unit. Part-time police officers who patrol the city after hours respond to alarms and break-ins at schools and form the CPS Night Stalkers Program. These efforts help to reduce burglaries, vandalism, and theft after school hours. The officers also give informational booklets to parents on the safe passage of students to and from school. The CPS Safe Passage booklet provided to principals and parents offers helpful tips to keep children safe on their way to and from school and in their neighborhoods during nonschool hours. Tips include using the buddy system, following a designated safety route, and knowing designated safe havens within the community.

Finally, metal detectors have been installed in middle and high schools. CPS has installed 277 metal detectors in all of the system's middle and high schools and in many elementary schools and have been responsible for recovering many weapons that may otherwise have gone undetected. Table 13–2 shows the outcomes of the 1997–1998, 1998–1999, and 1999–2000 (as of the time of this writing) CPS Random Metal Detector Program. It should be noted that during the 1997–1998, 1998–1999, and 1999–2000 school years, there were 59, 65, and 89 random sweeps, respectively; however, the number of weapons and other paraphernalia detected in CPS decreased each year. Such efforts create awareness between students and communities that the adult protective shield exists and that weapons and illegal contraband will not be tolerated.

TABLE 13–2.   Firearms, substances, and other paraphernalia detected in the Chicago Public Schools Random Metal Detector Program, 1997–1998, 1998–1999, and 1999–2000

	Number of detections per year		
	1997–1998	**1998–1999**	**1999–2000**
Firearms	0	1	1
Knives, box cutters, razors	107	96	54
Narcotics	75	63	51
Pagers[a]	816	649	534
Other weapons	158	200	29

Note.   For the three school years for which data are shown, the number of random metal detector operations by safety and security and Chicago Police Department personnel increased (number of random sweeps per year: 59 in 1997–1998, 65 in 1998–1999, and 89 in 1999–2000).
[a]No longer a legal violation in 1999–2000.
Source.   Office of Safety and Security of the Chicago Public Schools.

Parental Monitoring

Family-oriented intervention to change parenting style and practices can reduce risk for serious antisocial behavior and violence by increasing predictability and parental monitoring of children and decreasing negative parenting methods. Lack of parental monitoring, represented at its extreme by neglect and poor discipline methods and conflict about discipline, has been related to participation in delinquent and violent behavior for a range of populations (Farrington 1989; Gorman-Smith et al. 1996). One of CPS's initiatives to increase the monitoring behavior of parents of children in Chicago public schools was to require parents to pick up their youths' report cards during "a parent report card pick up day." CPS designed this activity to give parents and teachers an opportunity to collaborate on monitoring the student's academic performance and classroom behavior. In addition, 75% of CPS high schools have security cameras or complete surveillance systems, which allow staff to monitor hallways, stairwells, remote areas, and the perimeter of the campuses. These endeavors have significantly reduced vandalism. Further, the Chicago Board of Education provides monitoring of youth by providing truancy services, increasing summer school, and enriching school activities.

Table 13–3 compares the outcomes of CPS Uniform Discipline Code disciplinary actions in 1997–1998, 1998–1999, and 1999–2000 (as of the time of this writing). We propose there are fewer violations of the CPS Uniform Discipline Code, resulting in the reductions in suspensions, arrests, and expulsions. The downward trend of suspensions, arrests, and expulsions is interpreted as evidence of the success of CPS efforts to reestablish the adult protective shield.

TABLE 13–3. Uniform Discipline Code disciplinary actions: Chicago School System, 1997–1998, 1998–1999, and 1999–2000

	Number of actions per year		
	1997–1998	1998–1999	1999–2000
Suspensions	28,671	31,665	15,986
Arrests[a]	5,450	4,160	—
Expulsions	593	638	454

[a]Data on arrests not available for 1999–2000.
Source. Office of Safety and Security of the Chicago Public Schools.

REDUCING THE
EFFECTS OF TRAUMA

Behind all anger is hurt, and attached to the hurt is fear of being hurt again. Unfortunately, such emotions often cause individuals to engage in violence. Thus, in helping individuals to change their propensity for violence, the issue of traumatic stress that causes the original hurt must be addressed. Accordingly, Bell and Jenkins (1993) suggest developing a level of sensitivity to identify trauma in children. Crisis intervention teams are needed to address traumatic stress (Allen et al. 1999). Further, the effects of subtle long-term trauma need to be addressed with therapy (Pynoos and Nader 1988) (see Chapters 5 and 8, this volume). A major strategy of addressing issues of traumatic stress is to transform traumatic helplessness into learned helpfulness (Apfel and Simon 1996).

Mental health professionals at Chicago public schools have long observed the impact of traumatic stress on the youths they serve (Dyson 1990). Accordingly, CPS Specialized Services developed the CPS Crisis Intervention Services Program, which provides pupil support teams. In addition, partnerships with the religious community and community-based social and health services supplement the support teams. These services provide prevention, intervention, and postintervention counseling activities to reduce the possibility and impact of violent acts. All CPS schools have at least one counselor who can help students who are having difficulty in school or at home and a team that includes a nurse, psychologist, and social worker. Individual and small-group counseling are part of the school pupil support services program. However, whenever a student's needs are beyond the school's resources, he or she is referred to other programs or agencies. To expand CPS's network, 69 schools have received a grant to provide after-school mental health services by CPS or community-based mental health staff on the school site. In the 1999–2000 school year, the year of the initiative's inception, more than 3,500 sessions were held. To turn learned helplessness into learned helpfulness, CPS developed community service demands for students. As a required component of the high school curriculum, students are required to provide a minimum of 40 hours in service learning through activities such as tutoring, working with elders, and community beautification projects. Teens' learning is evaluated on the basis of presentations, papers, portfolios, and so forth.

Conclusion

We offer a model of violence prevention, including its theoretical under-pinnings, and summarize programmatic efforts used in the Chicago public schools. The principles necessary to promote violence prevention in an inner-city population are rebuilding the village; providing access to health care; improving bonding, attachment, and connectedness dynamics within the community and between stakeholders; improving self-esteem; increasing social skills of target recipients; reestablishing the adult protective shield; and reducing the residual effects of trauma. We do not maintain that what CPS has accomplished is easy or its methods foolproof, but its efforts are a significant start at curbing the epidemic of violence plaguing our schools and communities.

References

Ainsworth MDS: The development of infant-mother attachment, in Review of Child Development Research, Vol 3. Edited by Caldwell BM, Ricciuti HN. Chicago, IL, University of Chicago Press, 1973, pp 1–95

Allen SF, Dlugokinski EL, Cohen LA, et al: Assessing the impact of a traumatic community event on children and assisting their healing. Psychiatric Annals 29:93–98, 1999

American Psychiatric Association: Diagnostic and Statistical Manual of Mental Disorders, 4th Edition. Washington, DC, American Psychiatric Association, 1994

American Psychiatric Association: Practice guideline for the treatment of patients with nicotine dependence. Am J Psychiatry 153(suppl):1–31, 1996

Apfel RJ, Simon B (eds): Minefields in Their Hearts. New Haven, CT, Yale University Press, 1996, pp 9–11

Bean R: The Four Conditions of Self-Esteem: A New Approach for Elementary and Middle Schools, 2nd Edition. Santa Cruz, CA, ETR Associated, 1992

Bell CC: Promotion of mental health through coaching of competitive sports. J Natl Med Assoc 89:517–520, 1997

Bell CC, Jenkins EJ: Community violence and children on Chicago's southside. Psychiatry: Interpersonal and Biological Processes 56(1):46-54, 1993

Booth CL, Spieker SJ, Barnard KE, et al: Infants at risk: the role of preventive intervention in deflecting a maladaptive developmental trajectory, in Preventing Antisocial Behavior: Interventions From Birth Through Adolescence. Edited by McCord J, Tremblay RE. New York, Guilford, 1992, pp 2–42

Borduin C, Cone L, Mann B, et al: Changed Lives: The Effects of the Perry School Preschool on Youths Through Age 19. Ypsilanti, MI, High Scope Press, 1985

Bowlby J: Attachment and Loss, Vol 2: Separation. New York, Basic Books, 1973

Dryfoos JG: Adolescents at Risk: Prevalence and Prevention. New York, Oxford University Press, 1990, p 72

Dyson J: The Effect of Family Violence on Children's Academic Performance and Behavior. J Natl Med Assoc 82:17–22, 1990

Earls F: A developmental approach to understanding and controlling violence, in Theory and Research in Behavioral Pediatrics, Vol 5. Edited by Fitzgerald HE. New York, Plenum, 1991, pp 61–88

Elliott DS, Tolan PH: Youth violence prevention, intervention, and social policy—an overview, in Youth Violence: Prevention, Intervention, and Social Policy. Edited by Flannery DJ, Huff CR. Washington, DC, American Psychiatric Press, 1999, pp 3–46

Eron LD, Heusemann LR, Zelli A: The role of parental variables in the learning of aggression, in The Development and Treatment of Childhood Aggression. Edited by Pepler D, Rubin K. Hillsdale, NJ, Erlbaum, 1991, pp 171–188

Farrington DP: Early predictors of adolescent aggression and adult violence. Violence and Victims 4:79–100, 1989

Furstenberg FF, Brooks-Gunn J, Morgan SP: Adolescent Mothers in Later Life. New York, Cambridge University Press, 1987

Gorman-Smith D, Tolan PH, Zelli A, et al: The relation of family functioning to violence among inner-city minority youths. Journal of Family Psychology 10:115–129, 1996

Henggeler SW, Melton GB, Smith LA: Family preservation using multi-systemic therapy: an effective alternative to incarcerating serious juvenile offenders. J Consult Clin Psychol 60:953–961, 1992

Jenkins EJ, Bell CC: Violence exposure, psychological distress and high risk behaviors among inner-city high school students, in Anxiety Disorders in African-Americans. Edited by Friedman S. New York, Springer, 1994, pp 76–88

Klein RG, Abikoff H, Klass E, et al: Clinical efficacy of methylphenidate in conduct disorder with and without attention deficit hyperactivity disorder. Arch Gen Psychiatry 54:1073–1080, 1997

Lewis DO, Moy E, Jackson LD, et al: Biosocial characteristics of children who later murder: a prospective study. Am J Psychiatry 142:1161–1167, 1985

McCord J: A forty-year perspective on the effects of child abuse and neglect. Child Abuse Negl 7:265–270, 1983

Meloy R: Violent Attachments. Northvale, NJ, Jason Aronson, 1992

Moffitt TE: Neuropsychology, antisocial behavior, and neighborhood context, in Violence and Childhood in the Inner City. Edited by McCord J. Cambridge, UK, Cambridge University Press, 1997, pp 116–170

Pinderhughes CA: Managing paranoia in violent relationships, in Perspectives on Violence. Edited by Usdin G. New York, Brunner/Mazel, 1972, pp 111–139

Pinderhughes CA: Differential bonding: toward a psychophysiological theory of stereotyping. Am J Psychiatry 136:33–37, 1979

Pynoos R, Nader K: Psychological first aid for children who witness community violence. J Trauma Stress 1:445–473, 1988

Renken B, Egeland B, Marvinney D, et al: Early childhood antecedents of aggression and passive-withdrawal in early elementary school. J Pers 57:257–281, 1989

Resnick MD, Bearman PS, Blum RW, et al: Protecting adolescents from harm: findings from the National Longitudinal Study on Adolescent Health. JAMA 278: 823–832, 1997

Sampson RJ, Raudenbush SW, Earls F: Neighborhoods and violent crime: a multilevel study of collective efficacy. Science 277:918–924, 1997

Shaw CR, McKay H: Juvenile Delinquency and Urban Areas. Chicago, IL. University of Chicago Press, 1942

Tolan PH, Lorion RP: Multivariate approaches to the identification of delinquency-proneness in males. Am J Community Psychol 16:547–561, 1988

U.S. Department of Health and Human Services: Healthy People in Healthy Communities: A Guide for Community Leaders. Washington, DC, Office of Public Health and Sciences, Office of Disease and Health Promotion, U.S. Department of Health and Human Services, June 1998, pp 877–954

Weissberg RP, Elias MJ: Enhancing young people's social competence and health behavior. Applied and Preventive Psychology 3:179–190, 1993

Weissberg RP, Greenberg MR: School and community competence-enhancement and prevention programs, in Handbook of Child Psychology, 5th Edition, Vol 4: Child Psychology in Practice. Edited by Sigel E, Renninger KA. New York, Wiley, 1997, pp 877–954

14

A Social Systems–Power Dynamics Approach to Preventing School Violence

Stuart W. Twemlow, M.D.
Peter Fonagy, Ph.D., F.B.A.
Frank C. Sacco, Ph.D.

Deprived of the affective nourishment to which they are entitled, their only resource is violence. The only path which remains open to them is the destruction of a social order of which they are the victims. Infants without love, they will end as adults full of hate.

Rene Spitz

We live in a violent country: more people are incarcerated in the United States than in any other Western industrialized country. In fact, the number of people in United States prisons will soon exceed the number enrolled in colleges and universities! At a conference ("The School Shooter: A Threat Assessment Perspective") held by the Federal Bureau of Investi-

This work is an outgrowth of the Peaceful Schools Project of the Child & Family Center, The Menninger Clinic, Topeka, Kansas. Our grateful thanks are due to the many staff, students, and collaborators who are helping us.

gation (FBI) in July 1997 to discuss the problem of school shootings, it was mentioned that approximately three million crimes are committed in schools each year. More than 100,000 children carry guns to school each day. Homicide is the leading cause of death in children ages 5 to 14 years. The FBI considers the epidemic of severe school violence to be a form of domestic terrorism, developing in parallel with similar terrorism in our country at large.

We found, in a study of school shooters, that the idiosyncratic, obsessive, violence-focused mental state of these children and adolescents was very much affected by the social context (Twemlow 1999, in press). In virtually all cases, the youths were clearly existing in a social context that treated them as outsiders or that they felt treated them as such (see Chapter 1, this volume). Further, they felt justified in, even self-righteous about, their violent behavior. According to James Gilligan (personal communication, December 1997), the shame factor in violence is central. From this perspective, the crime is a restoration of justice, albeit in a bizarre and perverted way.

A POWER DYNAMICS THEORY OF SCHOOL VIOLENCE

In a study of 118 cultures reported by Garbarino (1999), among single factors, rejection had the highest impact on increasing violent tendencies in children (see Chapter 1, this volume). The core of this rejection is its humiliating impact in the context of the coercive power dynamics of the school climate. Our work strongly supports the centrality of coercive power dynamics, rejection, shaming, humiliation, and contempt as composing a prime etiological cluster in the epidemic of violence in our schools. Why shame generates rage of such cosmic proportions is not clear, and none of the contemporary psychodynamic explanations shed much light on this paradox.

We hypothesize that the power struggles in schools constitute one of the root causes of violence in children and adolescents (Twemlow, in press; Twemlow et al. 1996). Dreikurs (1957), from an Adlerian perspective, postulated that when the natural right of children for membership in the social group is abrogated through the operation of power dynamics, they feel excluded. Such children may become bullies or victims, whose power struggles represent a pathetic attempt to be accepted by their social group. In this context, youths present their frustration about group membership by attention-getting ploys. This frustration can develop into serious power struggles in which the roles of bully and victim interchange. If unchecked, these power struggles can lead to revenge-retaliation dynamics. Some youths become enraged by the failure of the group to accept them, and some withdraw in despair and give up the struggle for membership. The dilemma faced by these youths is summarized in Figure 14–1.

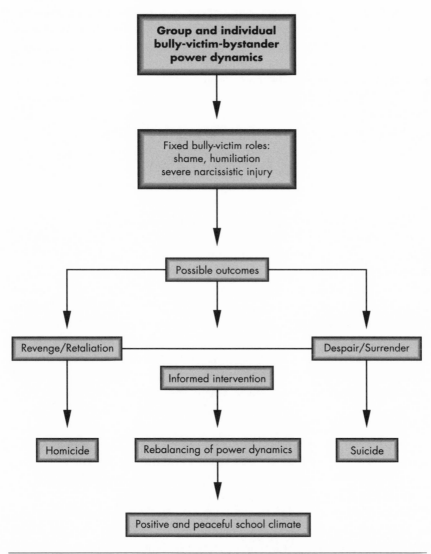

FIGURE 14–1.   Power struggles that can lead to lethal violence in schools.

In our social systems/dialectical theory of power dynamics, we hypothesize that the relationship between the bully and the victim is a dialectical one: the bully and the victim are co-created roles that would not exist without each other. If the coercive power dynamic is rebalanced, then these roles disappear.

An element unique to this theory is that the role of the bystanding audience facilitates the bullying and can intensify the misery and the humiliation of the victim, whose weakness and despair are displayed before the "applauding" bystanders. Thus, the concept of power dynamic here refers to conscious and unconscious coercive use of power in a system of domination and control of one individual by another or of one group by another.

The mind-sets of bullies and victims also undergo change. The cognitive mind-set of the victim is altered by autonomic nervous system activation and, as a result, is uncreative, preservative, overfocused, and sometimes sleepy (i.e., highly unconducive to survival) (Twemlow 1995a, 1995b). Similarly, a bully often can be trapped in a mind-set fueled by the interaction with the victim and the applause of the bystander, which promotes an intense grandiosity with heightening feelings of personal power. Such a bully may well have, according to Fonagy (1999), a mind-set that is nonmentalizing—that is, the bully is unable to see himself or herself reflected in the dehumanized victim. Fonagy's theories, which are based on investigation of early attachment patterns, suggest that violent individuals are incapable of representing the mental states of others and thus cannot see others as thinking, feeling human beings. Fonagy suggests that violent children often are brought up in families where there has been a fundamental failure of the parental capacity to recognize the child as a separate individual. Such a parental model does not foster an internal working model of self and other and may impair the individual's identity, feeling of responsibility for his or her own actions, and knowledge of the consequences of his or her actions. Thus, further humiliation of the victim may be seen as the only solution to the problem (Fonagy 1999; Fonagy et al. 1997).

The continuum of bully, victim, and bystander roles is summarized in Figure 14–2.

Depressed victims may be either despairing and suicidal or enraged and even homicidal, depending on which dynamic is closest to consciousness (see Chapter 5, this volume). In high schools, other forms of victimization are seen in girls who have a crush on macho, bullying boys and adopt the role of rescuer or martyr. The rescuing dynamic, less omnipotent than the martyring one, represents a denial of the fear of being hurt by treating

Victim		Bystander			Bully
Depressed–despairing	Victim type	Ambivalent type	Bully type		Sadistic bully
Depressed–enraged		Avoidant type	Puppetmaster		Bully–victim
Rescuing		Chameleon type	Variant		Physical taunter
Martyr					Teaser
					Rumor monger
					Ostracizer

FIGURE 14–2.   Continuum of interchangeable roles in populations with problems related to power dynamics.

the attacker as the helpless one. The martyr–victim, the more omnipotent response, usually results from a breakdown of the rescuing posture. The martyring victim often feels that there is some mystical hope that the bully will change and that the victim's proper role is to stand by him and protect him until the change occurs. Such a martyr often interprets for the bully, excuses him, and runs interference for him when problems with school authorities arise. The rescuing victim often compromises her own school performance by doing things to help the bully. In both instances, the intense emotionality of the state far supersedes any interest in academic and other intellectual pursuits.

Bullying may be of a sadistic type. Approximately 1% of the school population comprises youths whose behavior meets the definition of psychopathy (Hare 1998). Such youths have a frightening lack of empathy for others, have normal self-esteem, and are not made anxious by their sadistic actions, but, in fact, appear to enjoy the pain of their victims. A bully–victim is a youth who switches quickly from provocative bullying behavior to the pleading posture of a helpless victim when any recrimination or punishment is imminent. These roles can flip-flop with alarming frequency. The bully–victim is similar to what Olweus (1992) called the "provocative victim." However, we believe this behavior is a form of bullying rather than a victim role, since sadism is quite prominent in these youths. Some bullies have a variety of favorite methods for bullying, including physical taunting. The physical taunting is rarely injurious, because if the victim is injured, the bully will be blamed and the victim will get the sympathy.

Some bullies tend to tease, spread rumors, and ostracize. Rumor mongering and ostracizing are not uncommon in different developmental stages, especially among early adolescent girls. As they become aware of their sexual needs and sexual growth, girls can become very cruel to each other by forming groups that exclude certain girls who do not conform to the prevailing standards of "nonconformity."

These forms of bullying are present in the wide variety of social groups that exist within schools. Such groups have enormous power, sometimes focused around counter-culture music such as grunge, punk, or alternative; sometimes around sports, as with jocks; and sometimes around crime, as with gang bangers. There also are a wide variety of smaller social groups. Such complex social groups are more active in high schools and are virtually unknown in elementary schools. Thus, social bullying is a form of aggression that can be perpetrated not only by an individual but also by a group of youths (see Chapters 2 and 15, this volume).

Bystanders can be characterized on a continuum from victim to bullying type. Victim-type bystanders often are youths who have been abused and who are too frightened to refuse to assist the bully. Instead, they become an audience and helper for the bully and reluctantly but compliantly perform directed functions. The bully-type bystander is a youth who vicariously enjoys the pain of the victim but does not actually like to perform the bullying act itself. Such youths often mastermind the bullying. This type of youth has been implicated in more than one of the school shootings. We call the homicidal mastermind bully-type bystander a "puppet master," the one who pulls the strings of the whole school.

Avoidant bystanding often is seen in teachers and especially in school principals who, for a variety of reasons (including political ones), deny the serious nature of bullying and simply do not deal with it. Bystanders who are confused or ambivalent often are able to be recruited to interrupt this pattern of bullying, since they are not yet polarized into fulfilling one or other of the pathological roles. The chameleon-type bystander, often an "as-if" character, adopts the role of victim, bully, or bystander without any genuine involvement with these roles other than as a means to consciously manipulate the social climate.

It should be noted that these roles are interchangeable, and, with only a few exceptions, most youths are capable of alternating between them. It is when these roles become fixed that serious violence can occur.

We now can redefine bullying in schools as the repeated exposure of an individual or group to negative interactions (social aggression) by one or more dominant persons. This person(s) enjoys the discomfort and shame of the victim as if in a sadomasochistic ritual enacted for the perverse public enjoyment of an audience of bystanders who do nothing and may vicariously be aroused as bullies or victims.

SCHOOL VIOLENCE PROGRAMS

A sharp peak in the rates of antisocial and violent behavior occurs during the teenage years (Guerra et al. 1994). Aggressive behavior and peer rejection during early childhood predict later juvenile delinquency (Kupersmidt and Coie 1990). Kupersmidt and Coie (1990) make a strong case for early prevention efforts that attempt to deal with violent behavior before the adolescent years.

A growing array of programs have been developed to reduce violence in the school classroom, but few have been studied with good controls and outcome measures (Grossman et al. 1997). Few violence prevention programs target the school as a whole. Most tend to focus on at-risk, aggressive youths.

Bender and McLaughlin (1997) delineate a three-tiered practical approach to school violence. The first tier involves a prevention reduction strategy that is the least intrusive and costly of strategies. Instruction is built into the educational routines of the school, such as social-skills training, health education, and modeling safe behavior with strangers. These programs require little in terms of personnel and equipment and do not compromise civil liberties. A second tier of strategies focuses on assisting the student to understand his or her behavior through conflict management training, peer collaboration, and adult mentorship strategies (see Chapters 12, 13, and 15, this volume). The third tier of strategies involves intrusive strategies such as metal detectors, school security cameras, and employment of school-based police officers. These strategies are very expensive and involve loss of privacy for students and, therefore, are among the least desirable of the alternatives.

A few randomized, controlled studies of bullying prevention programs in school populations have been reported. Grossman et al. (1997) evaluated the effectiveness of the Second Step Violence Prevention Curriculum for elementary school children. Parent- and teacher-rated behavioral measures did not indicate significant change, but direct behavioral observations revealed a significant persistent decrease in physical aggression. Olweus (1991, 1992), in a series of studies of 42 schools in Norway over almost 20 years, reported on a bully-victim intervention program. Eliciting high cooperation of schools, Olweus found a generally significant decrease in pathological bullying and victimized behaviors, primarily in grades 4 through 7.

Versions of the Olweus program have been used as models for research in the United States. In particular, his findings formed the basis for an ongoing initiative in South Carolina (Melton and Limber 1998). The Second Step Violence Prevention Program is a time-limited, curriculum-based social skills and anger management program taught in the classroom by specially trained teachers. Other specific antibullying strategies include well-known programs like the Johnson Institute Program (Johnson Institute 1996) and the Bullying Proof Program (Garrity et al. 1996).

Approaches to coercive power dynamics in elementary schools usually use one of two main thrusts: they attempt to identify the bullies in the school and train students and staff to deal with them, or they focus on interpersonal problem-solving skills and the development of social skills, including the capacity to empathize with others (e.g., Greenberg et al. 1995). Another approach, of which our program is an example (see below), targets the school as a whole, without any individual focus on at-risk children. Thus, children without problems assist and modulate children with problems without the stigma and expense of formal medical referral.

THE CAPSLE PROGRAM: CREATING A PEACEFUL SCHOOL LEARNING ENVIRONMENT

Following our theory of power dynamics, clearly, any intervention should focus on the school as a whole—that is, the "climate" of the school—rather than on individual children. We hypothesized that more symmetrical power dynamics should result in reduction in disruptions in the classroom and produce fewer struggles on playgrounds. The ultimate hope was for a more compassionate and group-focused school climate, with improved academic performance. The school climate would become one in which the students and teachers help each other and serve group goals, rather than competing with each other, striving to achieve dominant status.

CAPSLE Program Components

The CAPSLE (Creating a Peaceful School Learning Environment) program consists of five components: zero tolerance for bullying, bystanding, and being a victim; discipline plan; Gentle Warrior program; Bruno Program; and peer mentorship.

Zero Tolerance for Bullying, Bystanding, and Being a Victim

The zero-tolerance approach assists in changing the language of the various participants in the school climate, including students, teachers, parents, school custodians, lunchroom workers, school security and resource personnel, coaches, school secretaries, and other administrative personnel. The program is coordinated by the school counselor, whose traditional role in dealing with individual problem children expands to include the school climate as a whole. In changing the language of the various participants in the school climate, we hypothesized that there would be heightened awareness of coercive power dynamics and an increase in skills to cope with them. One goal is to change the climate so that highly coercive roles—for example, that of the macho bully—would have less social status than more compassionate and respectful roles. Ideally, then, social status is achieved mainly in nonbullying, nonvictimized, and nonbystanding roles.

Posters are placed at strategic points around the school, depicting desirable behaviors to reinforce the central theme of the programs. The posters cover the following main ideas:

- Nine ways to handle bullies
- Are you a bully?
- Are you a victim?
- Are you a bystander?
- Right speech (a way of interacting with people noncoercively)
- Manners and social skills of a good elementary school student
- What is a gentle warrior? (emphasizing service to others and empathy)
- Are you getting angry?
- Self-protective response (a quick way of relaxing the body)

The posters are supported by regular discussion groups. Each class has an open discussion period about relationships among bully, victim, and bystander each semester. Teachers are encouraged in the daily classroom work to include frequent references to coercive power relationships.

Each semester, a workshop on family power struggles is conducted for parents and children. The workshop is designed to enable discussion of ways to handle specific family conflicts noncoercively by identifying the bully/victim/bystander roles and then shifting the power dynamics of the family group.

A system of rewards is developed for each class when the class succeeds in keeping the classroom and school free of fighting. First, each classroom has a banner that hangs outside the room for all to see. When there is a disruption judged by teachers to be serious enough, the students involved in the interaction take the banner down. There is a significant reward each month for the school with the smallest number of class banners taken down for fighting. In addition, the school as a whole has a peace flag that flies along with the Stars and Stripes and the state flag outside the school, prominently displaying the fact that the school has been free of fighting on that day. One hundred fifty consecutive days of peace in the school is rewarded by visits from local dignitaries. Other reinforcements include patches, buttons, magnets, and stickers depicting various aspects of the bully/victim/bystander relationships. Each school newsletter contains an article written by one of the program workers. The program leadership group meets once a month. This group includes, at a minimum, the principal of the school, the designated mental health worker (usually a social worker or counseling psychologist), and representatives from each area of the program, including children when appropriate. School morale, coordination of volunteers and progress, and evaluation are discussed.

The Discipline Plan

The discipline plan reinforces using more rewards than punishments, allowing a hierarchy of learning opportunities for teachers and students. It also encourages teachers and other personnel (including school custodians) who bully students to model noncoercive behavior.

Although teachers who are used to consequence-based discipline find this difficult at first, overall, teacher acceptance is very high, since the impact of such discipline is rather quick and dramatic. Each disturbance in the classroom is conceptualized within the bully/victim/bystander format. Attention-getting behavior, even if not aimed directly at humiliating an individual, bullies the class into losing learning time. Much behavior also is aimed at humiliating the teacher in front of the class. When an event occurs (e.g., a child throws spitballs), instead of punishing the child in the traditional fashion, the teacher has the whole classroom analyze the behavior and each member of the classroom becomes a bully, a bystander, or a victim, thus participating in and adopting some responsibility for the event.

The various bystander roles can be arranged in a hierarchy of usefulness, from the bystander who gains vicarious satisfaction from the behavior to the bystander who tends to intervene to stop it. A variety of discipline cards are given to reinforce the behavior of children. If a child cannot be handled in the classroom setting, he or she is sent with a power struggle referral alert to a school counselor, who again handles the event not with punishment, but with an intervention that provides an opportunity for insight and work. At this stage, parents may also be invited into the process. For example, in one school, two fifth-grade girls who were each leaders of their own subgroups ended up fighting rather viciously. One of them had a mother who sided with her daughter and attempted to split children at school functions into those who would sit with her and her daughter and those who were outsiders. When both girls were referred for counseling, they quickly realized that the goal of their behavior was not to humiliate each other, but to gain mutual respect. The mother was able to become involved in that process and accepted it with some reticence when she saw that her daughter agreed with that assessment.

Ultimately, children with behavior that does not respond to this approach (less than 1% in disciplinary situations) in our experience should be referred to the principal for more traditional consequence-based appraisal and possibly suspension. This approach gives a new, more central role to the school counselor, who is not usually so involved in class discipline. The extra work for the counselor is counterbalanced by freeing the principal for important attention to school policy and other matters that can improve the learning climate, rather than being endlessly preoccupied with disciplining children and dealing with angry parents.

The goal of this plan is to work toward fulfilling the ultimate goal of all discipline, which is to internalize controls. Coercive discipline, or what should be instead called control, is never internalized. Thus, when the outside agency, the teacher, is absent, the child will take the opportunity to misbehave even more creatively. A discipline system that is not perceived as coercive is far more likely to be internalized and transformed into self-discipline.

Gentle Warrior Program

The Gentle Warrior Program is a psychoeducational method designed to foster the psychological and physical skills of schoolchildren to enable them to deal personally with bullying and with their own tendencies to act as victims or as bystanders. This approach encourages the children to observe and to verbalize these behaviors in themselves and in others. Children's self-esteem and self-confidence increase. Children who tended to be quieter victims become much more assertive; sometimes their behavior initially is perceived as a classroom problem, until the whole school, including the teacher, learns the language of the program.

The Gentle Warrior Program comprises two 12-week training modules each year. Once a week, all classrooms in the school participate, and children are *not* identified on the basis of psychopathology or bully-victim-bystander ratings. The training period varies from 20 minutes for kindergarten to 1 hour for more advanced grades. The sessions are taught by martial arts–trained instructors, usually a female and male working together with the children. A lesson plan includes the following elements:

1. Sitting-down relaxation period (the self-protective response)
2. Question-and-answer time with discussion of the martial arts' Bushido Code of Conduct, stressing self-respect, self-control, and respect for others
3. Stretching and muscle strengthening exercises
4. Martial art techniques (No striking techniques are taught. Balancing, falling safely, defensive positioning, blocking, and release techniques are emphasized.)
5. Role playing (Bully/victim/bystander relationships are role-played by the children with instructor supervision.)
6. Reading stories (Stories are chosen from a variety of classical and historical sources to illustrate aspects of the Bushido Code. Sources include Aesop's fables, sayings of Thomas Jefferson, passages from Plato's work, etc.)
7. Tips for parents (These tips are circulated each week with the children's take-home folders, and parents are asked to reinforce the social and physical skills that have been emphasized in the program.)

The Gentle Warrior Program sessions are also open to parents and to teachers. Participation of parents and teachers is encouraged, and many participate quite frequently.

Bruno Program

The Bruno Program acknowledges the importance of the older individual in acting as a model for containment of the child's aggressiveness and competitiveness. Where possible, males are recruited for such activity, since in our culture males are associated with the development of children's capacity to control aggression. It is a well-known fact that our culture lacks male influence in children's upbringing. It has been estimated that some 20% of the families in the United States lack a functioning male; this figure approaches 90% among families in general assistance programs (Twemlow et al. 1996).

The Bruno Program is a collaboration between adult mentors and children to monitor the power dynamics of the school climate. Adult mentors, including parents of children and residents of retirement homes, are recruited from the local community, with as many males involved as possible. Adult mentors commit to a specific time each week to serve as monitors (e.g., before school, during recess and lunch, and immediately after school). They have limited involvement in traditional educational activities. Each adult mentor is paired with an honor patrol student, a fifth-grade child who assists the mentor in the intervention. The "Brunos" are clearly identified with T-shirts and function in an informal way, not only serving a surveillance function but also providing children with a consultant when they have conflicts. For example, conflicts can occur over play equipment and sports. The orientation manual given to Brunos captures the essential function of this group: "The Bruno is a metaphor, a way to communicate within the culture of the school that there is control and order that alters the atmosphere, so that everyone can have more fun and learn peacefully at school." The Bruno thus functions as a positive social control signal.

Peer Mentoring

Children often respond more positively to advice and assistance from those closer to their age, rather than from older individuals who remind them of parents and with whom they may have authority conflicts. We believe that involvement with peer mentors, usually from a local high school, can be beneficial both to the mentor and to the child in helping them sublimate aggressiveness and competitiveness and develop verbal and other skills for solving power struggles.

Students are recruited for this program from the high school that eventually most of the children at the elementary school will attend. These high school students generally have had problems with disruptiveness, attendance, and often violence and have been exposed to a variety of forms of remediation. The high school provides the peer mentors with academic credit for the work, which is carried out on a two- or three-times-a-week basis. Peer mentors sit with individual children to whom they are assigned and assist them in doing schoolwork, in mediating disputes, and, to a limited extent, in identifying personal problems and issues.

Peer mentors are oriented in a program that emphasizes the following:

1. Dealing with children's secrets and confidences
2. Dealing with physical violence in children
3. Committing to others, keeping one's word, not acting superior, showing forgiveness and compassionate self-control, and practicing honesty and sincerity in dealing with oneself and others.
4. Role-playing scenarios devised to address the various types of difficulties that the peer mentor may have with other children, such as an angry child, a child that will not stop crying, a child who will not cooperate, a child amid bully-victim-bystander dynamics

In addition, the group of peer mentors is usually supervised for 1 hour on a weekly basis to process their experiences.

CAPSLE Study Outcomes

Two self-selected schools participated in our study of the CAPSLE program beginning in 1994 (Twemlow et al., in press). Both schools had had serious disciplinary problems, with fighting necessitating police intervention. One of the schools had the highest out-of-school suspension rate in the school district. Both schools were located in an inner-city, low-income neighborhood and consisted of approximately 50% minority students, with a slightly lower percentage (58%) of single-parent families than in other schools. More than 60% of the students in each school were participating in the free or reduced-cost lunch programs. The demographic characteristics of the two schools did not differ significantly on any variable. For the purposes of this chapter, the school that received the CAPSLE intervention program is referred to as the experimental school, and the school that received the traditional school psychiatric consultation model from a senior psychiatrist is referred to as the control school.

A dramatic reduction occurred in notifications of serious discipline infractions to the principal, especially those involving aggression, but also those not involving aggression. Out-of-school suspension rates were computed as a percentage of the total number of students enrolled, because enrollment varied between the two schools. In the control school, suspension rates varied between 14% and 24% between 1994 and 1998, remaining relatively stable. In the experimental school, where there had been a dramatic rise in the suspension rate in the year before the program was initiated, there was a gradual and well-maintained reduction beginning in 1995–1996. From 1996 to 1998, the suspension rate was below 5%.

A dramatic increase in academic achievement occurred in the experimental school, with composite scores rising from the 40th percentile to the 58th percentile. In contrast, the composite scores for the control school did not change over the same period. Scores on reading and mathematics subtests also confirmed this pattern of findings. Interestingly, in the third through fifth grades in the experimental school, the composite score and reading score improved, but the mathematics score did not.

In the experimental school, the youngest group of children appeared to feel the most in danger initially (as seen on measures of school safety); however, their fears did subside somewhat. The older children felt less threatened and were quickest to benefit from the program. Teacher ratings of classroom behavior of the children showed a significant reduction in dependency and in withdrawal, and a trend toward reduction in hostility. There was a significant improvement in the victim factor (i.e., tendency to be victimized), with marginal improvement in the bullying factor. Both of these factors, and the changes seen, reflect a significant shift toward externalizing aggressiveness and becoming more assertive.

The CAPSLE program focuses on developing more self-confidence and assertiveness. We expected the program to have more of an effect on children with withdrawn victim behavior than on those exhibiting bullying behavior. Children with withdrawn victim behavior did become less dependent on others for their self-esteem and less withdrawn. Through group interaction, their victim behavior was reduced and, consequently, the bullying behavior was ameliorated. This process ultimately led to a normalization of power dynamics within the school climate. In this school, bullies now have less power over the victims because there is less submissiveness. Our intervention appears to shift children's mode of functioning to a less anxiety-provoking and more relational and compassionate level. As a result, the children become more reflective and less reactive (Fonagy 1998) and develop more response options that do not involve bulling, coercion, or anxious and/or depressed retreat.

Although this study was not randomized, the trends were sufficiently promising to attract significant funding for a definitive randomized study involving nine schools allocated to three experimental conditions: CAPSLE program for three schools, traditional school psychiatric consultation for three schools, and delayed intervention for three schools. In delayed intervention (no treatment condition), schools were promised that after 2 years the most effective of the other two programs would be given to them free of charge.

As part of a general investigation to see what components of the CAPSLE program are essential for success, the study was replicated in another elementary school in Topeka, Kansas. The school consisted of children from the white upper-middle-class professional community and children from the working class community, with a number of children on general assistance. The school had more than 400 students. The two components of the program chosen for the study were zero tolerance for bullying/victim/bystanding and the Gentle Warrior Program. After 1 year of the program, the number of suspensions in the school dropped dramatically and the composite Metropolitan Achievement Test scores rose significantly. These changes paralleled almost exactly the shift in the program in the original experimental school, although students in the replication school began the study functioning at a higher level.

CONCLUSION

Various components of the CAPSLE program can be used separately in different schools, depending on the location of the school, the specific problems, and the availability of parent volunteers. The martial arts–based Gentle Warrior Program, with its emphasis on physical action, is mainly of use in elementary schools, but could also be of use in middle schools; however, developmentally, children in middle school are more likely to be more interested in competitive sports as a vehicle for the program. In high school, as students develop more autonomy and the capacity for abstract thinking, more intellectual pursuits like forensics (public speaking and oratory) and debate can be used as an experimental approach for implementing this program. However, we suspect that the core of the program is the zero tolerance component and discipline plan, with the other components being add-ons depending on the circumstances in the school.

The CAPSLE program is seen as a foundation for academic excellence because it creates a psychologically comprehensive safe and pleasant environment for children, teachers, and service personnel. The program sets the scene for the success of components of the educational curriculum and for school governance and other programs that from time to time are used in school settings. Academic success, though not a direct result of the program, emerges naturally from an environment that is conducive to learning.

REFERENCES

Bender W, McLaughlin P: Violence in the classroom: where we stand. Intervention in School and Clinic 32:196–198, 1997

Dreikurs R: Psychology in the Classroom. New York, Harper & Brothers, 1957, pp 3–20

Fonagy P: An attachment theory approach to treatment of the difficult patient. Bull Menninger Clin 62:147–169, 1998

Fonagy P: Male perpetrators of violence against women: an attachment theory perspective. Journal of Applied Psychoanalytic Studies 1(1):7–27, 1999

Fonagy P, Target M, Steele M, et al: The development of violence and crime as it relates to security of attachment, in Children in a Violent Society. Edited by Osofsky J. New York, Guilford, 1997, pp 150–177

Garbarino J: Lost Boys: Why Our Sons Turn Violent and How We Can Save Them. Monroe, LA, Free Press, 1999

Garrity C, Jens K, Porter W, et al: Bully-Proofing Your School. Longmont, CO, Sopri West, 1996

Greenberg M, Kusche C, Cook E, et al: Promoting emotional competence in school-aged children: the effects of the PATHS curriculum. Development and Psychopathology 7:117–136, 1995

Grossman D, Neckerman H, Koepsell T, et al: Effectiveness of a violence prevention curriculum among children in elementary school. JAMA 277:1605–1611, 1997

Guerra N, Tobin P, Hammond W: Prevention and treatment of adolescent violence, in Reason to Hope: A Psychosocial Perspective on Violence and Youth. Edited by Eron L, Gentry J, Schlegel P. Washington, DC, American Psychological Association, 1994, pp 383–403

Hare RD: Psychopathy, affect and behavior, in Psychopathy: Theory, Research and Implications for Society (NATO Asi Series; Series D, Behavioural and Social Sciences No. 88). Edited by Cooke DJ, Forth AE, Hare RD. Dordrecht, the Netherlands, Kluwer Academic, 1998, pp 105–137

Johnson Institute: The No Bullying Program: Preventing Bully/Victim Violence at School. Minneapolis, MN, The Johnson Institute, 1996

Kupersmidt J, Coie J: Preadolescent peer status, aggression and school adjustments as predictors of externalizing problems in adolescence. Child Dev 61:1350–1362, 1990

Melton G, Limber S: Combating Fear and Restoring Safety in Schools. Edited by Annette JL, Walseleb MC. Juvenile Justice Bulletin, April 1998, p 5

Olweus D: Bully/victim problems among schoolchildren: basic facts and effects of a school based intervention program, in The Development and Treatment of Childhood Aggression. Edited by Pepler D, Rubin KH. Hillsdale, NJ, Erlbaum, 1991, pp 441–448

Olweus D: Bullying among school children: intervention and prevention, in Aggression and Violence Throughout the Lifespan. Edited by Peters R, McMahon P, Quincy V. London, Sage, 1992, pp 100–125

Spitz R: The First Year of Life. New York, International Universities Press, 1965, p 300

Twemlow SW: The psychoanalytical foundations of a dialectical approach to the victim/victimizer relationship. J Am Acad Psychoanal 23:545–561, 1995a

Twemlow SW: Traumatic object relations configurations seen in victim/victimizer relationships. J Am Acad Psychoanal 23:563–580, 1995b

Twemlow SW: Profile of a school shooter. Bulletin of the American Association of Psychoanalytic Physicians 87(2):3–9, 1999

Twemlow SW: The roots of violence: converging psychoanalytic explanatory models for power struggles and violence in schools. Psychoanal Q (in press)

Twemlow SW, Sacco FC, Williams P: A clinical and interactionist perspective on the bully-victim-bystander relationship. Bull Menninger Clin 60:296–313, 1996

Twemlow SW, Fonagy P, Sacco FC, et al: Creating a peaceful school learning environment: a controlled study of an elementary school intervention to reduce violence. Am J Psychiatry (in press)

15

The School in a Multicultural Society

Teaching Tolerance and Conflict Resolution

JAN ARNOW, B.F.A.

America is a country of immigrants. Although this has been acknowl-
edged as historical fact, many citizens fail to recognize the parallel truth: it
continues to be so. In fact, we are becoming so diverse a population that
the statistical meaning of the word "minority" is quickly losing its significance. Consider the following:

- Between 1980 and 1990, the white population grew by only 7.7% nationally. The African American and Hispanic populations grew by 15.8%
  and 34.5%, respectively.
- The fastest growing group during that decade was Asians, who make
  up about half of all new immigrants.
- Census projections indicate that by the middle of the twenty-first century, white Americans will become the nation's numerical minority.

Statistics in this chapter are based on information from the U.S. Census Bureau,
United States Department of Commerce (available at http://www.census.gov).

- The population is intermarrying with increasing frequency. By the middle of the twenty-first century, the "average" American citizen will trace his or her origins to Africa, Asia, Hispanic countries, the Pacific Islands—anywhere but white Europe.
- The rapid shift in demographics is already evident among our youth population. The number of linguistically different children is quickly rising, and our 25 largest city school systems have minority student majorities.
- More than 150 languages are represented in schools nationwide, and figures nearing this number occur in single large districts already.
- Children of color currently make up 30% of America's youths under age 18, and the percentage is increasing exponentially.
- It was estimated that as many as 5,000,000 children of immigrants would enter kindergarten through grade 12 in the 1990s.

These demographic changes are real, immutable, and accelerating. The continuing influx of immigrants has reverberated through every social institution in America, including our schools.

Making the equation more complex, ethnic identification is not the only criterion commonly used to denote differences in culture. Indeed, the term *culture* is increasingly a source of misunderstanding and confusion. In addition to its common usage regarding race or ethnic origins, the term is often used more generally to indicate a body of common understandings. Used in this way, culture can include everything that is part of everyday living, including customs, traditions, beliefs, morals, art, law, and knowledge. For example, people who are poor share a culture of poverty. It can be said that there is a culture of youth, because young people, by their nature, have many things in common. Religion, gender, lifestyle, and socioeconomic status all can and should be considered as having distinct cultural indicators.

In a country where one out of five children lives in a family with income below the poverty line, where huge numbers have been raised in non-English-speaking homes, where the characteristics of "different" can be applied to more children than not in any given classroom, it is imperative that we understand the depth and breadth of culture—and the extent to which many groups of people have been marginalized in this country—and be aware of its implications as it drives changes in our schools.

WHO FAILS AND WHO SUCCEEDS?

Contemporary laws, combined with our social norms and sense of justice, theoretically protect the educational rights of all children through equal access to education. These concepts and laws can allow diversity among students to be honored and their knowledge differences to be appreciated. Why, then, is the dropout rate for Hispanic students hovering at 45%, fully 20 percentage points above the already high national high school dropout rate of 25%? Why are there startling disparities by gender, race, and national origin in disciplinary referrals and suspensions in public schools? Why have minority students been suspended from school more often for "subjective" offenses and less often for serious offenses than their white peers? Why are poor children more likely to fail than children from economically advantaged homes? Why are these "at-risk" students more involved in unsafe activities either as victims or as aggressors than their majority peers?

One real answer is because American schools in general continue to both perpetuate and communicate the values, power relationships, and behavioral standards of those for whom schools in this country were originally intended: middle-class Europeans. As a result, students whose cultures are different from that of the school often feel alienated from and rejected by their school system.

Our schools, whether by law or by moral commitment, are responsible for the growth, development, and safety of all our nation's children. To accomplish this, our schools must create environments that are caring, safe, and secure for all children. Terms such as "ambience," "climate," "philosophy," and even "school culture" all reflect a process of humanizing education to make it more responsive to the needs of individuals and more affirming of the intrinsic value of human diversity. The reluctance or inability of schools to do this is at the heart of their failure to educate the racially, culturally, and otherwise "different" children of this country.

WHY KEEP KIDS IN SCHOOL?

In addition to the legal and ethical imperatives for educating all our children, two seemingly disparate phenomena now make it even more critical to provide such education: the increase in youth violence and the changing labor market.

Violence

Every day, quarrels among children that used to result in fistfights and bloody noses now end in gunshots. Every day, almost 135,000 students carry a gun to school. Every day, nearly 200,000 children miss school because of fear of attack by other students. Every day, some 2,000 young people are actually attacked in school. Every 2 days, 25 children—an entire classroom—are killed by guns.

The reasons for this raging brutality are clear. Neglected, rejected, cast-off kids turn into bitter, gun-toting criminals more often than not. Weaned on violent video games, toys, and media programming, they are desensitized to violence as never before. The presence of violence at school breeds more violence. The fear of attack escalates, more weapons are brought to school, and getting to the next class becomes a matter of survival. The unthinkable has become normal behavior for many children, who see no workable alternatives.

This fear of violence—and its resulting metal detectors, security guards, locked doors, fenced-in schoolyards, locker searches, and crisis drills—affects all children. The major consequences of violence and fear of violence are depression and anxiety, but additional effects include a sense of meaninglessness and emptiness, loss of self-esteem, feelings of humiliation, a sense of impotence because of a perceived loss of control over various aspects of life, and psychic numbing and emotional lethargy. Many children experience sleep disturbances, irritability, and excessive aggression. For others, action and decision making seem difficult. For all children, the energy that is spent on survival can no longer be spent on academics.

The Changing Workforce

Less than a generation ago, the term *workforce* conjured up visions of white men dressed in either ties or blue shirts. White males now compose only 15% of the net additions to the labor force. The other 85% are women and people from nonwhite and immigrant groups. This trend is reshaping both the color and cultural background of our workforce. Without training in learning to work cooperatively to achieve common goals among diverse groups of people, increasing linguistic and cultural problems between different ethnic and racial groups, and the resulting tensions, will be unavoidable.

At the same time, most companies face an extremely tight labor market as the baby bust of the 1960s and 1970s dramatically reduces the number of young people available to fill jobs. Yet, the decreasing labor pool needs to become more highly qualified as our businesses face growing competitive pressures—an impossibility if our young people continue their path of alienation and early exit from our schools.

It is economic suicide to let our children fail, for any reasons. They cannot be allowed to leave school without adequate knowledge of both academic and interpersonal skills. Whether or not educators have large minority populations in their schools, they must think about the wide diversity of people with whom their students will come into contact throughout their lives. They must then create school environments to retain their students and teach them how to build respectful partnerships with those who are different from them.

WHAT STRATEGIES CAN BE USED TO IMPROVE SCHOOL CULTURE?

Children who stay in school and who feel good about the experience and good about their classmates do so because their school is a safe and receptive environment for all children, both physically and psychologically. There are certainly many factors in the lives of students over which the schools have little or no control. But educators can do certain things to change the content and processes within our schools, improving the school climate to better serve this population. Adjusting the curriculum and other aspects of the educational structure to reflect the newest shifts in classroom composition is a step well taken toward ensuring that students and families from all cultures who are already in the system and immigrants new to our country and our social structures will have the skills to function together to build a peaceful future.

Multicultural Education

Mere mention of the term *multicultural education* immediately raises the hackles of some people, educators and noneducators alike. Those who question the validity or necessity of multicultural education mistakenly purport that it is a curriculum that attempts to discount and replace all things traditional, a cursory and largely ineffective nod toward pluralism, an inappropriate outgrowth of the Civil Rights movement, or simply a lame attempt at being "politically correct." Because of these misguided and uninformed indictments, multicultural education has been used, in some communities, as ammunition in the war between conservative and liberal groups. But multicultural education is not faction-specific, and, regardless of one's affiliation, it is critically important to understand the real goals of multicultural education and the positive effects it can have on race relations and effective teaching.

Significant multicultural education—that which is substantive in nature, process-oriented, and integrated throughout all of the school curricula and practices—is an approach by which children are prepared to live, learn, and work together to achieve common goals in a culturally diverse world. Through this process, children can

- Learn about and value the diversity that exists in the United States and the world.
- Become aware of and affirmed in their own cultural roots.
- Understand the social, historical, and psychological environments that cause people, including ourselves, to think and behave as we do.
- Become sensitive to other cultures, knowledgeable about other viewpoints, and able to accurately assess similarities and differences among people of the world.
- Understand their rights and responsibilities as citizens in a culturally pluralistic society.
- Become adequately prepared to live fruitful lives in an increasingly global society with shifting and permeable borders.

Unfortunately, much of the current effort in multicultural education in the United States is directed at teaching students bits and pieces of information about other cultures—"products"—through monthly celebrations, cultural posters, and world fairs. This additive approach, which can actually reinforce stereotypes by emphasizing exotic differences between people, seems to be used most often in school environments where there are few minorities in the system, or in places where assertions are made that "there are no problems here because everyone gets along." But true multicultural education is not a product at all. It is not a field trip to Taco Bell, the act of putting up a bulletin board about France, or a conversation with a foreign student. This simplistic approach undervalues the serious and complex social issues in our pluralistic society.

As with all public education, the goal of multicultural education is to maximize the potential for all students. This, of course, includes the minority child, for whom education must be made relevant. But multicultural education also benefits the majority child. Our schools have, in the past, focused nearly exclusively on the needs of majority students, propagating a monocultural view of society that is totally inconsistent with the past, present, and future realities of life in this country. Through a well-planned multicultural program, schools may be able to better prepare majority children for life in a pluralistic society, while offering children of diverse cultures a sense of belonging that can make their school experiences more positive and give them hope for the future.

Multicultural education should include, but need not be limited to, the following: 1) curriculum design, textbooks, and curricular materials that are bias-free and include ethnic and cultural content; 2) a commitment to ensure inclusive in-school and extracurricular activities, parent-teacher councils, and hiring practices, diverse staffing patterns, and continuing support for minority teachers and staff; and 3) adequate in-service training for teachers to provide them with information on how to make education multicultural.

According to Carl Grant, a long-term proponent of multicultural education, true multicultural education is visionary. Its objective is to help students acquire the skills and conceptual frameworks to pursue their own concerns, while removing the barriers that prevent them from achieving the best life has to offer. We have both an opportunity and an obligation to use the wealth of our diversity—our stories, folk literature, art, and music, as well as our experiences of our poverty, discrimination, and conflicts—to teach our children. Multicultural education is that type of education, and ultimately it can help all children develop the competencies they will need throughout their lives.

Human Rights Policies

On July 4, 1776, members of the Continental Congress that declared the United States an independent country signed a document. This statement of principles, the Declaration of Independence, subsequently became one of the most important legal and moral foundations for our country.

The second paragraph reads, "We hold these truths to be self-evident, that all men are created equal, that they are endowed by their Creator with certain unalienable Rights, that among these are Life, Liberty, and the pursuit of Happiness." These rights are alleged to be universal, to be held by people simply as people. This view implies that characteristics such as race, gender, religion, and nationality are irrelevant to whether one has human rights. Nowhere in this document does it say "but not for *those* people."

That we all display an enormous diversity is inescapable. A visible commitment to human rights within the school, however—a posted human rights policy statement, for example—is one of the most proactive approaches that a school can take to begin to ensure that the diversity of the school community is not ignored, devalued, or degraded. In making public a concise statement of policy, indicating that these rights are rooted in the dignity and worth of human beings and that adherence to these rights is the requirement of peace and security within the school, attention is focused on the intended good.

Human rights policies need to state clear guidelines against any form of infringement upon the rights of others, such as racism and sexism. The policy must be well publicized not only to students and staff but to parents, too. Most important, the leadership of the school must be willing to follow through on their policies. They must be able to punish behaviors that are counter to the policy, as well as reward behaviors of those in the school who actively promote the principles inherent within the policy.

Too often acts of racism and other infringements of human rights are addressed only after the school staff has been asked repeatedly to take action. Reasons for not wanting to face these sensitive issues head-on include not wanting to take time away from academic subject matter; not wanting to "rock the boat" and possibly incur the wrath of a wider spectrum of students and community members; not knowing how best to intervene in a positive and effective way; not thinking that there is a need to address the issues in a school system that is predominantly monocultural; and even having a complex psychological need to maintain the conflict.

But avoidance of human rights issues has damaging consequences for students. First, because violations of human rights are strong, negative experiences for children, they draw students' attention from academic pursuits as the children respond to them in nonconstructive ways. Second, evasion of the issues sends signals to all students that racism and other forms of human rights violations are trivial concerns or, worse, that they are acceptable forms of behavior.

Ignoring ethnic, racial, gender, and other differences and their potential for negative impact on children today, or even merely tolerating them, is no longer an adequate response for schools wishing to create safe and receptive environments for all children. A decent life, protected by basic human rights, is a modest standard. These rights do not supply everything that could contribute to making people's lives good or even wonderful, but they are an acceptable beginning. Educators would be wise to do more than simply acknowledge that human rights exist and conjecture about what they might mean in the lives of children. Proactively proclaiming a policy that supports basic human rights could go a long way toward counteracting the racism, bigotry, and other human rights violations, including physical violence, that are on the rise in today's schools.

Conflict Resolution Programs

Conflict is a daily reality for everyone. Whether at home or at school, the needs and values of people constantly and invariably come into opposition with those of others. Some conflicts are relatively minor, easy to handle, or capable of being overlooked. Others are not so easy to resolve. But it is a central fact of life that society is structured so that some individuals have more power and control than others do. The conflict that results is a natural phenomenon.

Children, too, need to work out their feelings about power and control. Many adults are concerned about the increasing levels of aggression children use with each other when conflicts occur between them. There should be little wonder about their predilection toward violence when they are bombarded with images of good triumphing over evil, often in violent ways, and when relatively few versions of power are represented to them in the mass media and toy markets other than the idea of power over rather than power with others.

From what they see and learn, children develop their own personal strategies for dealing with conflict. Given their general lack of awareness of nonviolent alternatives for resolving conflicts, how do we help them swap a combative attitude with a cooperative one? The Centers for Disease Control and Prevention has declared that violence has reached epidemic proportions and urges that nonviolent conflict resolution be taught to all students from preschool through twelfth grade as a response to the epidemic.

Conflict resolution training, included as a legitimate part of their curriculum, offers children a significant opportunity for developing some of the most important social skills needed in today's climate: on the cognitive level, the understanding that conflict is a normal part of everyday life, and, on the behavioral level, the ability to resolve conflict nonviolently.

A meaningful program to teach children how to mitigate discord allows them to study the causes of conflict, the different styles that people use to deal with anger and conflict, the process through which conflict escalates, and the skills needed to manage and resolve conflict creatively and nonviolently. They can explore conflict in a nurturing and cooperative classroom environment, through a number of different situations and perspectives. Through this type of program, they learn valuable life skills—verbal and nonverbal communication, listening, problem solving, critical thinking, decision making, and negotiation—and ultimately develop a productive response to conflict that helps build peaceful relationships in their classrooms, schools, and communities (see Chapters 12, 13, and 14, this volume).

In the contentious world climate today, we have come to think of these techniques as chiefly useful to adults. But it is essential that we redirect our efforts toward children for several reasons. First, our eagerness as adults to intercede in children's fights sends an implied message to them that we see them as fundamentally incompetent to settle their own disputes; we may inadvertently be giving them the impression that this whole business of conflict resolution is simply too difficult for them to master. But even the smallest children can understand many elements of arriving at outcomes where both sides win.

Second, children take into their adulthood the sense of self that they create in their childhood. It is during childhood that they form their world-views, as well as their methods of dealing with frustration and conflict. If they learn as children that dealing with conflict in violent, combative ways is the prevalent, if not the only, method, they will prolong that choice into their adulthood. At that point, it will not matter what types of arrangements our elder statespersons and gifted diplomats make to negotiate truces between warring factions, both overseas and in our own communities. There will be several generations of people who, by virtue of their training in childhood, will be willing, and more than able, to perpetuate the violence. If, instead, they learn as children a wide range of positive methods to resolve conflict peacefully in ways that are appealing and matched to their levels of development, they can spend less of their time as adults undoing destructive habits and more time contributing fully to society.

Cross-Cultural Counseling

As our schools address their urgent mission of helping prepare every child for life in a diverse society, the school counselor can be one of the most important links in the system. As much as anyone, counselors need to be aware of both the present reality and the direction of the future if they are to help children move more easily into a world filled with ever-increasing change.

The current concern for counseling the culturally different, like much of the recent focus on multiculturalism and equity in education, is a response to changing demographics. But counseling was not initially designed to treat students as individuals and help them maximize their capacity for growth. At the turn of last century, when the Industrial Revolution was in full swing, the aim of the fledgling counseling movement was, in fact, to assist in vocational training by matching a potential worker with a suitable vocation. Formal psychoanalytic methods were introduced into the United States in 1909, but counseling did not begin receiving widespread recognition until the 1940s.

By the 1950s, the aim of the counseling profession evolved to be one of assimilation. Group differences were minimized, and the goal of guidance and counseling was to assist various racial and cultural groups to become members of the larger society. Professionals were, for the most part, ethno-centric in their orientation, using the dominant culture as the standard to which all other groups were to aspire. It was not until the 1954 Supreme Court decision of *Brown v. Board of Education of Topeka*, and the Civil Rights movement that followed nearly a decade later, that the profession began to recognize the diverse counseling needs of various groups in our popu-lation. No longer was assimilation the desired goal. Recognition of and ap-preciation for cultural differences became major objectives.

But counseling is still primarily a white middle-class activity. Its practi-tioners, most of whom are white, are trained in European-centered counsel-ing programs that encompass Western-oriented philosophical assumptions. For example, the dominant culture of most schools values being "up front" about counseling issues; the students are expected to take a major role in the sessions. The traditions of most Asian Americans, Hispanics, and Native Americans, however, may preclude this pattern; their children have been raised to assume their positions within clearly defined traditional roles that include deference to their elders. Therefore, a minority student who is asked to initiate conversation may become uneasy and tense and respond with only short phrases or statements. The counselor may interpret this behavior as negative when it may actually be a sign of respect.

To successfully work with minority students, counselors must take into account each student's worldview, show respect for his or her history, and be as unbiased as possible. This requires them to learn new techniques and acquire new skills for understanding, motivating, and empowering each individual student regardless of race, gender, religion, or creed. At the same time, counselors also must be aware of the fact that the parame-ters of culture extend far beyond racial and ethnic categories.

To guide students effectively in a multicultural environment, a cultur-ally sensitive counselor will consider, at a minimum, these major points:

- Historical perspectives and the social support systems of diverse fami-lies
- Unique characteristics of the value systems of diverse families
- Any cultural communication barriers, either verbal or nonverbal, that may hinder the level of trust between the diverse student and the di-verse counselor
- Development of innovative treatment strategies based on cultural con-siderations that place a high priority on building a sense of personal worth in students and empowering them both as individuals within their particular cultural context and as an integral part of the larger school/ community setting

The degree to which counseling contributes to the development of a student's concept of his or her human potential is clear. All children in our schools today must receive the support and motivation that they need to identify and achieve their goals, regardless of their past histories, their present situations, or the sometimes limited expectations we hold for their futures.

THE CHALLENGE

The "melting pot" analogy that has been so prevalent in this country for generations is no longer appropriate. We are, in fact, in a superb position to benefit from the knowledge that comes from experiencing a confluence of cultures. After all, throughout our history, we have had representatives from most parts of the world living within our borders. Not all newcomers have been welcomed warmly by Native Americans, but the growth in population by immigration has surged forward. Without a doubt, future generations will be faced with living in an increasingly multicultural society, and our schools must play an essential role in the preparation of our children for life in this diverse, complex, and interdependent world.

Although cultures may mingle in the classrooms of our schools, it is not an indication that there is harmony in the hallways. If we change the culture of our schools to reflect and legitimize our human and cultural diversity, to respect and value each other regardless of our human or social differences, our children will be better prepared to live peacefully in this increasingly pluralistic world.

Index

*Page numbers printed in **boldface** type refer to tables or figures.*

Academic achievement, and CAPSLE Program, 286, 287. *See also* Tests of Academic Proficiency

Academic motivation, and school-based group therapy program, 182

Administration, school. *See also* School personnel
avoidant bystanding and, 278
school-based mental health programs and, 146
school environment and risk of school violence, 33

Adolescents and adolescence. *See also* Age; Children; High schools; Middle schools; Pregnancy; Violence and violent behavior
epidemiological literature on exposure to violence, 164
firearm injuries and, 220, 223–224
firearms and traumatic stress in, 221
homicide rate and, 7–9

increase in violent crime by, 9
psychiatric assessment of potentially violent, 91–103
psychiatric disorders and violence in, 60
suicide and, 9–10, 88–90
testosterone levels and, 55

Adulthood. *See also* Age
childhood and development of sense of self, 300
Columbine students and transition to, 160–161

Adult protective shield, and psychological first aid, 265

African Americans. *See also* Race; Racism
homicide as cause of death in males and, 29, 76
trauma theory and behavior of males, 235–236
violence in Southern culture and, 12–13

After-school programs, 242, 258–259

Age. *See also* Adulthood; Adolescence and adolescents; Children
  homicide rates and, 8
  as risk factor for violence, 76–77
Agent factors, and firearm violence, 222
Aggression and aggressive behavior. *See also* Behavior
  chronic exposure to violence and, 37
  serotonin dysregulation and, 56
  social systems–power dynamics theory and, 278, 286
Alaska Natives
  environmental influences on brain development, 68
  firearm violence and, 221–222
Alcoholics Anonymous, 106
Alternative Learning Center (Philadelphia), 237–238
Alternative programs, and prevention of school violence, 265–266
Alternative schools, and dropout prevention, 259
American Academy of Child and Adolescent Psychiatry (AACAP), 144, 224
American Academy of Pediatrics, 62, 63, 144, 223
American Indians, and firearm violence, 221–222. *See also* Alaska Natives
American Medical Association, 38, 62
American Psychiatric Association
  APA Alliance and essay contest on school violence, 37
  information on trauma and disaster response and, 144
  The Principles of Medical Ethics and, 194, 211
  on television and violent behavior in children, 62
American Psychological Association, 223–224

Amphetamines, 110
Animal models, and biological causes of violence, 55
Antisocial behavior, and suicide, 90. *See also* Behavior
Antisocial personality disorder, 60
Arizona. *See* Tucson, Arizona
Arkansas. *See* Jonesboro, Arkansas
Arrests, and risk factors for youth violence, 14. *See also* Law enforcement
Assessment. *See also* Diagnosis
  of potentially violent youths, 91–103, 112
  school-based group therapy program and, 168–172
  of threat in duty-to-warn situations, 204, 207, 208
Attachment behavior, and prevention of violence, 256–257. *See also* Behavior
Attendance, and Chicago public schools, **260.** *See also* Truancy
Attention-deficit/hyperactivity disorder (ADHD)
  parents and treatment of, 241
  psychopharmacology and, 110
  suicide and, 90
  violence and conduct disorder, 255
Australia, 13
Avoidance, of school, 37. *See also* Truancy
Avoidant bystanding, 278

Battle Creek, Michigan, 18
Beck Depression Inventory (BDI), 96
Behavior. *See also* Aggression and aggressive behavior; Antisocial behavior; Attachment behavior; Bonding; Violence and violent behavior
  assessment of adolescents for potential violence, 101
  prevention of violence and, 256–260

trauma theory and, 235
Behavior Management Training Program and Behavior Intervention Teachers (Chicago), 264–265
Big Brothers/Big Sisters of America, 45, 224
Biological causes, of violence, 54–60, 68–69
Bipolar disorder, 59, 110
Bomb threats, 81
Bonding
    parenting education and, 258
    school attendance and, 260
Borderline personality disorder, 111
Bosnia-Herzegovina, 185
Boston. *See also* Urban areas
    school violence prevention programs in, 44, 245–246
    youth homicide rate in, 9
Brain imaging studies, 58, 235
Brain structure, and biological causes of violence, 58–59, 68
Brown v. Board of Education of Topeka (1954), 301
Bruno Program, 284–285
Bullying, and school violence, 34, 234, 274–275, 277–278, 280–282, 287
Bullying Proof Program, 280
Bureau of Justice Statistics, 74, 75, 77
Bystanders, and bullying, 278, 280–282

California. *See* Los Angeles
California Supreme Court, 201–202
Canada, 8
CAPSLE Program (Creating a Peaceful School Learning Environment), 280–288
Carbamazepine, 110
Carneal, Michael, 5
Center for Epidemiologic Studies Depression Scale for Children, 166
Center on Juvenile and Criminal Justice, 78

Center for Mental Health Services (CMHS), 142
Center to Prevent Handgun Violence, 223
Center for the Study and Prevention of School Violence, 73
Centers for Disease Control and Prevention (CDC), 9–10, 15, 22, 26, 27, 29–30, 47–48, 299
Central nervous system dysfunctions, and psychopharmacology, 109. *See also* Neurological disorders
Character development, and self-esteem, 262
Chat rooms, and Internet, 66
Chicago. *See also* Urban areas
    community mental health centers and prevention of school violence in, 244–245
    homicide of children and homicide rates, 3–4, 7
    public school system and school violence prevention programs, 251–270
Chicago Tribune, 3–4
Child abuse. *See also* Domestic violence; Sexual abuse
    parenting education and, 247
    risk factors for youth violence and, 13
    serotonin dysregulation and, 57
Child Behavior Checklist (CBCL), 55, 95
Children. *See also* Age; Child abuse; Elementary schools and elementary school children; Infants and infancy; Middle schools; Preschool years and preschool-age children; Toddlers and toddlerhood
    attachment behavior and, 256–257
    as defendants in homicide trials, 19–21
    firearm injuries and, 220

Children *(continued)*
  homicides in Chicago of late 1980s
    and early 1990s, 3–4
  life experiences and schools,
    234–236
  psychiatric disorders and violence
    in, 60
  serotonin levels in aggressive, 56
  suicide and, 9–10, 88–90
Children's Aggression Scale (CAS), 96
Children's Depression Inventory
  (CDI), 96
Children's Depression Rating Scale
  (CDRS-R), 98
Children's Interview for Psychiatric
  Syndromes (CHIPS), 98
Chromosomal analysis, and biological
  causes of violence, 54
Cities. *See* Urban areas
Civil rights movement, 301
Class, socioeconomic
  child care and, 16
  media coverage of school violence
    and, 5–6
  multicultural society and, 293, 301
Classroom avengers, 34–35, 46, 224
Class size, and school violence, 31–32
Clinical practice. *See also* Psychiatrists;
  Therapists
  duty to warn and, 206–211
  influence of television on children
    and, 63–64
Clinton, Bill, 25, 78
Colorado, 142. *See also* Littleton,
  Colorado
Colorado Bureau of Investigation, 150
Colorado Child and Adolescent Psy-
  chiatric Society, 143–144
Colorado Organization for Victim
  Assistance, 136
Colorado Psychiatric Society, 143–144
Columbine Connections, 140–141, 142,
  153, 159
Columbine Crisis Chat Line, 139

Columbine High School. *See* Littleton,
  Colorado
Comer School Development Program,
  47
Commitment, and school-based group
  therapy program, 170
Communication, and Internet, 66
Community
  Columbine High School shootings
    and response of, 129–161
  public health interventions and
    rebuilding of, 252–255
Community mental health services.
  See also Mental health services
  resource allocation and, 157
  response to Columbine shootings
    and, 137–142
  school violence prevention pro-
    grams in Chicago and, 244–245
Comorbid diagnoses
  psychotherapy for potentially vio-
    lent youths and, 108
  suicide in children and adolescents
    and, 90
Conduct disorder
  depression and, 108
  serotonin dysregulation and, 56
  suicide and, 89, 90
Confidentiality. *See also* Trust
  duty to warn and, 92, 193, 205,
    211–212
  mental health services for students
    and, 38
  psychological autopsy of school
    violence and, 90
Conflict resolution, 43, 44–45, 262,
  298–300
Connectedness, and self-esteem, 262.
  See also School connectedness
Connecticut. *See* New Haven,
  Connecticut
Conners Parent Rating Scale—Revised
  and Conners Teacher Rating
  Scale—Revised, 95–96

Conscience, and assessment for potential of violence, 101

Conspiracy of silence, in schools, 37

Constitution, and Second Amendment, 225

Consultation, and psychodiagnostic assessment, 102–103

Contagion theory, of media and school violence, 64–65

Cook County (Illinois) Probation Department, 266

Coping, and chronic exposure to violence, 36–37

Cortisol, and aggression, 57

Cost. *See also* Funding
of firearm injuries, 67, 220
of long-term response to Columbine incident, 147

Counseling and counselors
CAPSLE Program and discipline plan, 283
community response to Columbine incident and, 139, 155
eyewitness account of school violence and, 117–127
multicultural education and cross-cultural, 300–302
parents and firearm violence, 223
traumatic stress in children and, 269
victims of school violence and, 45

CPS Near North Ministerial Alliance, 252, 254

CPS Region Anti-Violence Workshops, 254

Cradle to Classroom program (Chicago), 258

Crime. *See also* Homicide; Violence and violent behavior
decline in, 226
rates of in schools, 73
types of in schools, 75–76

Crisis Intervention Teams and Crisis Intervention Services Program (Chicago), 264, 269

Crisis services, and Columbine High School shootings, 138, 149–150

Cross-cultural counseling, 300–302

Culture. *See also* Multicultural society; Social factors
of disrespect, 38–39
emotional expression and, 38
increased number of teen parents and, 73
prevalence of violence and, 82, 232–233
of South and youth violence, 11–12
use of term, 292

Curriculum, of schools
multicultural education and, 297
programs for improving emotional climate and, 43–44

Cyclothymia, 110

Death, causes of
firearm injuries and, 67, 76, 219
homicide and African American males, 29, 76
prevalence of school-associated violence, 78–79

Debriefing, after incidents of school violence, 139

Declaration of Independence, 297

Delaware Supreme Court, 205

Demographics
historical comparisons of homicide rates and, 8
multicultural society and, 291–292

Denial, and duty to warn situations, 210

Depersonalization, and exposure to violence, 36

Depression. *See also* Major depression; Mood disorders
conduct disorder and, 108

Depression *(continued)*
  development of assessment and treatment for in children and adolescents, 87–88
  risk of after-school violent incidents, 150, 155, 159
Depression Self-Rating Scale (DSRS), 96–97
Development, and school-based group therapy program, 182, 183
Developmental history, and assessment of potentially violent children, 99–101
Deviance, and social disorganization theory, 265
Dextroamphetamines, 110
Diagnosis, suicide and postmortem psychiatric, 89. *See also* Assessment; Comorbid diagnoses
Diagnostic Interview for Children and Adolescents (DICA), 97
Diagnostic Interview Schedule for Children (DISC), 97–98
Discipline. *See also* Zero tolerance policies
  CAPSLE Program and, 282–283, 286
  child abuse and, 248
  prevalence of problems in schools and, 74–75
  zero-tolerance policies in schools and, 42–43, 280–282
Disrespect, culture of, 38–39
Divalproex sodium, 110
Divorce, 236
Documentation, and duty to warn, 198, 199, 208
Domestic violence. *See also* Child abuse; Family; Violence and violent behavior
  causes of school violence and, 232
  homicide and firearms, 222
  life experiences of children and, 234–235

Dosage, and psychopharmacology for children and adolescents, 109, 110–111
Dress code policies, 259
Dropouts and dropout rate
  Hispanic Americans and, 259, 293
  prevention of, 259
  teenage pregnancy and, 258
DSM-IV, and diagnostic criteria
  for posttraumatic stress disorder, 164, 166
  for schizotypal personality disorder, 195–196
Duty-to-protect doctrine, 203–205
Duty to warn
  assessment of potentially violent children and, 92
  legal perspective on, 189–199
  psychiatric perspective on, 201–213
Dysthymia, 89, 109–110

Early Warning, Timely Response: A Guide to Safe Schools (Dwyer), 42
Economics. *See* Cost; Funding
Edinboro, Pennsylvania, 78
Education. *See also* Psychoeducation; Schools
  impact of violence on, 73–74
  parenting and, 246–249, 258
  prevention of firearm violence and, 223, 224
  of teachers in behavior management techniques, 33
Education Week, 81
Elementary schools and elementary school children. *See also* Children; Schools
  developmental history and assessment of potential for violence in, 100
  prevalence of violence and, 80
Emotions
  costs of firearm injuries and, 220–221

culture and expression of, 38
programs for improving climate of
schools and, 43–48
Environment
biological causes of violence and,
68
firearm violence and, 222
Epidemiology, and youth violence,
10–19
Epilepsy, and violence rates, 58–59
Existential dilemma, 165, 178–179,
180–181
Expert witnesses, and homicide trials
of children, 19–21
Eye Movement Desensitization Reprocessing (EMDR), 159
Eyewitness account, of school violence, 117–127

Family. *See also* Domestic violence;
Family history; Family therapy;
Parents and parenting
characteristics of and risk factors
for violence in children, 94–95,
257
school-based group therapy programs and, 173, 182
Family history
assessment of adolescents for
potential of violence and, 101
of serotonin dysregulation and
aggression, 56
Family therapy, 111, 153
Fayetteville, Tennessee, 78
Fear
Columbine High School shootings
and, 131–132, 134–135
school-based group therapy program and, 179
of school violence, 74
Federal Bureau of Investigation (FBI),
7, 9, 273–274
Federal Emergency Management
Agency (FEMA), 141–142

Federal Rules of Evidence, 212
Fenfluramine, 56, 57
Firearms. *See also* Weapons
causes of death and, 67, 76, 219
causes of school violence and availability of, 232
children and access to, 21
cost of injuries from, 67, 220
culture of violence and availability
of, 82
emotional costs of injuries from,
220–221
legal issues and, 225–227
nonfatal injuries in children and
adolescents, 220
prevalence of in schools, 77
prevention of injuries by, 223–227
as public health problem, 221–222
social factors in school violence
and, 67–68
suicides and, 68, 219–220, 222
Youth Homicide Committee and,
239–240
youth violence and access to, 30
First aid, psychological for potentially
violent children, 91–92, 265
Fluoxetine, 108, 110
Follow-up
after treatment of potentially violent youths, 111
school-based group therapy program and, 184
Foothills Parks and Recreation District
(Colorado), 140
Forensic psychiatrists, 195, 196
Foreseeability, and duty to warn, 204
Freud, Sigmund, 235
Frontal lobe injury, 58
Full-service schools, 47
Funding, for community mental
health response to Columbine
incident, 141–142. *See also* Cost
Future, and school-based group ther-
apy programs, 183–184

Gangs
mentoring models and, 224
risk factors for youth violence and, 14
school-based group therapy programs and, 173–174
social factors in school violence and, 61, 82
Gender. *See also* Sexism
biological causes of violence and, 54–55, 57, 59
Bruno Program and, 284
rates of violence against women and, 82
social systems–power dynamics theory and, 276–277, 277–278
suicide among children and adolescents and, 9–10
teachers as victims of school violence and, 36
General Accounting Office, 67
Genetics, and biological causes of violence, 54
Gentle Warrior Program, 283–284, 288
Georgia, 78
Goals, of school-based group therapy program, 172, 174–175, 177, 180, 182, 183
Golden, Andrew, 14
Government. *See* Law enforcement; Legal issues; Legislation
Grief, and acute stress reactions, 150
Group therapy. *See also* Treatment
community mental health response to Columbine incident and, 156–157
for potentially violent youths, 111
school-based program
content and process of, 172–184
design of, 164–165
effectiveness of, 184–185
setting of and recruitment of members for, 165–172

Guidelines
for first aid for potentially violent children, 91–92
for mental health professionals in *Tarasoff* situations, 198–199
for psychiatric assessment of potentially violent children, 92–95, 112
for school violence prevention programs, 249–250
Guns. *See* Firearms; Weapons

Harassment, and school violence, 34
Harris, Eric, 5, 10, 131, 133, 134
Hawaii, 246–249
Head injury, and biological causes of violence, 58
Head Start programs, 246
Healing Fund, The, 142
Health care, and prevention of school violence, 255–256. *See also* Health insurance; Physical examination
Health insurance. *See also* Health care
access of children to health care and, 256
comprehensive psychological testing and, 102
psychopharmacology and, 108
Health maintenance organizations (HMOs), and psychopharmacology, 108
Healthy Kids/Healthy Minds, 256
Help-seeking, barriers to as risk factor for school violence, 38
High schools. *See also* Adolescence and adolescents; Littleton, Colorado; Schools; School violence
CAPSLE Program and, 288
prevalence of violence and, 80
Hippocampal atrophy, 58
Hispanic Americans, and dropout rate, 259, 293. *See also* Multicultural society

Homicide. *See also* Crime
　Chicago and children as victims of,
　　3–4
　children as defendants in trials for,
　　19–21
　decline in rate of youth, 29
　epidemic of youth violence and,
　　10–16
　firearms and, 67, 226
　schools and, 78–80, 82
　statistical patterns of, 7–9, 75–76
　suicide and, 10
Honor, code of and violence in South-
　ern culture, 12, 13
Hopelessness Scale, 168
Hospitalization, psychiatric
　duty to warn and, 207, 209
　increase of after Columbine inci-
　　dent, 132
　short-term for violent, homicidal,
　　or suicidal youths, 104–105, 111
Host factors, and firearm violence,
　221–222
Hostility, and chronic exposure to vio-
　lence, 37
Human rights policies, and multicul-
　tural society, 297–298
Humor, and school-based group ther-
　apy program, 179

I.C.E. Violence (I Can End Violence),
　242
Identifiable third party, and duty to
　warn, 203
Illinois. *See* Chicago
Imitation, of school violence, 80–81
Immigrants, and multicultural soci-
　ety, 291, 292, 302
Imminent threat, and duty to warn,
　203
Impact of Events Scale, 166
Individual psychotherapy. *See also*
　Treatment
　community mental health response

after Columbine incident and,
　156–157
for potentially violent youths,
　106–108
Infants and infancy. *See also* Bonding;
　Toddlers and toddlerhood
　developmental history and assess-
　　ment of potential for violence,
　　99
　firearms and traumatic stress in,
　　220–221
　risk factors for youth violence and
　　prematurity, 14–15
In re complaint of McLinn (1984),
　210
In re Estate of Heltsley v. Votteler (Iowa,
　1982), 210
Interdisciplinary programs, 242
Internet, and youth violence, 65–66.
　See also Web sites
Interpersonal disputes, and school
　violence, 27
Interpersonal relationships. *See also*
　Social skills
　assessment of adolescents for
　　potential of violence and, 100,
　　104
　school-based group therapy pro-
　　gram and, 171, 173, 182, 183
Interviews, with siblings and peers of
　potentially violent children, 99,
　103. *See also* Structured diagnostic
　instruments
Involuntary hospitalization, and duty
　to warn, 209
Iowa Supreme Court, 210
Iowa Tests of Basic Skills (ITBS), **263**
Ithaca, New York, 18
I-Thou relationship, 107

Jablonski v. United States (1983), 210
Jaffe v. Redmond (1996), 212
Jefferson Center. *See* Jefferson Center
　for Mental Health (Colorado)

Jefferson Center for Mental Health (Colorado), 135, 137–142, 151, 152, 154–155, 156

Jefferson County District Attorney's Office (Colorado), 136, 140

Jefferson County Sheriff's Office (Colorado), 136, 140, 159

Johnson, Mitchell, 5

Johnson Institute Program, 280

Jonesboro, Arkansas, 5, 14, 78

Kansas. *See* Topeka, Kansas

Kentucky. *See* West Paducah, Kentucky

Kid Care (U. S. Dept. of Education), 256

Kinkel, Kip, 4, 5, 10, 14

Klebold, Dylan, 5, 10, 131, 133, 134

Languages, and multicultural society, 292

Law enforcement. *See also* Arrests; Legal issues
   duty to warn and, 206
   gun control laws and, 225
   police in schools and, 233, 266–267
   probation officers and, 245–246
   truancy and, 239

Learning and learning disorders, 15

Legal issues. *See also* Expert witnesses; Law enforcement; Legislation
   children and homicide trials, 19–21
   gun control and, 224–225, 226–227
   liability and mental health professionals, 189–199
   multicultural society and, 292–293
   psychological aspects of youth violence and, 21–23
   truancy hearings and, 239

Legislation. *See also* Legal issues
   firearm violence and, 224–225
   immunity statutes and duty to warn, 203
   on school and youth violence, 25

Life experiences, of children, 234–236

Lighthouse Program (Chicago), 259

Lithium, 110

Littleton, Colorado (Columbine High School)
   background information on, 130–132
   conclusions on, 159–161
   conspiracy of silence and threats of violence, 37
   following school year and, 154–156
   impediments to treatment of victims, 149–152
   psychological impact of, 132–135, 152–154, 234
   reporting of in media, 5, 64–65, 78, 80–81
   retraumatizations and, 158–159
   school safety plan and, 41
   suicide and, 10, 78, 131

Liver function tests, and divalproex sodium, 110

Logan Square Neighborhood Association (Chicago), 254

Long-term residential placement, for potentially violent youths, 105–106

Los Angeles. *See also* Urban areas
   perceptions of high school students about teachers, 33
   school-based group therapy program and, 165
   school guidelines on media requests in, 149

Louisiana, 12

Major depression. *See also* Depression
   biological causes of violence and, 59
   psychopharmacology for potentially violent youth and, 109–110
   suicide and, 89, 90

Management, of violent and homicidal behavior in children and adolescents, 103–112
Martial arts, and Gentle Warrior Program, 283, 284, 288
Maryland, 46
Massachusetts. *See* Boston
McCormick Tribune Foundation, 142
Media. *See also* Television
 coverage of incidents of school violence, 5–6
 culture of violence and, 232
 firearm violence and, 222, 226
 negative impact of after Columbine incident, 149, 157–158
Medicaid, 256
Mental Health Association of Colorado, 139
Mental health professionals. *See also* Mental health services; Psychiatrists; Therapists
 liability as legal issue for, 190, 193–199
 response to Columbine High School shootings and, 135–147
Mental health services. *See also* Community mental health services; Mental health professionals; School-based mental health programs
 barriers to help seeking as risk factor in school violence, 38
 Columbine High School shootings and, 132
Mental retardation, and biological causes of violence, 60
Mentor Connection Program (Chicago), 262
Mentoring
 prevention of firearm violence and, 224
 prevention of school violence and, 45, 242, 284–285
Metal detectors, 41, 233, 267

Methylphenidate, 110, 241
Metropolitan Achievement Test, 287
Michigan. *See* Battle Creek, Michigan; Port Huron, Michigan
Middle schools. *See also* Adolescence and adolescents; Children; Schools
 CAPSLE Program and, 288
 firearms and, 67
 Philadelphia and summit meetings, 240–241
 prevalence of violence in, 80
Milwaukee, Wisconsin, 219
Miranda-type warnings, 212
Mission-driven philosophy, for school-community programs, 255
Mississippi. *See* Pearl, Mississippi
Missouri Assessment of Genetics Interview for Children (MAGIC), 97
Monitoring, by parents, 268
Mood disorders, and psychopharmacology, 110. *See also* Depression
Multicultural education, 295–297
Multicultural society. *See also* Hispanic Americans
 challenge of, 302
 demographics and, 291–292
 improvement of school culture and, 295–302
 legal issues and, 292–293
 school violence and, 293–295
Murder. *See* Homicide

Naidu v. Laird (Delaware, 1988), 205
Narratives, and school-based group therapy program, 179, 180–181
National Center for Education Statistics, 27, 41, 42, 74, 75, 77, 80
National Center for Injury Prevention and Control (CDC), 47–48, 76, 80
National Electronic Injury Surveillance System, 220

National Firearms Act, 224–225
National Rifle Association, 225
National School Boards Association,
    26, 42
National School Safety Center, 27, 76
National Spinal Cord Injury Statistical
    Center, 220
Neighborhoods. *See* Urban areas
Netherlands, The, 66
Neurological disorders, and risk
    factors for youth violence, 14–15,
    94. *See also* Central nervous
    system
Neuropsychiatric disorders, and vio-
    lent behavior, 255
Neurotransmitters, and biological
    causes of violence, 57–58
New Haven, Connecticut, 242–244
New Jersey, 224
Newsweek magazine, 225
New York State. *See* Ithaca, New York
Night Stalkers Program (Chicago), 267
Norepinephrine, 57
Normalization, of violence, 36–37
North Carolina, 220

Obsessive-compulsive disorder, 11, 235
Oklahoma City bombing, 145, 148, 149
Olanzapine, 111
Operation Jump Start (Chicago), 266
Operation S.A.F.E. (Schools Are for
    Education), 266–267
Oppositional defiant disorder, 90
Oregon. *See* Springfield, Oregon
Outcomes, and CAPSLE Program,
    286–287

Parents and Community Connecting
    Together (PACCT), 140
Parents and parenting. *See also* Family;
    Pregnancy
    attachment behavior and bonding
        with children, 256–257, 258
    children and television viewing, 63

culture of disrespect and, 38–39
    education in skills of, 246–249, 258
    firearm violence and, 222, 223
    Gentle Warrior Program and, 284
    increase in numbers of adolescents
        as, 73
    monitoring of students and, 268
    perceptions and reality of school
        violence and, 81–82
    prevention of violence and educa-
        tion for, 246–249
    school safety and security measures
        and, 266
    as teachers, 257
    treatment of child for attention-
        deficit/hyperactivity
        disorder and, 241
Parents as Teachers First program
    (Chicago), 257
Paroxetine, 108, 110
Pearl, Mississippi, 5, 117–127
Peer Leaders Program and Peer Medi-
    ation Program (Chicago), 263
Peer mediation, 44–45
Peer mentoring, 285
Pennsylvania, 81. *See also* Philadelphia
Pennsylvania Emergency Manage-
    ment Agency, 64
Perceptions, and reality of school vio-
    lence, 81–82
Personality profile, and risk factors for
    violence in children, 94
Pets, and psychotherapy for poten-
    tially violent youth, 107
Pew Foundation, 248
Philadelphia, 237–242, 248
Philadelphia Bar Association, 242
Physical conflicts, prevalence of in
    schools, 27
Physical examination. *See also* Health
    care
    assessment of adolescents for
        potential of violence and,
        101–102

psychopharmacology for children and adolescents and, 109

Physician-patient relationship, and duty to warn, 193

Physicians' Desk Reference, 195

Planning, of long-term response to Columbine incident, 147–149. *See also* Safety and safety plans

Police. *See* Law enforcement

Police Mental Health Collaboration (New Haven), 242–244

Police/Probation Sweep (Boston), 246

Pornography, and Internet, 66

Port Huron, Michigan, 81

Positron emission tomography (PET), 235

Posttraumatic stress disorder (PTSD) chronic exposure to violence and, 36

DSM-IV criteria for diagnosis of, 164, 166

Oklahoma City bombing and, 149

risk of after Columbine incident, 148, 150, 155, 158, 159

school-based group therapy program and, 176, 184

Poverty, and firearm violence, 222

Power, and self-esteem, 261

Prediction, of violence, 208

Pregnancy, teenage

parenting education and, 258

risk factors for youth violence and, 16

Pregroup clinical interview, and school-based group therapy program, 168–172

Premature infants, and risk factors for youth violence, 14–15

Preschool years and preschool-age children. *See also* Children

Chicago public schools and programs for, 258

developmental history and assessment of potential for violence, 99–100

firearms and traumatic stress in, 221

Parents as Teachers First program and, 257

Preventability, and duty to warn, 204

Prevention, of school violence

firearm injuries and, 223–227

basic premises for school and preschool interventions, 249–250

Chicago public schools and, 251–270

community mental health centers in Chicago and, 244–245

multicultural education and, 291–302

parenting education in Hawaii and, 246–249

Police Mental Health Collaboration in New Haven and, 242–244

programs for improving emotional climate of schools and, 43–48

public agencies in Boston and, 245–246

school-based strategies for, 233–234

social systems–power dynamics approach to, 273–288

Youth Homicide Committee and Philadelphia experience, 238–242

Principals. *See* Administration

Principles of Medical Ethics, The (American Psychiatric Association, 1981, 1998), 194, 211

Probation programs, 245–246, 266

Professional organizations, and community response to Columbine incident, 143–145

Project Exile (Richmond, Virginia), 225

Project on Human Development in Chicago Neighborhoods, 33–34

Prolactin, 56, 57

Psychiatric disorders. *See also*
  Comorbid diagnoses; *specific*
  disorders
  normalization of violence and,
    36–37
  rates of violence and, 59–60
  risk factors for violence in children
    and, 94
Psychiatrists, and community
  response to Columbine High
  School shootings, 143–147. *See also*
  Clinical practice; Mental health
  professionals; Therapists
Psychodiagnostic assessment, of
  potentially violent children,
  102–103
Psychoeducation. *See also* Education
  Gentle Warrior Program and,
    283–284
  school-based group therapy pro-
    gram and, 176
  for teachers after Columbine inci-
    dent, 146, 160
Psychological autopsy, of suicide in
  children and adolescents, 88–90
Psychological profile, of students at
  risk for school violence, 34
Psychological resiliency, indicators of,
  40
Psychology
  impact of Columbine High School
    shootings and, 132–135,
    152–154
  legal aspects of youth violence and,
    21–23
Psychopharmacology, for potentially
  violent youth, 105, 108–111. *See*
  also Psychostimulants; Treatment
Psychosis, and juvenile homicides,
  22
Psychostimulants, 108, 233. *See also*
  Psychopharmacology
Psychotherapy. *See* Group therapy;
  Individual psychotherapy

Public health
  community infrastructures and,
    252–255
  firearms and, 221–222
  response to school violence and, 69,
    130, 145
Public opinion, on gun control, 226
Public policy, and urban housing, 17

Quetiapine fumarate, 111

Race. *See also* African Americans;
    Multicultural society; Racism
  homicide rates and, 4, 13
  media coverage of school violence
    and, 5–6
  multicultural education and, 301
Racine, Wisconsin, 18–19
Racism. *See also* African Americans;
    Race
  human rights policies and, 298
  risk factors for youth homicide and,
    11
  segregation and urban neighbor-
    hoods, 17
Rape, and school-based group therapy
  program, 171
Rapid-cycling bipolar disorder, 110
Rapport, establishment of with
    potentially violent children and
    adolescents, 104. *See also*
    Therapeutic alliance
Rating scales
  assessment of potential violence in
    children, 95–98
  school-based group therapy pro-
    gram and, 166, 168
Red Cross, 136
Referral service network, 254
Rejection, and violence in children, 274
Religion
  Chicago public schools and part-
    nership with, 252, 254, 264
  violence in culture of South and, 12

Religious Institutions Partnership (Chicago), 264
Research, on school violence, 90, 149–150
Residential placement, for potentially violent youth, 105–106
Resource allocation, and community mental health services, 157
Rewards, and CAPSLE Program, 281–282
Risk factors
  for firearm injuries, 221–222
  for potential violence in children, 94–95
  for school violence, 31–40
  for suicide in children and adolescents, **89**
  for youth homicide, 10–11, 22
  for youth violence, 13–15, 76–77
Risperidone, 111
Road rage, 171
Role-playing, 106, 176, 284

Safe and Drug-Free Schools and Communities Act, 26–27
Safe and Gun-Free Schools Act (1994), 42
Safe Schools/Healthy Students Initiative, 25
Safe Schools, Safe Neighborhoods Summer (1998), 254
Safety and safety plans
  as approach to school violence, 41–42, 266–267
  prevalence of violence in schools and, 82
Salt Lake City, and gang violence task force, 18
Saturday Morning Alternative Reach Out and Teach Program (SMART), 266
Schedule for Affective Disorders and Schizophrenia—Child's Version (K-SADS), 98

Schizoaffective disorder, 111
Schizophrenia, 59, 111
Schizotypal personality disorder, 195–196
School Action Grant Program, 25
School-based mental health programs. *See also* Mental health services
  community response to Columbine incident and, 146, 155
  group psychotherapy and, 164–185
  prevention of school violence and, 46–47, 185
  Yale Child Study Center and, 244
School Climate Teams (Chicago), 264
School and Community Relations (Chicago), 264
School connectedness, 39–40, 262. *See also* Connectedness
School culture, and multicultural society, 293, 295–302
School Improvement Plans (Chicago), 264
School personnel, and community response to Columbine incident, 146, 151. *See also* Administration; Teachers
Schools. *See also* Curriculum; Discipline; Education; Elementary schools; High schools; Middle schools; Preschool years and preschool-age children; School-based mental health programs; School connectedness; School violence; Students; Teachers
  approaches and solutions to school violence and, 40–43, 233–234
  assessment of children and adolescents for potential of violence and, 103
  CAPSLE Program and learning environment of, 280–287
  community programs and activities in Chicago, 254

Schools *(continued)*
crime rate in, 74
difficulties at as risk factor in youth violence, 15
homicides in, 78–80, 82
life experiences of children and, 234–236
prevalence of weapons in, 77
programs for improving emotional climate of, 43–48
risk factors for school violence and environment of, 31–40
social factors and, 236–237
types of crimes in, 75–76
School violence. *See also* Schools; Violence and violent behavior
assessment and management of for children and adolescents with potential for, 87–112
community response to Columbine High School shootings and, 129–161
eyewitness account and, 117–127
school-based group psychotherapy and, 163–185
factors contributing to
biological and social causes of, 53–69
overview of contemporary problem, 3–23
school environment and, 25–49
trends in, 73–82
legal aspects of
attorney's perspective on duty to warn, 189–199
psychiatric perspective on duty to warn, 201–213
prevention of
basic premises for school and preschool interventions, 249–250
Chicago public schools and, 251–270

community mental health centers in Chicago and, 244–245
firearm fatalities and injuries and, 219–227
multicultural education and, 291–302
parenting education in Hawaii and, 246–249
Police Mental Health Collaboration in New Haven, Connecticut, 242–244
public agencies in Boston and, 245–246
school-based strategies for, 233–234
social systems–power dynamics approach to, 273–288
Youth Homicide Committee and Philadelphia experience, 238–242
Screening, for high-risk victims after Columbine incident, 152, 156
Second Amendment, of Constitution, 225
Second Step Violence Prevention Curriculum (South Carolina), 279, 280
Security, as approach to school violence, 41, 266–267. *See also* Law enforcement; Metal detectors; Safety and safety plans
Seizure disorders, and psychopharmacology, 110
Self
assessment of adolescents for potential violence and perception of, 101
conflict resolution training and, 300
Self-esteem
CAPSLE Program and, 287
psychotherapy for potentially violent youth and, 107
school violence prevention and, 260–268

Self-harm, and duty to warn, 206
Self-help groups, for potentially violent youth, 106
Self-mutilating behavior, and serotonin dysregulation, 56–57
Semistructured diagnostic instruments, 98
Serious harm, and duty to warn, 203
Serotonin dysregulation, and biological causes of violence, 55–57
Serotonin reuptake inhibitors (SRIs), 108
Sertraline, 108, 110
Severe violence, 26
Sex differences, and biological causes of violence, 54–55
Sexism, and human rights policies, 298. *See also* Gender
Sexual abuse, and *Tarasoff* duty, 210–211. *See also* Child abuse
Short-term psychiatric hospitalization, 104–105
SHOUTS (Students Helping Others Unite Together Socially), 141, 142, 154
Side effects, and psychopharmacology for children and adolescents, 109
Social disorganization theory, of deviance, 265
Social factors. *See also* Culture; Social skills; Social systems–power dynamics theory
etiology of violence and, 61–69
schools and, 236–237
Socialization, of children, 234
Social skills. *See also* Interpersonal relationships; Social factors
conflict resolution training and, 299
education in and school violence prevention, 262–265
school-based group therapy programs and, 176

Social systems–power dynamics theory
CAPSLE Program and school learning environment, 280–287
explanation of theory, 274–278
school violence prevention programs and, 279–280
South, and culture of violence, 11–13
South Africa, 13
South Carolina, 280
South Dakota, 12
Springfield, Oregon, 4, 14, 78
Standard of care, and legal issues, 198, 212–213
STOP program, 223
Straight Talk About Risks (STAR), 224
Stress. *See also* Trauma
firearms and, 221
grief and acute reactions to, 150
Stroop Color-Word Test, 58
Structured diagnostic instruments
assessment of potentially violent children and, 95–98
school-based group therapy program and, 166, 168
Students, and risk factors for school violence, 34–35. *See also* Schools; Victims
Substance abuse
biological causes of violence and, 60
causes of school violence and, 232
firearms and, 220
posttraumatic stress disorder and, 164
risk factors for youth violence and, 14, 94
suicide and, 89
Suicide
of Columbine High School student, 159
firearms and, 68, 219–220, 222
follow-up care and, 111

Suicide *(continued)*
  prevalence of among children and
    adolescents, 9–10
  psychological autopsy of in chil-
    dren and adolescents, 88–90
  statistics on child and adolescent,
    75
  television and copycat, 64, 65
Summer programs, and Chicago public schools, 258–259
Support groups, and community mental health response to Columbine
  incident, 153, 155
Surgeon General's Scientific Advisory
  Committee, 62
Survey of Children's Exposure to
  Community Violence, 166

Tarasoff v. Regents of University of
  California (1976), 189–199, 201–213
Teachers. *See also* School personnel;
  Schools
  as avoidant bystanders, 278
  CAPSLE Program and discipline
    plan, 282
  efforts of schools to prevent vio-
    lence and, 233–234
  multicultural education and, 297
  parents as, 257
  psychoeducation for after Colum-
    bine incident, 146
  social factors in school violence
    and, 237
  as victims of school homicides, 79
  as victims of school violence, 35–36,
    73
Teen Court Program (Chicago), 263
Telephone calls, and duty to warn, 209
Television. *See also* Media
  Columbine High School incident
    and, 80–81
  social factors in violence and,
    61–65
Temporal lobe epilepsy, 58–59

Tennessee, 68. *See also* Fayetteville,
  Tennessee
Termination, of school-based group
  therapy program, 184
Testosterone, and biological causes of
  violence, 55
Tests of Achievement Proficiency
  (TAP), **264**
Texas Supreme Court, 202
Thapar v. Zezulka (Texas, 1999), 202
Therapeutic alliance. *See also* Rapport
  duty to warn and, 210
  school-based group therapy pro-
    gram and, 169
Therapists. *See also* Clinical practice;
  Mental health professionals;
  Psychiatrists
  duty to warn and relationship with
    patient, 211
  school-based group therapy pro-
    gram and, 168–169
Thioridazine, 111
Third-party liability cases, 190,
  191–193
Third-party payers. *See* Health
  insurance
Thought process, and assessment of
  potential for violence, 100
Threats, of violence
  duty to warn and assessment of,
    204
  following media coverage of school
    violence incidents, 81
Time limitations, on duty to warn, 205
Time magazine, 159
Tipping point, and epidemiology of
  youth violence, 16–17, 18, 19
Toddlers and toddlerhood. *See also*
  Children; Infants
  developmental history and assess-
    ment of potential for violence,
    99
  firearms and emotional stress in,
    220–221

Topeka, Kansas, 287

Torts, 191

Trails B test, 58

Trauma. *See also* Stress

chronology of chronic exposure and, **167**

Columbine High School shootings and, 131, 158–159

as etiological factor in emotional disturbance and mental illness, 233

individual psychotherapy for traumatized youths, 106–107

reducing effects of, 269

school-based group therapy programs and reminders of, 175–176, 184

understanding of behavior and, 235

Trauma Management Consultants (Jefferson Center), 137–142

Treatment. *See also* Group therapy; Individual psychotherapy; Psychopharmacology

community response to Columbine incident and, 140–141, 142

impediments to after Columbine incident, 149–152

of potentially violent children and adolescents, 103–112

Truancy. *See also* Attendance; Avoidance

Juvenile Court of Philadelphia and, 239

prevention of, 259

Trust. *See also* Confidentiality

duty to warn and, 211

research on school violence and, 90

Tucson, Arizona, 244

TV Guide, 62

UCLA Grief Inventory, 166

UCLA Traumatic Expectations, 168

Uniform Discipline Code (Chicago), 265, 268

Uniforms, school, 41, 259

Uniqueness, and self-esteem, 261–262

United Way, 142

University of California at Los Angeles, Trauma Psychiatry Program, 165, 185

University of Colorado, Department of Psychiatry, 135, 143–147, 148, 151, 152, 156

University of Oklahoma, Department of Psychiatry, 148

Urban areas. *See also* Boston; Chicago; Los Angeles

epidemic of youth violence and, 10, 11, 12–13, 16–19

neighborhoods and safety of schools, 29, 33–34

U. S. Department of Education, 42, 61, 74, 77, 256

U. S. Department of Justice, 60, 61, 74, 76, 142

U. S. Office of Juvenile Justice and Delinquency Prevention, 26, 224

U. S. Public Health Service, 142

U. S. Supreme Court, 212

Value systems, 237

Victim Compensation (Colorado), 137

Victims, of school violence. *See also* Students; Witnesses

characteristics of, 35

counseling for, 45

impediments to treatment of in Columbine incident, 149–152

school homicides and, 79–80

social systems–power dynamics theory and, 274–275, 276–278, 287

teachers as, 35–36

Victim Services (Colorado), 135, 136–137, 155

Victims of Crime Act, 142

Video games, and youth violence, 65–66

Violation of the Uniform Firearms Act (VUFA), 240
Violence and violent behavior. *See also* Crime; Domestic violence; School violence
assessment of risk for, 208
biological causes of, 53–60
culture of, 232–233
data on youth, 26–27
definition of, 26
epidemic of youth, 10–19
epidemiological literature on adolescent response to, 164
health care and, 255–256
interaction of psychological, biological, and social factors in, 53–54
prevalence of problems in schools, 74–75
psychiatric disorders and rates of, 59–60
psychiatric effects of chronic exposure to, 36
psychological and legal issues in youth, 21–23
social factors and, 61–69
Violence Prevention Strategic Plan (Chicago), 245
Virginia, 225

Warning signs, for school violence, 42, 133–134. *See also* Risk factors
Washington State, 68, 220
Weapons. *See also* Firearms
prevalence of at schools, 77

risk factors for youth violence and, 14
students and carrying of in schools, 22
Web sites, and community response to Columbine High School shootings, 139. *See also* Internet
West Paducah, Kentucky, 5
White House Conference on School Safety, 25
Wisconsin. *See* Milwaukee, Wisconsin; Racine, Wisconsin
Wisconsin Card Sorting Test, 58
Witnesses, of school violence, 45. *See also* Victims
Woodham, Luke, 5, 118, 119, 123, 125
Workforce, and multicultural society, 294–295
Wounded adolescence, 163
Wurst, Andrew, 5

Yale Child Study Center, 242–244
Young Negotiators Program (Chicago), 263
Youth advisory boards, 141
Youth Homicide Committee (Philadelphia), 238–242, 243
Youth Outreach Workers program (Chicago), 254
Youth Risk Behavior Surveillance Survey, 77, 78, 79, 80

Zero Tolerance/Alternative Programs (Chicago), 265
Zero-tolerance policies, 42–43, 280–282. *See also* Discipline
Zung Depression Scale for Adults, 96